8th Edition

Wilderness and Rescue MEDICINE

WILDERNESS MEDICAL ASSOCIATES INTERNATIONAL

Eighth Edition
Wilderness and Rescue Medicine
Jeffrey Isaac, PA-C
David E. Johnson, MD
Wilderness Medical Associates International
2022 Printing

Wilderness Medical Associates International
1 Forest Avenue
Portland, ME 04101
www.wildmed.com

Production Credits
Cover Image: Josh Kling
Printing and Binding: Penmor Lithographers
Cover Printing: Penmor Lithographers
Designed and Edited by: Laura Lee

ISBN
Hard Copy: 978-0-9814831-9-1
E-Book: 978-0-9814831-8-4

Library of Congress Control Number: 2020902926

In Memory of

John Robert Isaac, MD

Physician, Surgeon, and Father

Brief Contents

Expanded Contents

Section VI: Backcountry Medicine 193

Acknowledgments

We would like to express our sincere appreciation for the efforts of all the instructors and staff of Wilderness Medical Associates International. Having a stadium full of experts to consult with is a rare privilege and a considerable benefit, not to mention a challenge. All of you have contributed to the success of the company and the continued production of this text, now in its 8th edition, and its associated materials. In particular, we would like to thank Deborah Hayes, Abby Rowe, Ted Mahar, Debra Ajango, Doug Cameron, Molly Charest, Justin Childs, Tom Clausing, Samanta Chu, Anne Dunphy, Erik Forsythe, Greg Friese, Judi Alberi, Sawyer Alberi, Jobi Hansen, Stephen Halvorson, Emily Hinman, Will Hooper, Ármann Höskuldsson, John Jacobs, Rachel Jamieson, Fay Johnson, Denis Langlois, Laura Lee, Sun Lingye, Rick Lipke, Mike Motti, Aaron Orkin, Takuya Ota, Bradford Sablosky, Dugg Steary, Cabot Stone, Sarah Strickland, Dave Vanderburgh, Mike Webster, Laura Wininger, and Isamu Yokobori.

We would also like to thank the Medical Library staff at Central Maine Medical Center for its prompt, accurate, and enthusiastic efforts to find and organize medical reference materials. We sincerely appreciate Drs. Douglas Casa, Peter Hackett, William Mills, Mary Ann Cooper, Gordon Giesbrecht, Martin Hoffman, and Frank Walter for sharing their insight and experience. And, as always, we owe a great debt of gratitude to Dr. Peter Goth for having the wisdom to recognize a good idea and the courage to promote it.

Our appreciation is extended to the Crested Butte Professional Ski Patrol, Crested Butte Mountain Rescue, and the GVH Mountain Clinic for providing a solid base of practical experience and an unparalleled opportunity to test protocols, equipment, and technique.

We also wish to acknowledge that the only real way to create a useful text is to respond to the people who are using it. We will be most grateful for any comments and critique from our readers, students, and instructors.

With deep gratitude,

Jeffrey Isaac, PA-C and David E. Johnson, MD

About the Authors

Jeffrey Isaac is a physician associate and WEMT with a particular interest in backcountry and marine medicine. His 40 years of experience includes service as a fire/rescue crewman, professional ski patroller, mountain rescue team leader, and medical practitioner in hospital emergency departments and remote clinics. He has been an instructor for Wilderness Medical Associates International since the inception of the company and has served as its Curriculum Director for more than 25 years.

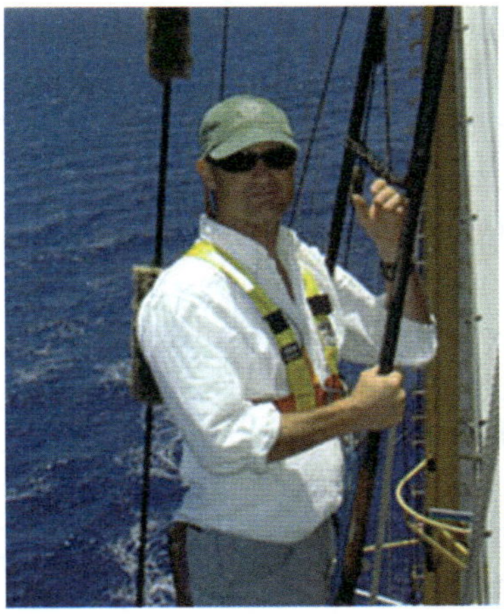

Jeff is also a licensed captain and an experienced mariner, having logged thousands of miles in the Atlantic and Pacific Oceans and the Caribbean Sea. His outdoor resume includes 20 years as an instructor and course director with the Hurricane Island Outward Bound School, as well as numerous backcountry misadventures by foot, horse, canoe, bicycle, raft, and old trucks.

David Johnson is a retired emergency physician with a lifetime of experience in a variety of outdoor pursuits. He has spent the last 40 years applying his experience as a physician and wilderness traveler to consulting, curriculum development, and teaching focused on remote and low-resource environments around the world. He currently serves as the Medical Director for Wilderness Medical Associates International.

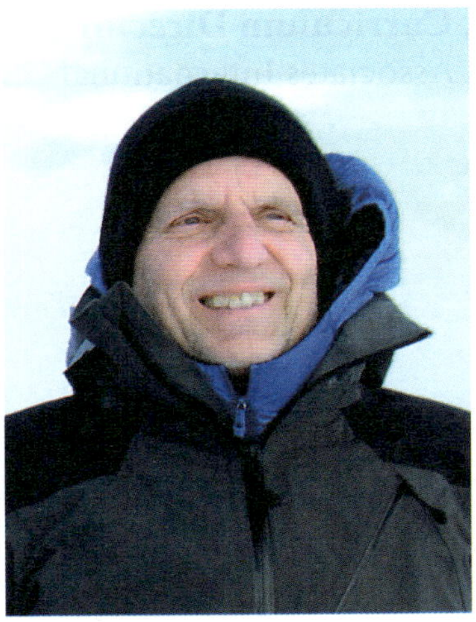

David is known for being firmly committed to the science behind the subject, as well as its practical application at all levels of medical training. For these efforts, David has been recognized by Outward Bound USA with the McGory Award for outstanding contributions to experiential education, and is a recipient of the Charles (Reb) Greg Wilderness Risk Management Award.

Preface

This edition of *Wilderness and Rescue Medicine* (WARM) represents our continued efforts to keep it lean but comprehensive, relevant, and practical for professional and lay practitioners who find themselves working, living, and playing in remote and low-resource settings.

Like many other educational institutions, Wilderness Medical Associates International (WMAI) has struggled with how to continue operating under the constraints imposed on us by the COVID-19 pandemic. We have endeavored to take advantage of the shutdowns to look at how we offer educational opportunities and work to broaden the reach and upgrade the content and format. For example, we wrote a companion text, *Wilderness and Rescue First Aid* for our Wilderness First Aid and Advanced First Aid courses. We continue to develop our dream of a dynamic bibliography and periodic updates online.

Even before COVID-19, WMAI was working to script and produce teaching materials specifically for online use to supplement the course materials primarily used on face-to-face courses. Serendipitously, these proved invaluable for the online recertification options we offered prior WMAI graduates when COVID-19 forced us to postpone courses. Rather than give a blanket extension, these were free online educational opportunities designed to refresh and extend their knowledge. These are now being modified and expanded for use on our growing number of hybrid courses.

People learn in different ways, and using different tools and approaches to education enhance learning and retention. But the COVID-19 experience has reminded us again that nothing beats a face-to-face learning environment where a well-trained and experienced instructor can guide and challenge learners, allowing them to make mistakes, test assumptions, and ultimately succeed in an inclusive and supportive environment.

In the autumn of 2020, Abby Rowe became the new owner and President of WMAI. A detailed biography is posted at https://www.wildmed.com/about-us/meet-the-team. Abby came to her roles familiar with WMAI and is prepared to move the company forward. She is a WMAI course graduate and instructor. She also directed a program that has been a long-term sponsor of WMAI courses. Abby has redoubled the efforts of her predecessors and is committed to serving WMAI clients, supporting instructors, and providing high-quality curriculum and programing for WMAI learners. The future continues to look bright as more and more people who work and play outdoors seek the kind of training that can enhance their safety and personal responsibility.

We continue to be grateful to learners, instructors, and course hosts for their trust and support as we redouble our efforts to evolve and make our curriculum accessible, practical, and accurate. We hope you find this 8th Edition of WARM a challenging, informative, interesting, and worthwhile successor.

David E. Johnson MD, Medical Director
Jeffrey Isaac PA-C, Curriculum Director
Wilderness Medical Associates International

Introduction

Wilderness and Rescue Medicine (WARM) is composed for use as the primary text for Wilderness Medical Associates International (WMAI) courses. As such, it was conceived to be a clear, concise, and user-friendly guide to medical care in remote and low-resources settings. In this, our 8th Edition, we have remained focused on knowledge and techniques that are practical and useful in field medicine while updating from the current medical literature and our own evolving base of experience. The content will be appreciated by practitioners at all levels of training, but it is aimed at learners in our Wilderness First Responder and Wilderness EMS courses.

WARM is more practical than encyclopedic and is written to be read from front to back. We have tried to structure it in a way that is logical, with one section building on to the next. The general principles described in the beginning will enhance your appreciation of the systems and problems discussed later. Your initial understanding of the body systems will guide the process of developing accurate and useful assessments leading to appropriate and realistic treatment plans for evermore complex problems. One of our goals is to offer assessment criteria that are logical and practical for field application. To apply competently, one only needs to integrate the information acquired from listening and observing with the principles that we have outlined in WARM and the classroom.

Although this text can be understood as a standalone resource, it is best accompanied by the *Field Guide of Wilderness and Rescue Medicine* as well as case studies provided by Wilderness Medical Associates International. The Field Guide is designed for your first aid kit as a quick-reference alternative packaged in a weather resistant format. The case studies offer an opportunity to review important principles in realistic settings.

Within these publications you will find certain procedures identified as Wilderness Protocols. The procedures described expand the scope of practice for traditional first aid and many EMS practitioners. They are meant to address specific problems often encountered in a wilderness and rescue environment. WMAI graduates have been trained and certified in these techniques, but the authorization to use them comes from the patient's informed consent and, where relevant, practitioner's licensing agency.

The Wilderness Protocols are freely offered for modification and use for the wilderness and rescue setting. Each carries the acknowledgment that the practitioner is appropriately trained and that the protocol is employed only in situations where transport to definitive care would result in unacceptable risk to the patient or rescuers or where field treatment offers a clear benefit in improved outcome and diminished pain. The Wilderness Protocols require a clear diagnosis and a specific action.

Not all situations, however, can be so clearly addressed. As you train for medical care in remote and low-resource settings, you must be prepared to do some unconventional thinking. Mainstream medical practice may have little relevance to you as the skipper of a small boat hundreds of miles from shore or as the leader of a rescue team on a high mountain ledge. There are many cases where applying conventional EMS protocols and equipment will substantially increase the risk to the patient and entire rescue effort. For some of you, especially those with years of emergency medical services training, this perspective may be difficult to adopt. Others among you may find that it validates opinions formed by experience.

Within the text and presentations, these issues take the form of wilderness perspective notes and risk versus benefit discussions. While you may have been taught that the ideal plan for traumatic brain injury is evaluation in a hospital, what if the route to get there is extremely dangerous for you and your patient? How do you balance the risk versus the potential benefit? These types of decisions are not easy, but they are necessary.

This text and the courses it serves are designed to provide you with some background with which to make tough choices and to provide the most effective medical care possible in unique and challenging circumstances. In addition to understanding principles and learning procedures, you will need to keep an open mind. The ability to innovate and adapt will serve you far better than trying to memorize a protocol for every circumstance.

Finally, if you are new to the study of medicine, you may feel overwhelmed by abbreviations, mnemonics, and acronyms. Even experienced practitioners are occasionally baffled by their colleague's documentation shortcuts. To help with some of this we have included a list of abbreviations and a glossary in the back of the text.

All of us at WMAI hope that you find WARM interesting, relevant, and useful. We plan to continue updating and revising this text and our curriculum regularly, and we welcome and encourage your comments and critique.

office@wildmed.com
www.wildmed.com

Section I: General Principles

Chapter 1: General Principles of Physiology and Pathology

Most emergency medical assessment and treatment is based on a few general principles of pathology and physiology. If you can understand these basic human responses to injury and illness, you will be in a much better position to adapt your medical skills and experience to the remote and extreme environment. These principles are fundamental and will surface frequently in your study of wilderness and rescue medicine. The ideal result is that you will never forget what to do because you will *understand* what needs to be done.

Oxygenation and Perfusion

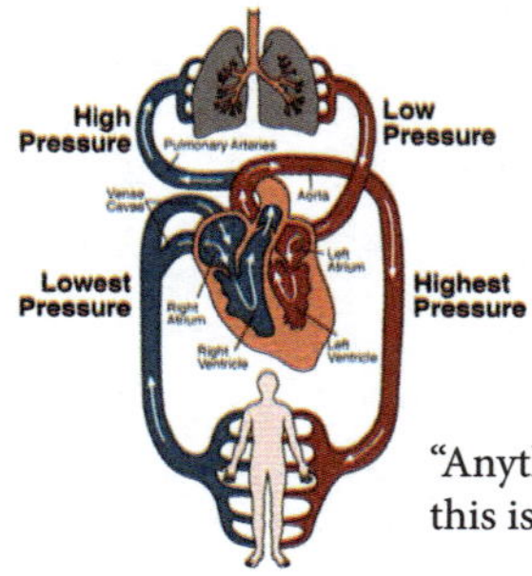

"Anything that interferes with this is a serious problem."

Oxygenation and Perfusion

All living tissue must be continuously perfused with oxygenated blood to function normally. For each cell in the body to be adequately oxygenated, a continuous flow of fresh air to the lungs and a continuous flow of blood to the body tissues are required. Anything that interferes with these processes is a serious problem. The preservation of oxygenation and perfusion is the fundamental goal of emergency medical care.

The basic function of the respiratory system is to bring outside air into the alveoli of the lungs where only a thin membrane separates air from blood. This allows oxygen from the air to diffuse into the blood and combine with hemoglobin in red blood cells. Adequate oxygenation of the blood requires adequate respiration.

The basic purpose of the circulatory system is to perfuse the lungs with blood in need of oxygen, and to perfuse the rest of the body tissues with the newly oxygenated blood. Adequate perfusion requires that the circulatory system generates enough pressure to force the blood through the capillary beds in body tissues where oxygenation of the cells and removal of carbon dioxide and metabolic waste occurs.

Three Critical Systems, Three Serious Problems

The organs of the circulatory, respiratory, and nervous systems perform the functions most essential to life. A serious problem with any one of these systems is considered an immediate threat to life. Your first steps in patient examination are focused on evaluating the function of these three systems. Your priority in patient care is to quickly correct any serious problems with oxygenation and perfusion.

The serious problem called shock is inadequate perfusion pressure in the circulatory system resulting in inadequate tissue oxygenation. Respiratory failure is the term for inadequate oxygenation of the blood due to a serious respiratory system problem. A serious nervous system problem causing brain failure can inhibit normal control and function of the other two critical systems.

The circulatory, respiratory, and nervous systems are interdependent. A problem with one quickly affects the functions of the other two. For example, shock from blood loss stimulates an increase in the respiratory rate and causes changes in brain function. Because the critical systems affect each other in a variety of ways, it can be a challenge to determine in which critical system the original problem lies.

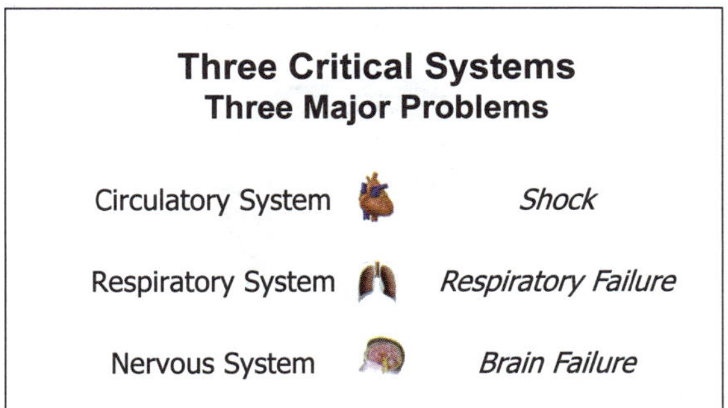

"Recognizing…a major problem with a critical body system is the key to recognizing a life-threatening emergency."

Recognizing or anticipating the development of shock, respiratory failure, or brain failure is the key to recognizing a serious problem. This skill is especially helpful in recognizing when the problem is not serious, which is most of the time.

Patterns and Trends

The nervous system regulates the function of the circulatory and respiratory systems to maintain adequate oxygenation and perfusion under a variety of conditions.

The system also compensates for the effects of an injury or illness by adjusting cardiac output, respiratory rate and effort, and tissue perfusion. Measuring vital signs reveals the compensation mechanisms at work.

We routinely look at pulse rate, respiratory rate and effort, level of consciousness and mental status, blood pressure, skin perfusion, and body core temperature. Minor changes occur as the healthy body adapts to the various stresses of normal life.

A pattern of substantial, progressive, or persistent changes in vital signs indicates an evolving problem. The volume shock pattern is a good example.

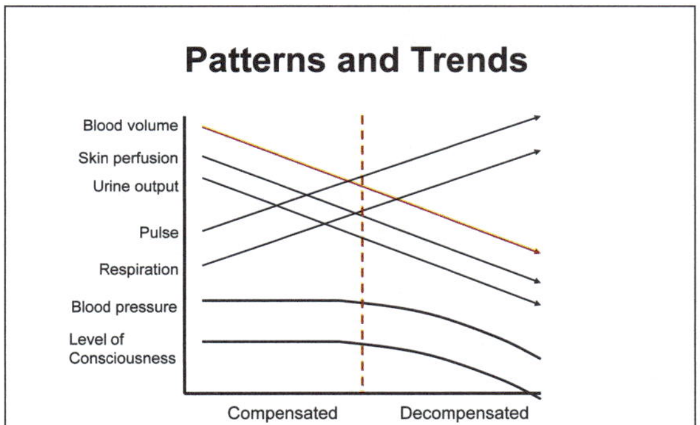

"Accurate assessment of critical system function involves the recognition of patterns and trends."

Mental Status and Level of Consciousness

Mental status is the most useful vital sign in emergency medicine. Nervous system tissue, especially the brain, is exquisitely sensitive to oxygen deprivation. Subtle changes in brain function are often your earliest indicator of a problem with oxygenation and perfusion. Patients remain conscious and alert but may become anxious and confused early in the pattern of shock or respiratory failure. The severity of the signs and symptoms correlates well to the severity of the problem.

Picture the brain like the layers of an onion with increasingly complex layers of function from the inside out. The basic physiological functions that control consciousness and heart and respiratory rates extend from the innermost layers in the brain stem. Higher brain functions such as speech, behavior, judgment, and problem solving are controlled by the outer layers of the brain. These outer layers are usually the first to be affected by a developing problem with oxygenation and perfusion, causing changes in mental status.

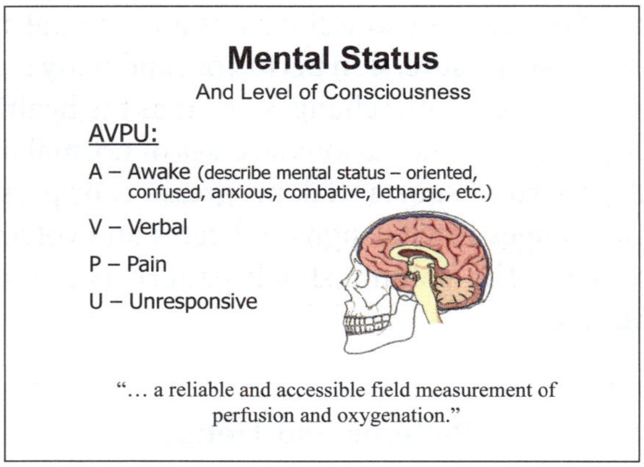

As critical system problems become more serious, mental status worsens and the deeper layers of the brain begin to fail, causing a decrease in the level of consciousness. Students often refer to this pattern as "peeling the onion." The progression can be reversed if the underlying problems are corrected.

In the absence of shock or respiratory failure, changes in mental status can indicate a problem within the brain itself such as intoxication, infection, or stroke. Again, the severity of the symptoms correlates well to the severity of the problem. Being a little tipsy after a beer is not serious, but being unconscious after a night of drinking is. If the deeper layers of the onion stop working, the patient will stop breathing. Monitoring consciousness and mental status offers a reliable and accessible field measurement of the quality of oxygenation and perfusion.

Swelling and Pressure

Swelling is a common, generic response to injury and illness. Swelling can interfere with oxygenation and perfusion. Many of our emergency drugs and procedures are used to prevent and control swelling or reduce the associated problems and risks.

Swelling is caused by the accumulation of excess fluid in body tissues. It can develop quickly as blood escapes from ruptured arteries or slowly as serum oozes from damaged or inflamed capillaries, causing the condition known as edema. It may be localized, such as the swelling of a sprained ankle, or systemic, such as the swelling of the whole body that occurs in allergic reactions.

Swelling is bothersome when it causes pain, and dangerous when it causes problems with oxygenation and perfusion. Swelling that develops inside a restricted space, such as the skull or a muscle compartment, can result in enough pressure to restrict perfusion causing the condition known as ischemia. This is exactly what happens to the brain with the development of increased intracranial pressure due to head injury. It is also responsible for the damage caused by compartment syndrome that develops in the muscles of the lower leg or forearm. Swelling in the confined space of the upper airway can cause obstruction, whereas swelling lower in the respiratory system can cause lower airway constriction or fluid in the alveoli. Swelling can evolve over hours or days, or nearly instantly with severe internal bleeding.

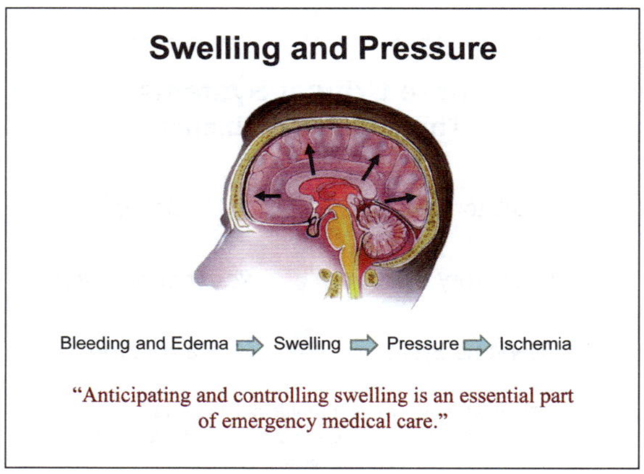

Obstruction to Infection

The human body is full of hollow organs that store, transport, or excrete liquids of all types. These include sweat glands, intestines, the bladder, and all their associated ducts. If the drainage from these organs is obstructed by swelling, deformity, or a foreign body, the accumulation and pressure causes inflammation and pain.

If the obstruction lasts long enough, any bacteria present can begin to grow out of control in whatever substance is trapped, and infection will develop. The most common example is the average pimple. This is an infection in an obstructed sweat gland. Appendicitis is a more serious example of the same pattern. Many illnesses have their origins in obstruction—and their cures are in relieving it.

Wounds also create cavities prone to obstruction and infection. Closing a wound with staples or sutures will obstruct drainage, which is part of the natural healing process. Infection becomes more likely, especially in wounds treated in less than ideal conditions.

Ischemia to Infarction

Ischemia is a localized problem of inadequate tissue perfusion, as opposed to the whole body problem with perfusion, which is known as shock. Blood flow is blocked by a clot, deformity, or swelling causing symptoms including pain, numbness and tingling, and impaired function. The chest pain of a heart attack, for example, is caused by ischemia of the heart muscle. Numbness of the hand, for example, can be caused by the deformity of a dislocated shoulder.

Prolonged ischemia inevitably leads to infarction, which is the term for tissue death. Some tissue, such as the brain, can die from just a few minutes of ischemia. The skin, however, can live for hours without adequate perfusion. Essentially, the more important an organ is to immediate survival, the more sensitive it is to the loss of perfusion.

Ischemia to Infarction

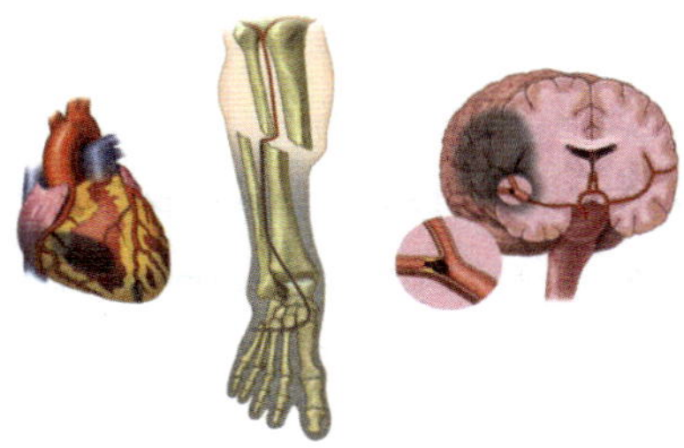

"Ischemia that you cannot fix will lead to infarction."

Ischemia can be complete or partial. It can develop from an internal problem such as a blood clot or compartment syndrome, or from external pressure such as a tight splint or lying on an unpadded backboard. The symptoms of ischemia are an early warning of the serious and permanent problems caused by infarction.

Anticipated Problem

Ischemia is just one example of a serious problem that can become an emergency if it cannot be fixed. A dislocated shoulder, for example, causes ischemia of tendons and muscle and represents a limb-threatening problem. Fortunately, field reduction is often successful, avoiding any need for an urgent evacuation.

The pattern of respiratory distress to respiratory failure is another example of a serious pattern that will progress to an emergency if you can't fix it. Other examples include compensated shock to decompensated shock; mild hypothermia to severe hypothermia; and local infection to systemic infection.

Fortunately, you will learn how to fix or stabilize some of these serious problems, but it is equally important to know when you can't. Recognizing the progression and gauging your ability to slow it down or reverse it helps to simplify treatment and evacuation decisions and the sense of urgency surrounding them.

Anticipated Problem

- Ischemia to Infarction
- Obstruction to Infection
- Compensated Shock to Decompensated Shock
- Respiratory Distress to Respiratory Failure
- Mild Hypothermia to Severe Hypothermia

"A serious problem that you cannot fix will become an emergency."

Most People Live

- First, do no harm
- Watch critical systems and body core temperature
- Keep yourself and your team safe

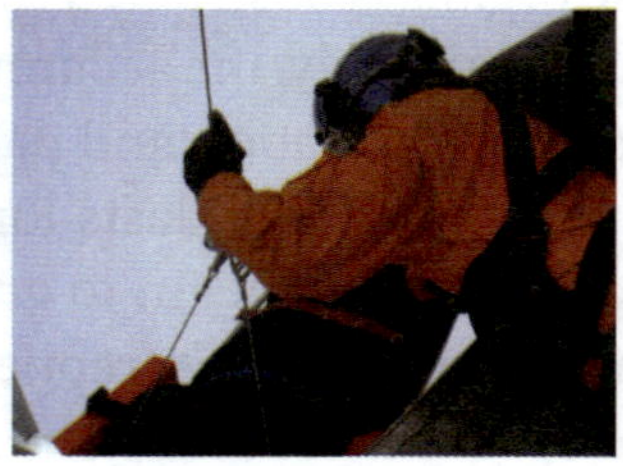

For example: *My patient is in respiratory distress progressing toward respiratory failure. This is serious. I can't fix it. This is an emergency. We need to move fast and accept greater risk in evacuating this patient to medical care.*

Most People Live

Curiously, the development of hospital-based imaging technologies like computed tomography (CT), magnetic resonance imaging (MRI), and ultrasound (US) have been very helpful to wilderness and rescue medicine. The ability to detect a spleen or kidney laceration and watch it stop bleeding and heal without surgery tells us that not everybody who ruptures an internal organ dies. As a result, very few injured spleens or kidneys are removed these days.

With CT and ultrasound, we can watch appendicitis stabilize and even resolve on oral antibiotics. Brain scans after trauma often reveal intracranial bleeding that causes no symptoms and resolves without permanent injury. While we don't have such imaging equipment in the wilderness, what we have learned from its use in the hospital helps with our decision making, especially in more remote and dangerous places.

Critical system injury is not a death sentence. If your patient survives the initial insult and the first few minutes thereafter, they have a good chance of living to see another day. The body has an incredible ability to compensate for significant injury and overcome devastating illness. Our job is to support that effort without doing additional harm.

Critical system injury does not always demand a high-risk rescue. A hospital might be the ideal destination, but good basic life support and careful handling will give your patient a better chance for survival than a high-risk evacuation that kills them in the process. Although an emergency evacuation is often the ideal plan, it is not always the real one.

Chapter 1 Review:
General Principles of Physiology and Pathology

- Anything that interferes with the oxygenation and perfusion of a critical system is potentially life threatening.
- Shock is inadequate perfusion due to inadequate perfusion pressure in the circulatory system.
- Respiratory failure is inadequate oxygenation of the blood due to a respiratory system problem.
- Brain failure can be a primary problem causing inadequate circulatory or respiratory control, or a symptom of shock or respiratory failure.
- Altered mental status is often the earliest vital sign change when oxygenation and perfusion are impaired.
- Swelling is a common cause of problems with oxygenation and perfusion. Anticipating and controlling swelling are important parts of emergency medical care.
- Ischemia is local loss of perfusion due to swelling, deformity, or obstruction. Ischemia that is not corrected will result in infarction.
- A serious critical system problem that cannot be corrected will become an emergency.
- Obstruction of a hollow organ due to swelling, deformity, or mass will result in infection.
- Most people live. There will be situations where good basic medical care on scene offers a better chance for survival than a high-risk rescue.

Chapter 2: General Principles of Wilderness Rescue

There are countless examples of high-risk solutions to low-risk medical problems. This is nowhere more apparent than in backcountry and marine rescue. The reasons are not difficult to understand: Information about the scene is often unreliable, rescuers can become emotionally involved in the patient's plight, and the operation itself can be an exciting, powerful, and distracting experience. Risk affinity often increases well out of proportion to the actual need.

As a medical officer your primary responsibility is to reduce risk to your patient, the public, other rescuers, and yourself. This is not easy. Flexibility, innovation, and a certain amount of courage are required to cope with the varied and constantly evolving nature of medicine and rescue in the wild and remote setting. There are, however, a few guiding principles of wilderness rescue that can help to impose some degree of order on chaos.

Serious or Not Serious

There are only three things that will kill you or your patient: shock, respiratory failure, and brain failure. Anything causing these critical system problems is serious and an invitation to immediate action. Any concern for the development of critical system problems in the near future is serious and requires early treatment to prevent the pattern from progressing.

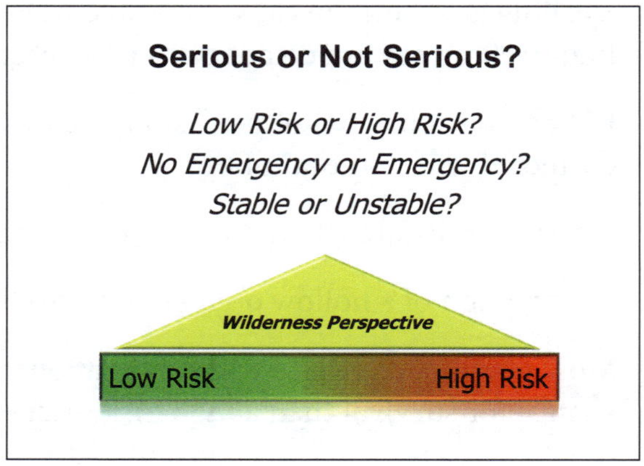

Based solely on the diagnosis of *serious,* you can begin basic supportive care and protection and summon help or initiate an evacuation. Conversely, no evidence of shock, respiratory failure, or brain failure, and no reason to anticipate these problems, means *not serious*. You may have time to treat and observe, and perhaps avoid evacuation altogether.

Serious or not serious is the most generic and important diagnosis of all in field medicine. It is only a serious problem that we cannot fix in the field that we label a true *emergency*. Everything else is just a logistical dilemma.

The Risk/Benefit Ratio

Every treatment (or decision not to treat) and every emergency evacuation (or decision to stay in the field) involves the risk that the medical problems will become worse because of what we have done. We also run the risk of causing injury to the rescuers themselves or to other people who may be involved. Against this risk, we balance the potential benefits of our actions. Good decisions increase benefit and decrease risk.

Risk/benefit decisions in medicine are usually reserved for licensed practitioners. In the wilderness setting, this kind of critical thinking becomes a required skill at any level of medical training. It is often up to the person in charge of medical care on scene to convey the appropriate sense of urgency, determine the type of care needed next, and figure out how to access it safely and efficiently.

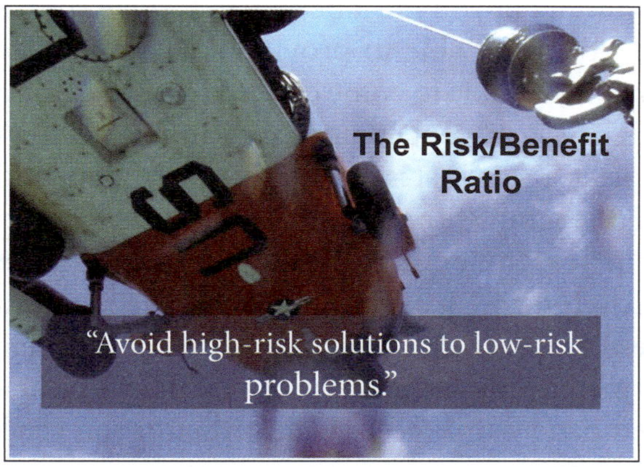
The Risk/Benefit Ratio
"Avoid high-risk solutions to low-risk problems."

A good risk/benefit judgment may be the result of a gut feeling or the product of a more formal group process. Whatever form it takes should replace emotion, obligation, panic, and established protocol if necessary. The beneficiaries include the rescuers and bystanders, as well as the patient.

Probability and Consequence

We tend to look at the risk associated with any decision or activity as a function of chance. We may know or guess that there is a 10%, 5%, or 0.005% probability of a bad outcome, but we seldom give much thought to the bad outcome itself. Treatment failures, falls, and crashes during rescue are considered tragedies, mistakes, or serendipitous events. But risk is really a function of probability *and* consequence. Both elements are important to overall risk assessment.

You may choose, for example, the faster evacuation route down a ridgeline because the probability of a lightning storm is low and there are good escape routes available if one does develop. We like low probability and low consequence choices. This is good risk management.

A more complex example is the ubiquitous use of helicopters in rescue work. Although air medical helicopters experience the highest rate of accidents in civilian aviation, the probability of one crashing is still quite low. However, the consequences of a helicopter crash are usually extreme, which elevates the overall risk considerably. Good weather, a safe landing zone, and a conservative pilot will all contribute to keeping the probability of an accident low. But a significant change in any one of these factors can quickly change the risk profile. Whenever possible, avoid the combination of high probability and high consequence.

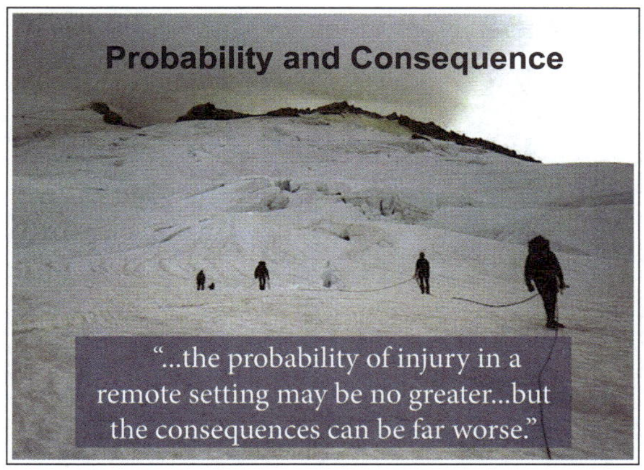
Probability and Consequence
"...the probability of injury in a remote setting may be no greater...but the consequences can be far worse."

In medical care, an example of a good risk/benefit profile is the use of epinephrine in the field treatment of anaphylaxis. The risks associated with injectable epinephrine are very low while the risks associated with untreated anaphylaxis are very high. This is a low-risk treatment for a high-risk problem. All of our wilderness medical protocols are examples of this principle.

Generic to Specific

In a hospital, the process of diagnosis and treatment moves from generic to specific. The generic complaint of abdominal pain, for example, can quickly become the specific diagnosis of appendicitis with a few lab tests and a CT scan. But, if your examining room is the salon of a small boat 200 miles offshore, it is nearly impossible to distinguish an ectopic pregnancy from appendicitis or any one of a dozen other problems. The practitioner is often left working with a generic diagnosis of serious abdominal pain for the duration of field treatment and evacuation.

Nevertheless, an important component of this generic-to-specific principle is the need to consider and treat, if possible, all likely causes of a problem until a specific diagnosis can be rendered. This is especially important when a critical body system is involved. For example, altered mental status in an alpine climber could be caused by high-altitude cerebral edema, hypothermia, intoxication, brain injury, or low blood glucose. Some of these problems may be treatable on scene.

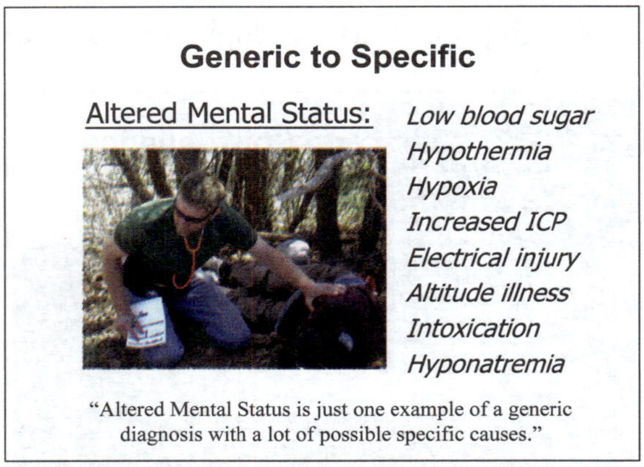

As further investigation is conducted, and the results of treatment are observed, some of the possible causes can be ruled out and the treatment directed at those that are left. Considering the generic diagnosis first avoids the oversight caused by puddle vision—that is, inappropriately focusing on one specific diagnosis or puddle of blood to the exclusion of everything else.

Ideal to Real

Medical practitioners are fond of the excuse, "If I just had my jump kit, or nurse, or defibrillator..." In a wilderness rescue situation, you are not being quizzed on the ideal hospital or ambulance treatment for the condition you have identified. You are being challenged to come up with a plan that makes sense for the environment in which you are operating.

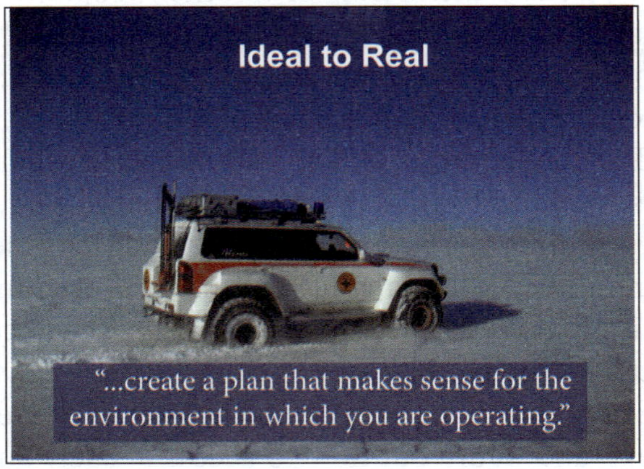

It is certainly helpful to have the ideal treatment in mind, but you must be able to forgive yourself for not being able to provide it. In some cases, you may be able to come close. In most cases, you will have to accept compromise and be willing to execute a plan that is real for the patient's situation.

For example, the ideal treatment for a trauma patient with neck injury might involve spine stabilization with a cervical collar and vacuum mattress; however, if your problem list includes being 20 meters down a crevasse in an Antarctic glacier, your patient may freeze to death before this can be accomplished. Helping the patient climb out may be the only real treatment for a situation like this.

Focus on Important

"The patient is the one with the disease." This time-honored medical school quip is another way of saying don't panic, you are not the one injured and in need of help. You *are* the help. You will function more efficiently and safely by remembering this important fact, and by remaining objective and task oriented. The more confusing and complicated the problem, the more important this behavior is. This can take considerable self-discipline.

Rescue scenes are full of distractions courtesy of radio traffic, bystanders, fellow rescuers, and anyone suffering pain and acute stress reaction. Your attention will be drawn in a dozen different directions. Learn to focus your attention on the problems that are truly urgent and important and those that are going to be urgent and important if you do not address them. Avoid addressing anything that is not important to the care and safety of your patient and crew. To an untrained or uninformed observer, you may appear detached or overly concerned with your own safety. Their perceptions are not your problem—the execution of a safe and competent rescue is.

The Problem List

Practitioners familiar with the SOAP format (Subjective, Objective, Assessment, and Plan) for medical documentation will recognize the problem list as the A, or Assessment. Using this tool will allow you to render order from the chaos of an accident or disaster scene.

The Problem List
SOAP

Assessment:
- Existing environmental problems and threats
- Existing medical problems
- Anticipated problems and threats

Plan:
- Risk vs Benefit analysis
- A plan for each problem
- Action to prevent anticipated problems

"Constructing a succinct list of problems…begins a well-ordered process of treatment and evacuation."

Constructing a succinct list of problems identified by the scene size-up and examination of the patient begins a well-ordered process of treatment and evacuation. For each problem identified, the practitioner establishes a priority and plans treatment. The problem list is also a primary tool for communicating the patient's condition and treatment to other people.

In the wilderness or disaster setting, the patient's medical condition may be just a small part of a much larger problem list that includes adverse weather, difficult terrain, and hazardous working conditions.

These factors can create new medical problems as well as determine the plan for dealing with the existing ones. For the wilderness medical practitioner, the problem list includes the environmental issues along with the medical. SOAP is discussed in more detail in the Patient Assessment and the SOAP Format chapter.

Medicine Is Dynamic

Everything in medicine, from general principles of care to specific treatment, carries some degree of uncertainty. Fortunately, some of what we do is validated by extensive experience and good science. We must remember, however, that our practice setting bears little resemblance to the conditions under which most medical studies are performed.

Medicine is Dynamic

What we know:
- Good science
- Solid experience

What we think:
- Incomplete science
- Tangential experience

Educated speculation:
- What seems to make sense

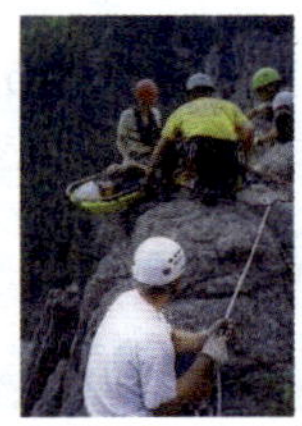

"We should be prepared to improvise, adapt, and to keep an open mind."

Although laboratory science and medical center practice has plenty to teach us, those lessons must be measured against the irreducible reality of providing care in a remote and dangerous place. Some of our practice must be based on anecdotal experience and incomplete scientific evidence. Where even less experience is available, we are left to rely on educated speculation supported only by what seems to make sense. As more data becomes available, some widely accepted medical practices will be debunked and others validated. Medical practitioners at every level of training must be willing to reevaluate the standard of care whenever new information and field experience suggests a better way. We should be prepared to improvise, adapt, and keep an open mind.

Chapter 2 Review:
General Principles of Wilderness Rescue

- Risk/benefit decisions can be considered a form of medical judgment usually reserved for licensed practitioners. In the wilderness setting, this type of critical thinking becomes a required skill at any level of medical training.
- Risk is a function of probability and consequence. Avoid high-risk solutions to low-risk problems.
- *Serious* or *not serious* is the most generic and important diagnosis in field medicine and is the beginning of risk versus benefit analysis. The only true emergency is the serious problem that you cannot fix in the field.
- The wilderness practitioner is often left working with a generic diagnosis for the duration of field treatment and evacuation.
- It is helpful to have the ideal treatment in mind, but you must move forward with treatment that is realistic for the situation you are in.
- The patient is the one with the disease. You are the help. Focus on the important problems.
- The SOAP process allows you to render order from the chaos of an emergency scene.
- Medicine is dynamic. Flexibility, innovation, and a certain amount of courage are required to cope with the varied and constantly evolving nature of medical care in the wild or remote setting.

Chapter 3: Patient Assessment and the SOAP Format

The Patient Assessment System (PAS) is a tool for organizing your response to any situation involving an ill or injured person. The more complicated and difficult the situation is, the more valuable a well-rehearsed PAS will be. Properly applied, the PAS will lead you to a concise description of the problems you are facing and what you are going to do about them.

The PAS consists of three important steps: gathering information, creating a problem list, and planning treatment and evacuation. Information is collected in a series of surveys, which is summarized as three triangles.

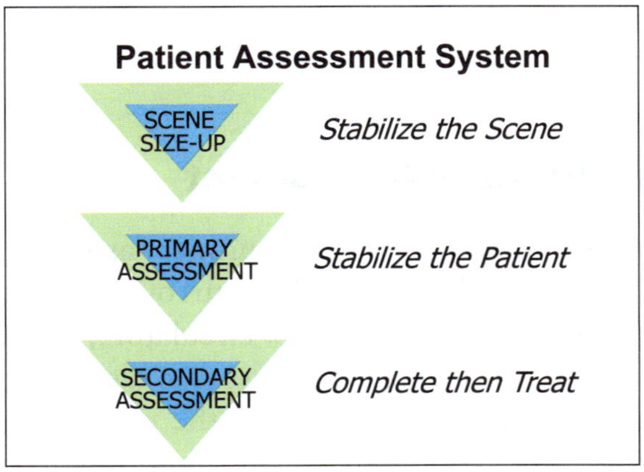

These steps allow you to gather the necessary information systematically, act on what is urgent and important, and organize your ongoing response. Becoming competent and comfortable with the PAS requires lots of practice, but it is one of the best tools that you have available for reducing risk and improving outcome.

Gathering Information

The Scene Size-Up

For Search and Rescue (SAR) teams, the scene size-up begins with the call out. While the team is getting organized, the team leader will usually delegate a member to collect data from dispatch, the reporting party, and people on scene, if possible. By adding a weather report and local knowledge, it is sometimes possible to form a near-complete picture of the situation and the associated risks. More often, however, it is the rescuer on scene who performs this vital function.

The scene size-up is designed to keep you alive and effective. It also serves to protect other rescuers, bystanders, and the patient from further harm. If you are among the first on scene, a complete scene size-up is your first responsibility. It is also your first opportunity to assess the number of people affected and the forces and factors involved.

Stabilize the Scene

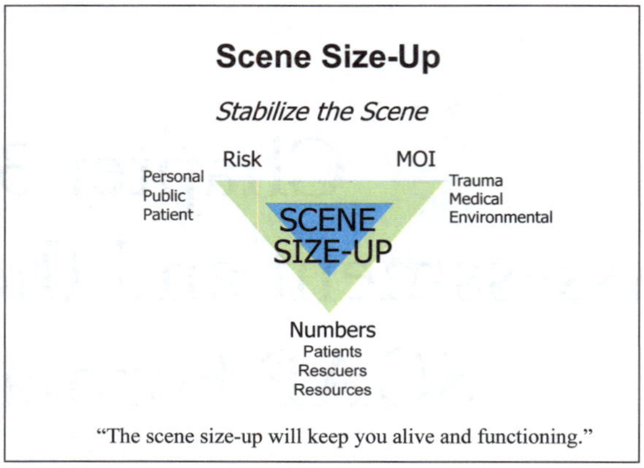

It can take tremendous discipline to overcome the urge to rush to the aid of a person in trouble, but this is exactly what you must do. Stop, look around, and assess the risk to yourself and your team. The threats may be environmental, such as frigid water or a hang fire avalanche, or generated by the activities of other people. If it can harm you or your fellow rescuers, it must be stabilized before you can do anything else.

Once you are safe, or relatively so, look for any further threat to bystanders and the injured person. Stabilize the scene by either moving danger from the patient or the patient from the danger.

This has priority over everything else that follows. You must get the patient out of the water or out from under the cornice and clear the area of well-meaning (but potentially unsafe) bystanders.

Determine Mechanism of Injury

As you approach the scene, try to evaluate the mechanism of injury (MOI). How the problem developed is usually obvious, but occasionally more investigation will be necessary. For example, how far did the patient fall? Was it enough of a tumble to cause significant injury? Are there other factors, such as exposure to weather, that might contribute to the patient's condition? You may be able to ask the patient or others on the scene for additional information about the MOI.

Determine the Number of Patients

Your scene size-up also determines how many people are injured or at risk. This is especially important in harsh environments where all field personnel may be at risk for hypothermia or dehydration. In multiple-casualty incidents, more seriously injured people are often overlooked in the rush to treat the noisiest and most uncomfortable patients.

Standard Precautions

Included in this survey of dangers is the potential for exposure to bodily fluids. Several diseases can be transmitted via bodily fluids, including human immunodeficiency virus (HIV) and hepatitis B and C. The use of standard precautions is now standard in all areas of medicine where bodily fluid contact is possible. Standard precautions include the use of gloves, eye protection, face masks, hand washing, antiseptics, and proper disposal techniques.

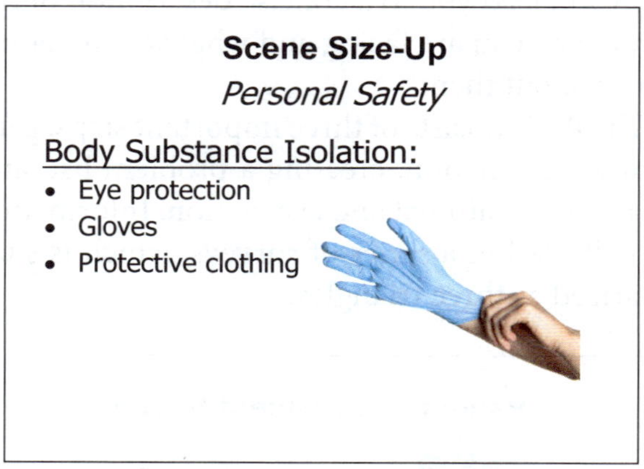

The Primary Assessment

The second part of PAS is the primary assessment, which is a quick check on the status of the patient's three critical body systems: circulatory, respiratory, and nervous. The purpose is to identify and correct immediate threats to the patient's life. These three systems are equally important to survival, and major problems associated with them are equally dangerous. The order in which you check and stabilize them should be determined by the situation, not by the order in which they appear on any list.

Stabilize the Patient

Make sure that the patient's airway is clear and that there is sufficient respiratory effort to oxygenate their lungs. Check for a pulse and perform a quick sweep for severe bleeding or other problems capable of causing shock. While you are doing this, assess brain function by noting mental status and level of consciousness.

Primary Assessment

Stabilize the Patient

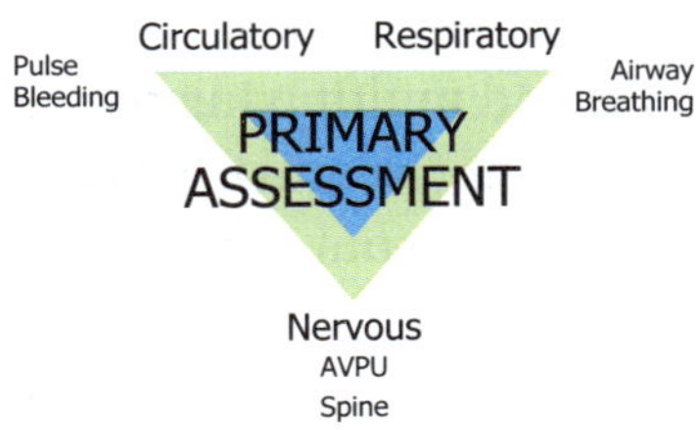

"The initial assessment is your quick check on the status of the patient's three critical body systems."

Your primary assessment might be as simple as asking, "How do you do?" and getting a "Fine" and a smile. Or, you might be on belay in a crevasse listening for breath sounds and looking inside bulky clothing for blood on an unresponsive climber. Whatever form it takes, the primary assessment is a critical step in your organized approach to the situation. Any serious problems encountered in the primary assessment must be immediately stabilized before worrying about anything else.

Your immediate treatment of life-threatening problems found in the primary assessment is referred to as Basic Life Support (BLS) and may include cardiopulmonary resuscitation (CPR), airway control, bleeding control, and protection from extremes of heat or cold. Advanced life support (ALS) adds medications and specialized tools to manage these same critical system problems. You may not get any further than BLS or ALS with your assessment and treatment if the injury or illness is severe. In most cases, however, you will be able to rule out or stabilize serious problems and go on to the secondary assessment.

The Secondary Assessment

The secondary assessment involves gathering a relevant medical history, investigating the patient's chief complaint, and systematically assessing the patient. Speed and detail change with circumstance. It is not necessary or efficient to stop and treat problems as you find them. Get the whole picture, complete your list, and then return to treat each problem in order of priority.

Secondary Assessment

Complete Then Treat

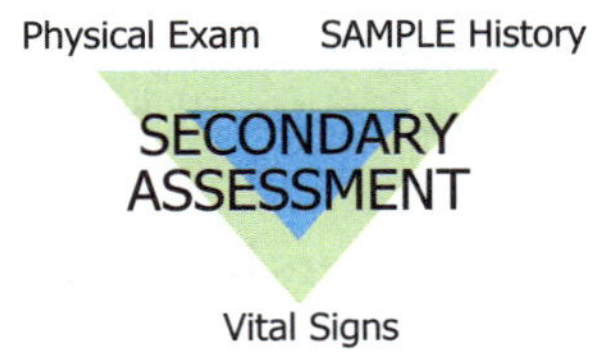

"Get the whole picture, complete your list, then return to treat each problem in order of priority."

Most practitioners in the civilized setting are accustomed to patients sitting quietly on an exam table and prefer to start their exam with the head and neck and then move to the chest, abdomen, pelvis, legs, arms, and back. It is comforting to have a routine, making the process more efficient and reassuring for both the examiner and the patient.

A well-rehearsed routine will be even more valuable in the backcountry situation when you are challenged by wind, cold, radio traffic, and scene management. You may not yet know what the problem is, but you know what to do: examine the patient. Conducting your exam will calm you down, focus your attention, and give you the information that you need.

Your exam should be as comprehensive as the situation requires and allows. Realistically, the order in which you perform your exam makes no difference. Start where it makes sense to start. If the patient is lying face down, examine their back first. It is not necessary to see or feel every body part if no symptom or MOI suggests involvement. It *is* important that the rescuer go through a complete head-to-toe checklist, mentally if not physically.

The complaint of a sprained thumb by an otherwise healthy person does not warrant a complete survey with vital signs and a full physical examination; however, a person with altered mental status and a mechanism for significant injury certainly does. The less information the patient can give you, the more information you will need from your exam.

Your secondary assessment catalogs anything abnormal, such as tenderness, discoloration, swelling, and deformity. You do not have to be an experienced anatomist to recognize a deformed long bone or bruises and abrasions. If your patient is at all responsive, you will be able to find out what hurts.

Advanced practitioners listen for breath sounds with a stethoscope, look in ears, and peer down throats. The abdominal exam might also include listening to bowel sounds or palpating specific spots for tenderness. The secondary assessment of the nervous system may be as simple as talking to the patient to determine mental status or as complex as testing cranial nerves and deep tendon reflexes. The complexity of your exam will depend on your level of comfort and training. In all but the simplest case, any exam is better than no exam.

In an unresponsive or unreliable patient, your exam should also include the patient's pockets, wallet, and pack. A medication bottle, insulin syringe, or medical identification bracelet or card can provide valuable information in a confusing case. Respect privacy but get the data you need.

Vital Signs

During the primary assessment we look at pulse, respiratory effort, and mental status as part of our quick look for serious problems. During the secondary assessment, the measurement of vital signs provides a more complete view of critical system function and compensation. Decay or improvement in the patient's condition is revealed by changes in the vital sign pattern over time. This can serve to reassure you that the patient is okay or provide an early warning of developing trouble. The detail with which you measure vital signs will depend on the equipment available and your level of training. How often you measure vital signs will depend on the logistical situation and your level of comfort with the patient's condition.

Pulse rate (P) is usually easy to measure accurately and reflects almost any change in the circulatory system. During the primary assessment, we were concerned only with the presence of a pulse and the estimation of fast, slow, or normal. During our secondary assessment, we have the time to measure pulse rate more accurately in beats per minute—quickly obtained by counting the pulse for 15 seconds and multiplying the count by four. Noting the rhythm (irregular or regular) can be helpful in some cases, but subjective assessments like weak, thready, or bounding are rarely useful in the field setting. You can find the pulse in any artery, but the radial (wrist), carotid (neck), and temporal (temple in front of the ear) are the most accessible.

Blood pressure (BP), like pulse, is a measurement of circulatory system function. A reading of 120/80 mm Hg is considered normal for a healthy adult. The systolic reading (top number) indicates the pressure produced by the force of each heart contraction. The diastolic reading (bottom number) reflects the resting pressure of the system maintained by arterial muscle tone. The systolic pressure is the most useful and the easiest to measure in the emergency setting.

Systolic BP is usually measured by inflating a blood pressure cuff around the arm and applying enough pressure to stop arterial blood flow completely. The cuff is then slowly deflated while the examiner watches the gauge and feels for the return of a pulse in the wrist. The reading on the gauge when the first beat is felt is the systolic BP. Diastolic BP is obtained by listening to arterial flow with a stethoscope or Doppler device. Portable automated BP cuffs capable of measuring systolic and diastolic are often used in ambulances and emergency departments, and now appear in the jumps kits used by some ski patrols and backcountry rescue teams.

Respiratory rate (R), expressed in breaths per minute, is a direct measurement of respiratory system function but can be difficult to measure accurately. It is more valuable to note the *effort* involved in respiration. An increased respiratory rate may be a compensatory response to shock, which is a circulatory system problem and not an indication of respiratory distress. Labored and noisy respiration would confirm a respiratory system problem and true respiratory distress.

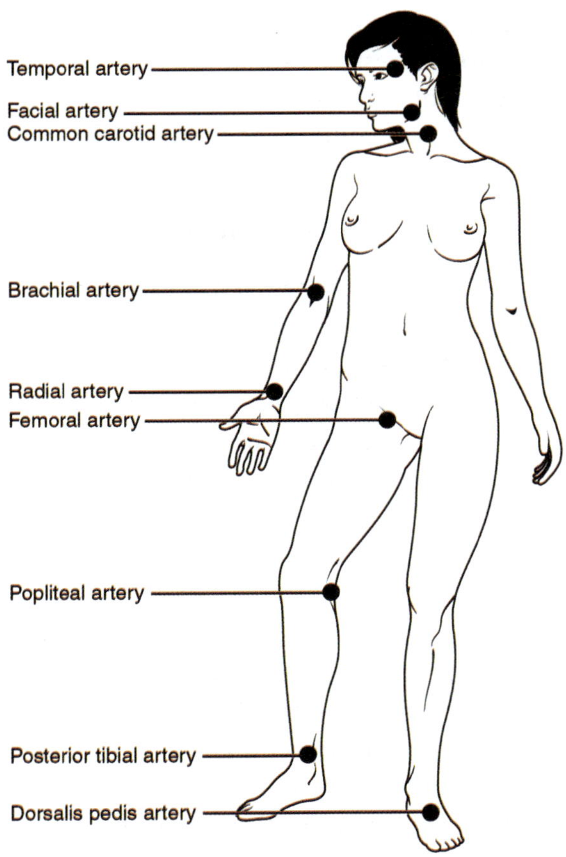

There are a number of places where arteries lie just under the skin where the pulse can be felt and the rate counted.

Temperature (T) refers to the temperature of the body core. This can be quite different from skin temperature, especially when exposed to extremes of heat or cold. The rectum is the most accurate place to measure core temperature in the field. Oral temperatures are certainly more convenient, but are affected by eating, breathing, and talking and may be lower than core temperature. The more accurate esophageal or bladder probes are generally not available or practical for field use.

Skin color and temperature (S) reflects the perfusion of the body shell. Reduced skin perfusion may indicate compensation for loss of blood volume in illness and injury. Or, cool and pale skin might just be part of the normal response to cold weather. Warm, dry, and pink skin is normal. The perfusion status of dark-skinned patients can be assessed by observing the palms and soles and the mucosa of the lips.

Oxygen Saturation (O2) measures the percentage of the blood's oxygen carrying capacity that is currently in use. At sea level, a healthy circulatory and respiratory system will oxygenate to 98–100%. This drops to 90–95% at 3000 meters of elevation. Some chronic respiratory problems will result in an O2 saturation as low as 85%, which may be normal for that person. Generally, anything below 89% indicates a problem, unless other factors such as altitude are considered.

Oxygen saturation is measured in the field with a small device that fits on a finger, toe, or earlobe. Called a pulse oximeter, it measures the color of the blood from which it calculates the percentage of hemoglobin molecules that are combined with oxygen. Some smartphones also have this measuring capability. An accurate reading depends on good circulation to the digit being used for measurement.

Placing the probe on a cold or ischemic extremity may result in an artificially low oxygen saturation reading. The presence of carbon monoxide, which produces a bright red color when combined with hemoglobin, will result an artificially high reading. Fingernail polish has also been shown to effect the device.

Consciousness and mental status (C) is a measure of brain function. No special instruments are required. Consciousness is described as relating to one of four letters on the AVPU scale:

- A is awake, with the patient's condition further described in terms of mental status using terms like oriented, disoriented, confused, combative, etc.

- V on AVPU refers to a patient who appears unaware but responds to verbal stimulus. The response may range from eye opening to just a grunt or turn of the head.
- P indicates a response only to pain. The patient may localize to pain by pushing your hand away from an injury or respond with just a groan or nonspecific movement.
- U describes a patient who is completely unresponsive.

When measuring vital signs, it is most useful to take them all together at regular intervals, allowing you to observe change over time. Even without a blood pressure cuff, thermometer, oximeter, or a watch, a valuable assessment of vital signs can still be made. Measurements become relative: Pulse is fast or slow; temperature is cool or warm. Blood pressure and oxygenation can be assessed as normal or low based on such signs as mental status and skin color.

It is important to remember that each vital sign contributes to a pattern.

Vital Signs

P – Pulse
R – Respiration
BP – Blood Pressure
T – Temperature
S – Skin: color, temperature, moisture
O – Oxygen Saturation
AVPU - Level of Consciousness
- A - awake (further define mental status)
- V - responds to verbal stimulus
- P - responds to painful stimulus
- U - completely unresponsive

A single vital sign taken out of context can be misleading. For example, an O2 saturation measurement of 68% would not be expected in a patient whose vital signs are otherwise normal. Something is probably wrong with the meter or the placement of the probe. A single vital sign that does not fit the rest of the pattern should motivate further investigation before making a judgment based on that finding.

SAMPLE History

A good history can be the most useful part of the whole assessment. Initially, at least, it should be focused on the immediate problem. Details about your patient's abdominal surgery in 1983 are not relevant to the assessment of their sprained knee.

However, the history of surgery would certainly be relevant in evaluating a complaint of abdominal pain because surgical scars can increase the risk of bowel obstruction. A history of allergy is especially important if you are thinking of giving medication. Questions about last food and fluids are important where extreme weather is an issue or if you suspect volume shock from dehydration.

SAMPLE History

S – Symptoms; as described by the patient.
A – Allergies; and nature of reaction.
M – Medication; Rx and non-Rx.
P – Pertinent History; to current problem.
L – Last Ins and Outs; food, fluids, meds.
E – Events; leading to current problem.

The history can be taken before or after the exam. Beware of the common mistake of taking a history while performing the exam. "Does this hurt?" and "Have you ever had abdominal surgery?" asked at the same time may produce a useless answer to both questions. In the ideal situation, your history will be gathered separately.

The *events* question pertains specifically to what happened that directly led to the problem with which you are dealing. This could be a description of a fall, a long hike leading to heat exhaustion, or being stung by a wasp. Careful attention here can reveal undiscovered problems or help make the difference between diagnosing a critical system problem like a traumatic brain injury and reassuring yourself that you're looking at a simple scalp contusion.

Creating a Problem List: SOAP

The information you have gathered in your surveys should be organized in a format abbreviated SOAP: Subjective, Objective, Assessment, and Plan. This is a common way to organize medical information and will be recognized by practitioners worldwide. Using this method, information regarding the patient assessment and history are divided into two groups: what you learn from your survey of the scene and talking to the patient and witnesses (subjective) and what you learn from your examination of the patient (objective). This report also provides the answer to the all-important question: What's wrong here and what you are going to do about it (assessment and plan)?

SOAP Note

Subjective:
- Story
- SAMPLE history, if relevant

Objective:
- Exam findings
- Vital signs

Assessment:
- Problem list (A)
- Anticipated problems (A′)

Plan:
- Treatment for each existing problem
- Evacuation and/or monitoring for anticipated problems

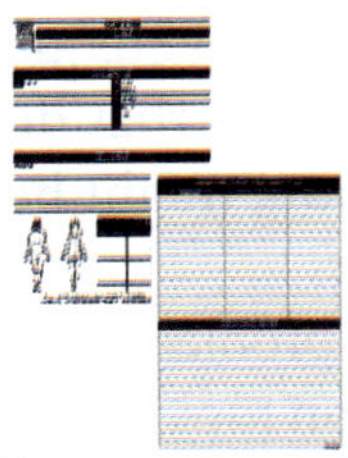

Using this system, a typical brief SOAP for an emergency room case might look like this:

S: A 19-year-old man fell off his bicycle when he rode over a curb at slow speed. He complains of pain in his right wrist and tingling of his fingers. He has no complaints of pain anywhere else. He was not wearing a helmet but did not hit his head and has full memory for the event. No allergies, no medications, no history of previous wrist injury; last meal 12:00.

O: An alert, oriented, but uncomfortable man. The right wrist is swollen and tender to touch. There is no other obvious injury. The patient refuses to move the wrist voluntarily. The fingers are warm and pink and can be wiggled with slight pain felt at the wrist. The patient can feel the light touch of a cotton swab on the end of each finger. X-ray shows a non-displaced mildly angulated fracture of the distal radius. Vital signs: P: 80; R: 18, easy; O2: 99%; BP: 122/72; S: warm, dry, pink; T: 37.1°C; C: awake, alert, and oriented.

A: Fractured right radius.

P: Wrist splint. Rest, ice, and elevation. Acetaminophen 500 mg every 6 hours for pain. Follow up with an orthopedic surgeon within 3 days. Return to the hospital if fingers become blue or cold, or if the tingling becomes at all worse.

This format paints a clear picture of the situation. In just a few words, you get a sense of who the patient is, what happened, and what the practitioner is going to do about it. There is also a brief description of problems that might develop and what the patient's response should be.

The SOAP format is perfectly adaptable to the backcountry setting. It performs the same vital function that it does in the emergency department. SOAP organizes your thoughts and allows you to communicate your ideas and plans.

Now, let's take this same case into the backcountry:

S: A 19-year-old man performed a slow fall over the handlebars on a mountain bike ride near Horse Thief Canyon about 1 hour ago. He complains of pain in his right wrist and tingling of his fingers. He has no complaints of pain anywhere else. He did not hit his head and has full memory of the event. No allergies, no medications, no history of previous wrist injury, last meal 12:00. He feels cold and hungry. It is now 18:30 and getting dark. The air temperature is 48°F. It is raining lightly. The scene is a 3-hour bike ride from the trailhead. There is no good off-road vehicle access.

O: At 18:30: An alert, responsive, but uncomfortable man is found sitting on a rock holding his right arm. He is cool and wet but inadequately dressed. His right wrist is deformed and tender to touch; he is unable to move it.
He can wiggle his fingers and feel the light touch of the examiner's hand. His skin color is pale. There is no other obvious injury. Vital signs: P: 80; R: 18, easy; BP: 122 systolic; O2: 99%; S: cool and pale; T: 37.1°C; C: awake and oriented.

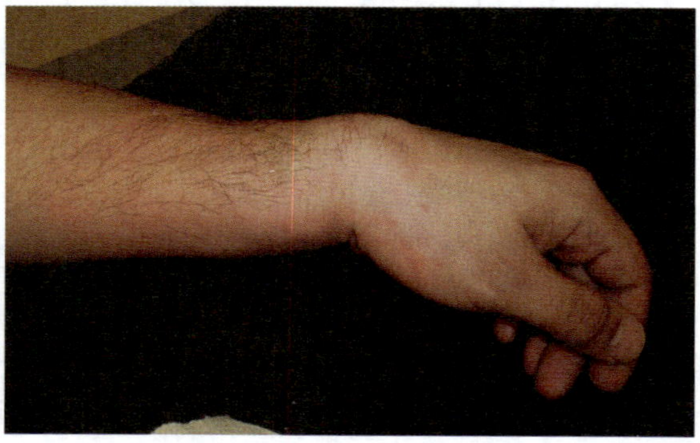

A:

1. Unstable injury; right wrist
   A': Swelling and ischemia
   A': Pain
2. Cold response
   A': Hypothermia
3. Dark, wet, unsafe riding or hiking conditions.

P:

1. Wrist splint. Elevation and rest. Acetaminophen. Monitor distal CSM.
2. Dry clothes, food, and shelter from the rain and wind.
3. Stay on scene tonight, walk out tomorrow.

We have expanded SOAP to include environmental and logistical factors. Sometimes these are more of a threat than the original injury or illness. In long-term care, we also add a list of anticipated problems (A'), which could be complications of the injury itself or the result of exposure to environmental conditions. By listing the anticipated problem of hypothermia, for example, we are reminded to take measures to prevent it.

In more complicated cases where a patient may have more than one problem, the format remains the same. Under A (Assessment), we would list the problems in order of priority, and be sure that we have a plan for each one. By checking each problem for a plan and each plan for a problem, we can avoid missing anything. We can also avoid the common mistake of making plans for problems that don't exist.

As our patient's condition and evacuation logistics change, our problem list and plans will need to be revised. Backcountry rescue is rarely straightforward and predictable. Monitoring the condition of the patient and crew is essential. SOAP is a dynamic process.

Patients with anticipated critical body system problems should be reassessed most often, at least every 15 minutes, if possible. The status of injured extremities in a reliable patient can be checked less frequently, at 1- to 2-hour intervals. Conditions that develop slowly, such as wound infection, might be adequately monitored every 6 hours.

Our problems list also becomes a useful communication tool. "The problem list is as follows: One, unstable right wrist. Two, cold response" gives the relevant information in just a few words in a text message, brief radio transmission, or while updating rescuers arriving on scene. This format can be especially useful in a multiple-casualty incident or other high-stress operation.

When time and technology allow, more complete information can be relayed. Still, the practitioner should keep the message concise. The essential points can be lost in too much information. Try to paint a picture of your situation, including your problem list and plan: "This is Search and Rescue on the scene of a mountain bike accident mile 42, White Rim Trail. One male patient: Problems are unstable right wrist and cold response. Current weather is cold rain and wind. We will stay here tonight and evacuate in the morning." In this case, relaying specific exam findings and vital signs is unnecessary. The receiving station knows your location, situation, problem list, and plan.

Radio SOAP

1. Location, situation, scene.
2. Plan and support requested.
3. Patient and problem list.
4. Additional information as needed.

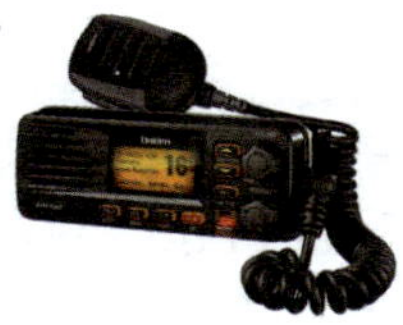

"This format paints a nice picture of the situation…who the patient is and what happened, and what the practitioner is going to do about it."

In the ideal setting your SOAP note would be a well-organized written document, but we realize that this is impossible to do in a life raft or on a mountainside during a storm. But it is just these challenging situations that are most in need of critical thinking and an organized response. Reviewing the SOAP, especially the assessment and plan, even if it is all done in your head, can help render order from chaos, improve communication, and save lives. Practice it. Use it.

Chapter 3 Review: Patient Assessment and the SOAP Format

- The patient assessment system consists of the scene size-up, primary assessment, and secondary assessment.
- The scene size-up includes identifying the number of patients and available resources, hazards to rescuers and patients, and the mechanism of injury.
- The primary assessment identifies serious problems with the circulatory, respiratory, or nervous systems requiring immediate treatment.
- Basic and advanced life support is the immediate care rendered to stabilize or correct serious problems identified by the primary assessment.
- The secondary assessment includes a more complete patient examination and medical history to identify all relevant problems.
- The SOAP format is used to organize and present information obtained by the scene size-up and patient assessment.

Case Study 1: Fall While Climbing

SCENE

A mountain rescue team responds to the scene of a climbing accident. A 24-year-old man has fallen 5 meters off a cliff, impacting and rolling 30 meters down a steep scree slope. The report was called in by cell phone at 1700 hours by his climbing partner. Mountain Rescue arrives on scene at 1900 hours. The weather is clear and calm with a temperature of 18°C. The scene is at the base of a granite cliff at an elevation of 3300 meters. The evacuation will require a descent of a 35% slope of loose scree and trees to the valley floor at 2750 meters.

S: The patient is found sitting upright on a steep scree slope. He complains of a mild headache and severe right ankle pain on attempted movement and weight bearing. He reports full memory for the event. He denies neck or back pain, difficulty breathing, abdominal pain, or distal numbness or weakness. His history is remarkable only for infrequent exercise-induced asthma. He describes himself as otherwise healthy and using no medication. His last meal was lunch at 1300. He last drank 500 ml of water just before the fall. He reports his normal resting pulse rate as 64. He lives at 3000 meters.

O: Awake and calm with normal mental status. Scalp with several superficial lacerations and contusions. Other superficial abrasions and contusions noted over trunk and extremities. Right ankle is markedly swollen and tender. Distal circulation, sensation is intact. There is no respiratory distress. There is no significant chest wall, abdominal, or pelvic tenderness. There is no tenderness to firm palpation of the spine, and the distal motor and sensory exam is fully intact (exception for R ankle motor exam). Vital signs at 1915: P: 106, R: 16 and easy, O2: 93%, BP: 126 systolic, S: normal, T: normal, C: awake and oriented.

A:

1. High risk MOI with elevated pulse; concern for volume shock
   A': Decompensated volume shock
2. Unstable right ankle injury
   A': Ischemia
3. Numerous superficial abrasions, lacerations, and contusions
   A': Infection
4. Difficult and dangerous evacuation
   A': Delayed transport, rescuer fatigue and injury

P:

1. Proceed with emergency evacuation. Bolus of 500 mL IV fluid. Monitor vital signs.
2. Ankle splint, litter evacuation. Monitor distal CSM. Pain medication.
3. Wounds irrigated with water, deeper wounds dressed.
4. Mutual aid for more technical rescuers and logistical support.

Discussion:

This was an arduous and hazardous night evacuation. Mountain Rescue transferred the patient to EMS at the trailhead at 0300 the following day. Fortunately, only minor injuries were experienced by the rescuers during the process. The patient's pulse rate remained between 106 and 120 throughout. No critical system problem was ever identified.

This case is interesting because the concern for shock was made based on the mechanism and pulse rate alone. The emergency response might have been usual in the ambulance context but was not appropriate in this high-risk backcountry scene. The rest of the volume shock pattern was not present. There was no severe external bleeding, or pain and tenderness that suggested internal bleeding. Removing volume shock from the problem list would have allowed the medical officer to make a better risk/benefit decision, perhaps to remain on scene until the evacuation could be carried out in daylight with more equipment and personnel.

Case Study 2: Offshore Illness

SCENE
A 40-meter sail training vessel located 500 nautical miles east of Bermuda bound for the Azores. A trainee has reported ill and unable to stand watch. The medical officer is called to evaluate. The weather is overcast with occasional squalls. Winds are west at 25 to 30 knots with seas of 2 to 4 meters.

S: A subdued and ill-looking 18-year-old woman is found lying in her berth. She admits to being sea sick for the past three days with nausea and vomiting. She has been able to eat and drink very little. She last urinated eight hours ago. She complains of almost fainting on trying to stand, a mild headache, and abdominal pain. History reveals that her last menstrual period was eleven weeks ago and that there is the possibility of pregnancy. She describes herself as otherwise healthy and using no routine medications. She denies difficulty breathing.

O: Awake and subdued with normal mental status. Her skin appears pale and her lips and mouth are somewhat dry. Breathing appears easy and lung sounds are clear on auscultation with a stethoscope. There is mild abdominal tenderness and subdued but present bowel sounds. There is no kidney tenderness. There is no other obvious abnormality on physical exam. Vital signs at 1300: P: 122, R: 22 and easy, O2: 98%, BP: 96/62, S: pale and cool, T: normal, C: awake and oriented.

A:

1. Compensated volume shock due to sea sickness and dehydration
   A': Decompensated shock
2. Possibility of pregnancy
   A': Complications due to shock, limits medication options
3. No early evacuation options

P:

1. Begin oral hydration. Consider intravenous or subcutaneous hydration if not successful.
2. Urine pregnancy test when patient can produce urine.

Discussion:

Compensated volume shock is a serious problem. When the MOI is dehydration from a treatable cause, it may be a problem you can fix in the field. A positive urine pregnancy confirmed the potential complication, but was not a serious problem at this point. An electric Relief Band for nausea was suggested by a shoreside doctor and offered by another trainee. The nausea was reduced, and rehydration was successful without medication. The patient elected to leave the ship when she made port five days later.

Section II: Critical Body Systems

Chapter 4: The Circulatory System

One of the three critical body systems, the circulatory system, is responsible for perfusing all body tissues with blood. This requires a complex arrangement of connected structures, including a four-chambered heart, arteries, arterioles, capillaries, venules, and veins conducting a fluid consisting of millions of suspended and dissolved particles and chemicals. Failure of the circulatory system to perfuse body tissues adequately is called shock, and it is a serious critical system problem requiring immediate and aggressive life-saving treatment.

Circulatory System

Structure:
- Blood
- Vessels
- Heart

Function:
- Maintain perfusion pressure
- Circulate oxygenated blood

Problem:
- Shock: inadequate perfusion pressure

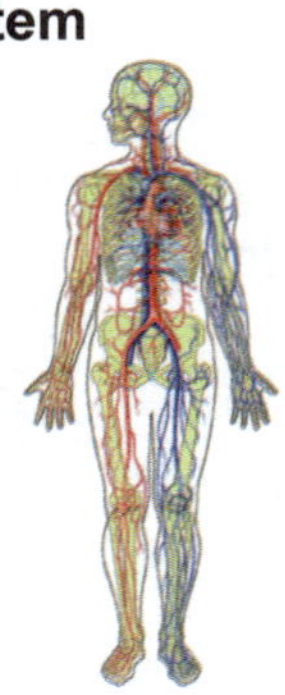

Structure and Function

For field purposes, we can simplify the structure of the circulatory system to three basic components: the blood, the blood vessels, and the heart. These components work together to distribute oxygen and nutrients and to remove waste.

Blood, the primary transport medium of the circulatory system, is composed of fluid, cells, and dissolved gases. The fluid component of the blood consists of water, proteins, electrolytes, and the various chemical mediators of body function called hormones. The cellular component includes red blood cells to carry oxygen, white blood cells to fight infection, and platelets to effect blood clotting.

The average human body contains about 5 liters of blood; however, this volume is not contained in a closed system. The fluid component can migrate between the interior of body cells (intracellular space), the space between the cells (extracellular space), and the blood itself (vascular space). This ability to shift fluid explains how a patient can lose blood volume by losing water and electrolytes from sweat glands. It also explains how blood volume can be restored by consuming water and electrolytes.

The blood is distributed to all living cells in the body (except for the cornea of the eye) by traveling within a system of arteries, veins, and capillaries. There are two zones in the system; one circulating through the lungs (pulmonary circulation) and the other through the rest of the body (systemic circulation). As the blood leaves the right ventricle of the heart, it flows into the pulmonary circulation in the lung, where oxygenation of the blood occurs and carbon dioxide is released to be exhaled. Oxygenated blood returning from the lungs enters the left side of the heart where the left ventricle pumps it to the rest of the body.

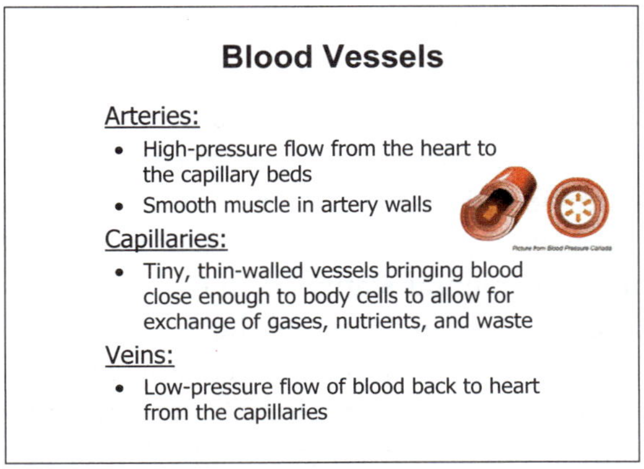

From the thoracic aorta, which is about the diameter of a garden hose, the blood flows through progressively smaller vessels into the capillary beds. The capillary beds consist of a dense matrix of tiny vessels about the diameter of a red blood cell. This is how blood is brought into very close proximity to individual body cells, allowing for cellular oxygenation and the removal of carbon dioxide. Exiting the capillaries, the blood enters the veins to be returned to the right side of the heart.

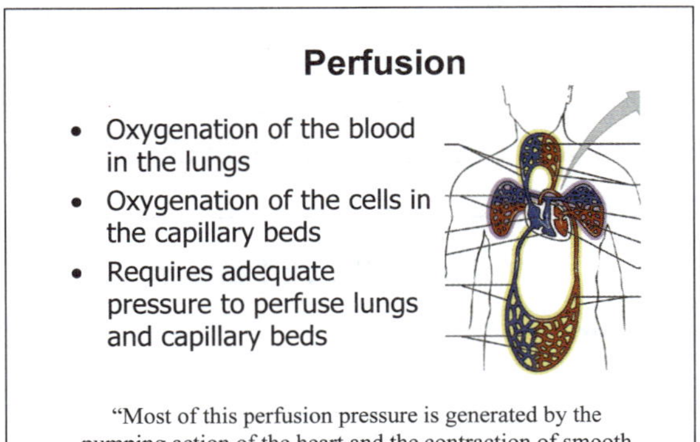

"Most of this perfusion pressure is generated by the pumping action of the heart and the contraction of smooth muscle in artery walls."

To keep you alive, your 5 liters of blood are pumped through approximately 14 kilometers of blood vessels about a thousand times per day. Considerable pressure is required to overcome the natural resistance to flow and to ensure perfusion of all body tissues. We can measure the perfusion pressure generated by the circulatory system in the form of arterial blood pressure.

Most of this perfusion pressure is generated by the pumping action of the heart and the contraction of smooth muscle in artery walls. Blood circulation is augmented by the elasticity of arteries, the system of one-way valves in the veins and the contraction of skeletal muscles as you move about. In a healthy individual, these work together to keep blood pressure relatively constant throughout a variety of activities and environmental conditions.

Shock

Shock is the term for inadequate perfusion pressure in the circulatory system resulting in inadequate oxygenation of body cells. While even a small drop in pressure can cause poor oxygenation of tissues in the extremities and skin, compensatory mechanisms will usually adjust blood flow to preserve the oxygenation and perfusion of vital organs. If pressure continues to drop, even vital body tissues will suffer. Shock that is not corrected will inevitably result in circulatory system failure and death.

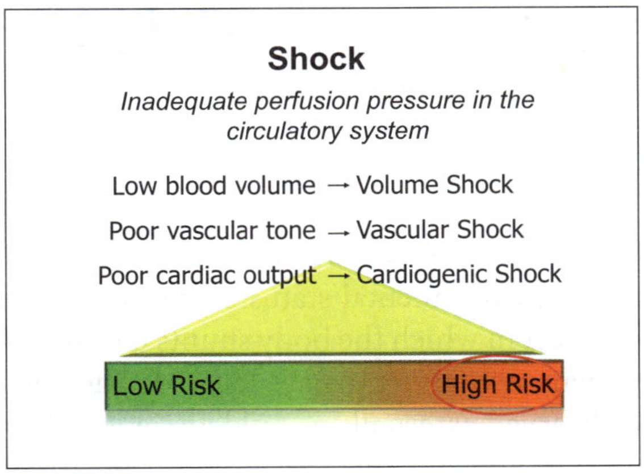

There are three basic types of shock that correspond to the three major components of the circulatory system. Volume shock (also called hypovolemic shock) is caused by blood or fluid loss from blood vessels. Vascular shock results when the blood vessels lose muscle tone and dilate due to injury or illness. Cardiogenic shock is caused by inadequate pumping action of the heart. The basic problem caused by all three is inadequate perfusion pressure resulting in inadequate oxygenation.

Volume Shock

A history of trauma sufficient to cause severe internal or external bleeding should alert you to look for evidence of volume shock. A more common mechanism in the wilderness environment, however, is dehydration from diarrhea, vomiting, or sweating. Regardless of the mechanism, the problem is the same: inadequate perfusion pressure due to low blood volume.

Severe external bleeding is usually easy to spot. But in cases where fluid loss is not so obvious, watching the body compensate may be the only way to detect the onset of volume shock from slow internal bleeding or dehydration. We observe compensation by measuring vital signs.

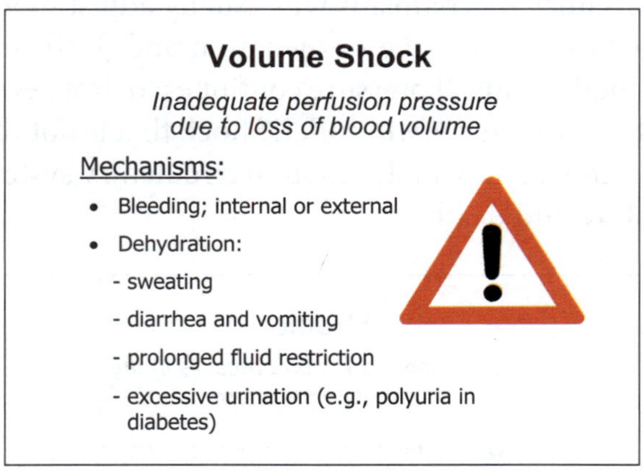

As shock develops, the first vital sign changes to occur are early mental status changes and shell/core effect in which the body shunts blood to the core where vital organs are located. The effects are observed externally as mild anxiety and cool, pale skin and mucous membranes. A little further into the pattern compensatory efforts will include an increase in pulse and respiratory rate. This accounts for the classic symptoms of shock described as cool, pale skin and rapid pulse and respiration.

Early on, perfusion is maintained to the vital organs of the body core through this combination of increased cardiac output and respiratory effort and shell/core effect. It is augmented by fluid shifting into the blood from body cells and tissues, although this compensatory mechanism is difficult to observe directly. Dizziness may occur with standing or sitting up as brain perfusion is temporarily impaired because the circulatory system is unable to compensate quickly for the effects of gravity.

If you can measure blood pressure, you may observe that the compensatory mechanisms keep it near normal in the very early stages of volume loss. Because the brain is still enjoying near-normal perfusion, the patient may exhibit only mild mental status changes. This stage is called compensated volume shock.

This serves to remind us that a single measurement of blood pressure alone is not particularly useful. It offers only an approximation of perfusion pressure at one place on the upper arm or leg. It does not reliably indicate low blood volume or the status of cellular oxygenation. Unless you are alert to the entire vital sign pattern for volume shock, you may miss the diagnosis until it is too late.

In the long-term care situation, monitoring urine output is a good way to monitor the status of the circulatory system. Reduced blood volume will result in greatly reduced urine output as the kidneys do their part to conserve fluid. The urine that is produced will be more concentrated and appear dark yellow or brown. These are important signs to watch for when you're concerned about the slow loss of fluid with burns, vomiting and diarrhea, and other forms of dehydration.

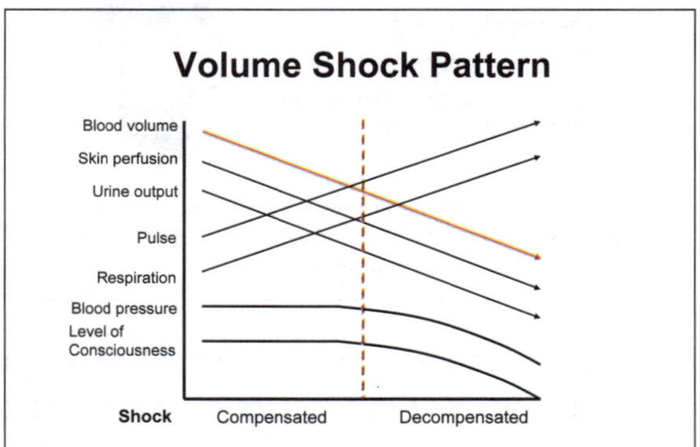

"Fast or slow, bleeding or dehydration, it looks the same."

As volume shock progresses and the compensation mechanisms are overwhelmed, oxygenation and perfusion of the brain will be further reduced resulting in more profound brain failure. The patient's level of consciousness will decrease and the brain's ability to control the circulatory and respiratory systems will become impaired. Cardiac output will decrease as heart muscle is deprived of oxygen. Circulatory collapse and respiratory failure are imminent. This is called decompensated shock.

The rate of progression of volume shock will be directly related to the rate of fluid loss, but the vital sign pattern and trend will be the same: altered mental status, increasing pulse and respiratory rate, and decreasing skin perfusion and urine output. In the case of severe bleeding, the patient may progress from compensated volume shock to decompensated shock within minutes. Dehydration, on the other hand, can progress over many hours or days. Either way, if volume shock cannot be reversed, the patient will die.

Field Treatment of Volume Shock

Stop the Fluid Loss. Severe bleeding is a critical system problem identified during the primary assessment and treated as part of basic life support (see the basic and advanced life support chapter). Dehydration is a more common mechanism for volume shock in the wilderness or offshore setting. It is less urgent, but no less important, and is also initially treated by stopping the fluid loss. You will need to reduce heat stress to reduce sweating or use medication to stop diarrhea or vomiting. This may or may not be easy to accomplish in a high-risk situation.

Restore Blood Volume. The first aid treatments of reassurance, elevating the feet, and keeping the patient warm do nothing to address the real problem of low blood volume. A patient in volume shock from uncontrolled blood loss needs a surgeon and a hospital, and blood. Intravenous therapy with normal saline or other crystalloid solution is only a temporary treatment that may buy time, but can also cause harm.

When blood loss can be controlled or where shock is caused by dehydration, field treatment with oral, IV, or subcutaneous fluids may be definitive. Oral rehydration can take hours or days and is not ideal but may be your best option in a high-risk situation. The return of normal vital signs, along with normal urine output, is the best indication of success. If the patient is not improving within a reasonable period, evacuation must be considered. Shock that you cannot reverse in the field is a life-threatening medical emergency regardless of its cause.

Volume Shock Treatment

Stop the fluid loss:
- Control bleeding
- Reduce sweating
- Treat diarrhea and vomiting

Replace fluid volume:
- IV blood and electrolyte solutions
- Oral electrolyte solutions or water and food
- Rectal or sub-cutaneous rehydration

Maintain calories and body core temp

Position and Protection. Regardless of the cause of volume shock, it is important to protect the patient from heat loss. The patient in shock will not be generating much heat through metabolic processes or muscle activity, and hypothermia will greatly reduce the chances of survival. Contact with the ground, water, or cold IV solutions and bottled oxygen will exacerbate the problem. Be sure to add heat to the patient package in all but the warmest of conditions.

A patient in shock should be carried horizontally because an upright orientation can inhibit perfusion of the brain and can be fatal. Avoid a vertical hoist into a helicopter or onto a ship, or a technical evacuation with the litter belayed in the vertical position.

Oxygen. Supplemental oxygen may be brought to the scene by rescue teams. Adding more oxygen to the air the patient is breathing increases the efficiency of a limited blood supply. In the field setting, oxygen is usually administered by nasal canula at a rate just adequate to reduce symptoms and maintain oxygenation of the brain. A flow rate as low as 0.25 liters per minute can make a difference. Improved mental status and an increased oxygen saturation are a good indication of success. High-flow oxygen by mask is rarely necessary and may result in depletion of the supply before the mission is over.

Vascular Shock

With the loss of muscle tone in the arteries or the inflammation and dilation of capillaries due to injury or illness, the pressure exerted on the blood volume drops. The pattern of vital sign changes as the body compensates will include the typical increase in pulse and respiratory rate and reduction in urine output. However, you may not see shell/core compensation as you do in volume shock because the blood vessels in the skin may be unable to constrict normally. This is where the appearance of vascular shock might differ from that of volume shock.

Vascular shock is most commonly seen in the severe, systemic allergic reaction called anaphylaxis. It can also be part of a syndrome caused by systemic infection (septic shock) or due to the loss of nervous system control in severe spinal cord injury. The result is the same: inadequate perfusion pressure in the circulatory system resulting in inadequate cellular oxygenation.

Field Treatment of Vascular Shock

Field treatment for vascular shock includes keeping the patient horizontal because the ability to compensate for the effects of gravity is impaired. Treat the cause if possible. Anaphylaxis, for example, can be reversed with injectable epinephrine (see the Allergy and Anaphylaxis chapter). If vasodilatation is not reversible with field treatment, as in spinal cord injury or infection, evacuation and IV fluid to expand blood volume and maintain perfusion are indicated. ALS providers may also use vasoactive medications like norepinephrine to temporarily boost perfusion pressure pending definitive treatment.

An awake and responsive patient is a sign of adequate perfusion pressure and a good target for fluid resuscitation in the field. If you can measure blood pressure, work toward a systolic reading of 90–100 mm Hg. As with volume shock, hypothermia is an anticipated problem in the wilderness setting.

Vascular Shock Treatment

Reverse vasodilation:
- Medications for anaphylaxis
- Vasoconstrictors and antibiotics for infection

Increase fluid volume:
- IV blood or electrolyte solutions
- Oral electrolyte solutions or water and food

PROP and Evacuation as Needed

Cardiogenic Shock

Cardiogenic shock is most often caused by myocardial infarction or cardiac dysrhythmia (i.e., heart attack), resulting in reduced cardiac output. Symptoms include chest pain or pressure accompanied by the signs and symptoms of shock. The pattern of compensation will resemble that of volume shock, except that the heart rate may be very fast, slow, or irregular since abnormal heart function is the root of the problem.

The symptoms of a heart attack may be very severe or quite subtle. Heart attack with the anticipated problem of cardiogenic shock should be on your problem list whenever a patient complains of chest discomfort without an obvious mechanism of injury. This is especially true when the patient's history includes several risk factors for coronary artery disease, such as smoking, obesity, hypertension, or diabetes.

Cardiogenic shock from trauma generally occurs when blood or fluid accumulates in the pericardial sack around the heart, inhibiting heart filling and reducing cardiac output. It can also develop because of poor function in a contused heart. It should be suspected or anticipated whenever a trauma patient complains of persistent chest pain. Cardiogenic shock from trauma is as serious a problem as a heart attack. In either case the problem is the same: inadequate perfusion pressure due to inadequate pumping action of the heart.

Field Treatment of Cardiogenic Shock

Field treatment options for cardiogenic shock are limited and the patient really needs a hospital. Suspected myocardial ischemia is treated with oxygen, aspirin, and the patient's own nitroglycerin if the drug has been prescribed. Even advanced life support (ALS) treatment is very temporary. This is covered in more detail in the Chest Pain chapter.

Cardiac trauma requires urgent evacuation to surgical care. ALS field treatment is limited to pericardiocentesis, which is the aspiration of excess blood or fluid from the pericardial sack. Definitive care may require cardiovascular surgery. This should be considered in planning your evacuation route and destination. Not all hospitals offer this level of surgical care.

> **Cardiogenic Shock Treatment**
>
> Heart Attack:
> - BLS; oxygen, aspirin, nitroglycerin as prescribed
> - Urgent evacuation to ALS and hospital
> - Coronary care unit
>
> Trauma:
> - BLS and oxygen
> - Urgent evacuation to ALS care and hospital
> - Cardiothoracic surgery

Acute Stress Reaction

Acute stress reaction (ASR) is discussed here because it can look like shock, but it has none of the serious consequences. ASR is the term for the frequent and normal response to emotional stress caused by fear, disappointment, surprise, pain, grief, or any number of other influences. Some texts use the term psychogenic shock for this phenomenon. However, ASR does not cause a significant loss of perfusion pressure or serious critical system problems.

The sympathetic form of ASR is the "speed up" response you feel when you are anxious or scared, produced by the release of the hormones epinephrine (also known as adrenaline) and norepinephrine. It speeds up the pulse and respiratory rate, shunts blood to the muscles, dilates the pupils, and generally gets the body ready for action. It also stimulates the release of natural hormones that serve to mask the pain of injury.

This type of ASR certainly has value to human survival. It allows for extraordinary efforts even in the presence of significant injury. Unfortunately, it also makes the accurate assessment of the patient difficult for the rescuer by hiding pain and altering vital signs. The elevation in pulse and respiratory rate and change in mental status can mimic the volume shock pattern resulting in high-risk evacuations for low-risk problems.

The parasympathetic form of ASR is the faint and nauseous feeling some people experience with pain or the sight of blood. Its effect slows the heart rate enough to cause a temporary loss of perfusion pressure. The evolutionary value of this response is unclear. This form of ASR is also harmless except in its ability to mimic the shell/core compensation seen in true volume shock or the change in mental status seen in brain injury.

> **ASR**
>
> Sympathetic:
> - Mediated by epinephrine
> - Increases pulse, respiration, reduces skin perfusion; increases anxiety
> - Can look like shock or respiratory distress
>
> Parasympathetic:
> - Multiple chemical mediators
> - Slows pulse, causes fainting
> - Can look like TBI or other mechanism for mental status changes

The key to recognizing ASR is in the mechanism of injury and the progression of symptoms. ASR can look like shock but can occur with or without any mechanism of injury to cause shock. We have all seen people with only minor extremity sprains or superficial wounds become lightheaded, pale, and nauseous. Although they appear to be in shock, there is no cause for alarm. They have no mechanism for significant volume loss.

It is important to remember that ASR can coexist with shock. In cases where the patient has both a mechanism of injury for true shock and the signs and symptoms to go with it, you must treat it as such. Within a short time, ASR will improve—shock will not.

Field Treatment of ASR

Allowing the patient to lie down, providing calm reassurance, and relieving pain should result in immediate improvement in symptoms. Note that this is the traditional treatment for shock described in many first aid texts. In the ambulance setting, the difference between ASR and shock is less important because both are managed as shock during the short period of treatment and transport. For long-term management in the remote setting, recognizing ASR for what it is can save a lot of resources and risk, not to mention your peace of mind.

Risk Versus Benefit in Shock

Shock is a serious critical system problem that will kill the patient if it is not corrected. The ideal treatment is emergency evacuation to definitive medical care, but in the wilderness or offshore setting it is reasonable to anticipate improvement with treatment on scene when the mechanism is reversible. Dehydration and anaphylaxis are the most obvious examples. Care may be definitive and evacuation unnecessary.

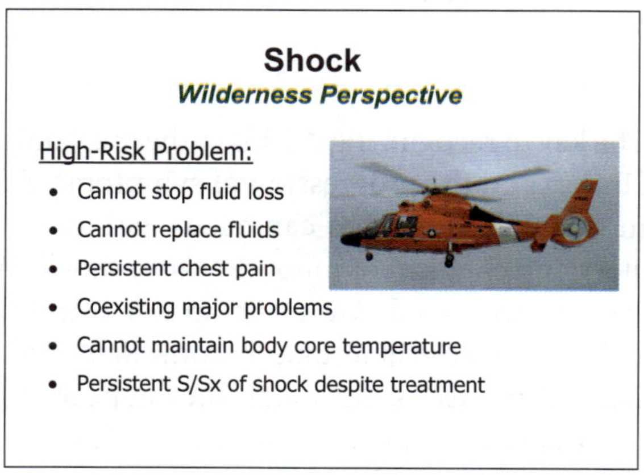

Cases where you cannot reverse the progression of shock, such as internal bleeding or heart attack, may be worth a high-risk evacuation, but beware of committing to a process during which you will be unable to maintain oxygenation, perfusion, and body core temperature. You must balance the risks associated with an unstable evacuation against the benefits of moving fast. A desperate sprint for the hospital is one option, but rarely the best.

Critical thinking about a critical system injury in a difficult and dangerous place requires time and effort. Consider stabilizing and protecting the patient on scene while advanced care is brought to you. Consider a slower carry out during which bleeding can be monitored and controlled rather than risking loss of control during a helicopter hoist. Remember that a cold patient has a much lower chance of surviving shock.

Consider the possibility that even a severely injured patient may have a better chance of survival by remaining aboard the boat rather than being dunked in the ocean during a difficult extrication at sea. And, finally, remember that most people live.

Chapter 4 Review:
The Circulatory System

- The circulatory system is one of the three critical body systems. The basic components include the blood volume, the blood vessels, and the heart.
- The primary function of the system is to circulate blood under pressure adequate to perfuse all body tissues.
- The major problem that can develop in the system is inadequate perfusion pressure caused by low blood volume, inadequate blood vessel constriction, or inadequate heart function. This is called volume shock, vascular shock, or cardiogenic shock respectively.
- Shock should be suspected or anticipated with mechanisms including severe bleeding, dehydration, systemic infection, anaphylaxis, or heart attack.
- Shock is recognized by a mechanism of injury coupled with the characteristic pattern of vital sign changes.
- Shock that cannot be fixed in the field is an emergency.

Chapter 5: The Respiratory System

One of the three critical systems, the respiratory system, is responsible for oxygenating the blood as it perfuses the capillaries in the lungs. Respiration involves a complex arrangement of muscle, bone, airway tubes, semipermeable membranes, and the adjacent capillaries and larger blood vessels. Respiratory failure occurs when the respiratory system is unable to supply enough air to the alveoli of the lungs to adequately oxygenate the blood or remove the accumulated carbon dioxide. Respiratory failure is a serious critical system problem requiring immediate and aggressive lifesaving treatment. Caring for someone in respiratory distress or failure is the scariest thing you will ever do in emergency medicine.

Respiratory System

Structure:

- Upper Airway
- Lower Airway
- Alveoli
- Chest Wall and Diaphragm
- Neuro Drive

Function:

- Oxygenation of the blood
- Regulation of blood pH

Problem:

- Respiratory Failure

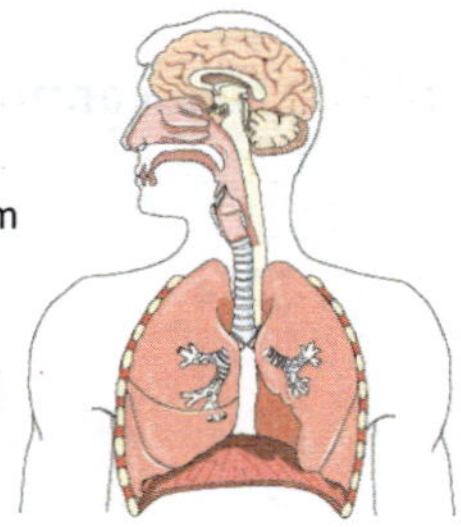

Structure and Function

The structure of the respiratory system is designed to bring air into the alveoli where only a thin semipermeable membrane separates air from blood.

The combined surface area of the millions of alveoli in the lungs would cover a tennis court, offering an extensive membrane through which oxygen can diffuse to bind with the hemoglobin in the red blood cells and for carbon dioxide to diffuse passively from the blood plasma into the air to be exhaled. The efficiency with which the system works is measured as oxygen saturation.

A healthy person at sea level would measure 95% to 100% on a pulse oximeter, indicating that the oxygen-carrying capacity of the blood is met. In the presence of respiratory problems, oxygen saturation will fall, indicating less efficient respiration. It is also possible to measure the efficiency of the respiratory system by assessing mental status and skin color.

Like the circulatory system, the structure of the respiratory system can be described in basic terms for field use: upper airway, lower airway, alveoli, chest wall and diaphragm, and nervous system control. The upper and lower airways consist of the semi-rigid tubes that conduct air into the alveoli. These passages are lined with mucous membranes designed to continuously remove contaminants and bacteria from the system. The upward flow of mucus is generated by tiny hair-like structures called cilia. You are continuously swallowing the resulting mixture, usually without thinking about it.

The chest wall and diaphragm act like bellows to draw the air in and out. The rate and depth of breathing is under nervous system control. In a healthy person, the brain regulates breathing by measuring the carbon dioxide concentration of the blood. Too much carbon dioxide in the blood causes an increase in acidity. The brain responds by increasing the rate and depth of respiration to "blow off" the carbon dioxide until normal acidity is reestablished. Conversely, alkalosis (decreased acidity) is corrected by decreasing the rate and depth of respiration to retain carbon dioxide.

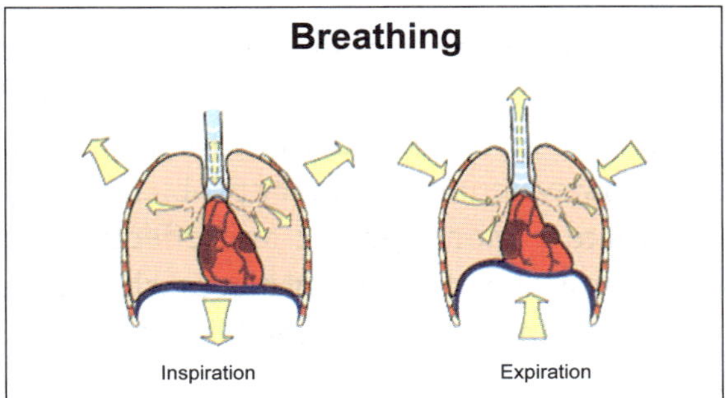

"...the brain regulates breathing by measuring the pH (acidity) of the blood. This is actually a reflection of the amount carbon dioxide dissolved in the blood plasma."

This acid–base regulation system is very precise and results in a smooth and regular respiratory pattern. However, in some disease conditions, such as emphysema, the amount of carbon dioxide in the blood is high all the time because the lower airway is chronically constricted and cannot ventilate properly. Conversely, in a metabolic condition like diabetic ketoacidosis, the patient may be breathing fast to blow off carbon dioxide to keep the pH under control even though the carbon dioxide concentration is already low. Conditions like these can result in respiratory regulation that is much less precise, more easily upset, and results in a more irregular pattern.

Respiratory Problems

Respiratory distress is the generic term for difficulty breathing. Symptoms include increased respiratory rate, increased respiratory effort, anxiety, wheezing, and coughing. One of the most obvious signs of respiratory distress is the use of accessory muscles.

Normally, a person at rest uses only the diaphragm to breathe. When work is increased, oxygen demand increases, and the respiratory system will use muscles in the chest, shoulders, and neck to increase the depth of respiration. You would expect to see this as a normal response in someone who is running or hiking hard; you would not expect to see it in someone sitting still. Accessory muscle use at rest indicates respiratory distress.

A more subtle sign is shortness of breath on exertion. This patient has a compromised respiratory system that can supply enough oxygen only if the demand is low. Sitting and resting are fine, but any level of increased exertion, such as hiking, causes severe shortness of breath. This symptom is often an early sign of respiratory distress due to pneumonia, high-altitude pulmonary edema, or asthma.

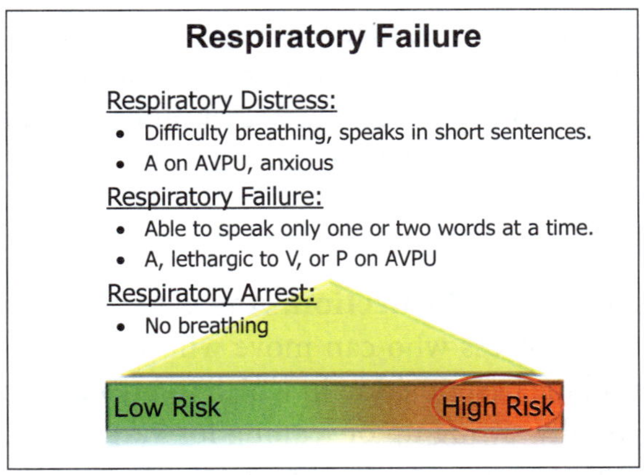

Regardless of the cause of respiratory distress, the condition will eventually progress to respiratory failure if not corrected. Respiratory failure means that the system cannot supply enough oxygen to the blood to keep the brain functioning normally. The primary distinction is made by the decay in mental status and level of consciousness.

If respiratory failure is not corrected, the patient will inevitably deteriorate into respiratory arrest.

An early sign of respiratory failure is the inability to speak more than a few words between breaths. This is called one- or two-word dyspnea. To illustrate what this looks like, imagine trying to speak easily after sprinting hard for 500 meters or so. A patient in this condition at rest, without having sprinted anywhere, is in serious trouble. Conversely, patients who can talk at length about their shortness of breath are probably okay for the time being.

Respiratory distress that you cannot fix in the field is a serious problem. The progression to failure may be rapid or slow. The treatment and evacuation may be a desperate emergency or a careful and low-stress process depending on the rate of progression.

Generic Treatment for Respiratory Distress

Respiratory distress is one of the most frightening problems you will encounter in emergency medicine. Your immediate response should be to initiate treatment while you develop a more specific assessment and plan. You can use the acronym PROP to help you remember the generic treatment for all forms of respiratory distress: Position and protection, Reassurance, Oxygen, and Positive pressure ventilation.

PROP

Position and Protection. Any patient in respiratory distress who can move will have already found the best position in which to breathe. This is usually sitting up or leaning forward to allow gravity to assist the diaphragm and to help keep fluids out of the upper and lower airway. In unconscious or immobile patients, special care must be taken to position them in a way that protects the airway from obstruction or aspiration of vomit, blood, and secretions.

Reassurance. Encourage the patient to breathe slower and deeper, rather than panting like a dog. This brings in fresh oxygen rather than simply moving the old carbon dioxide back and forth in the airways.

Oxygen. If available, giving supplemental oxygen from a tank or concentrator may increase the amount of oxygen getting into the blood, and ultimately to the brain.

Positive Pressure Ventilation. A patient in respiratory distress will fatigue rapidly. You may need to provide positive pressure ventilation to assist the patient's efforts. You do not need to wait until the patient goes into respiratory arrest to use this technique.

Specific Treatments for Respiratory Distress

Although PROP may significantly improve symptoms in some cases, it may be nearly ineffective in others. If you can identify in which part of the respiratory system the primary problem lies, you can initiate a more specific and effective treatment. This is one of the many places where a well-practiced, calm, and disciplined exam will really pay off.

Respiratory Problems

Upper Airway:
- Choking, stridor, or not being able to inhale at all

Lower Airway:
- Prolonged expiration, wheezing, cough

Alveoli:
- Crackles, cough

Chest Wall:
- Pain, history of trauma

Neuro Drive:
- Slow respiration, altered level of consciousness

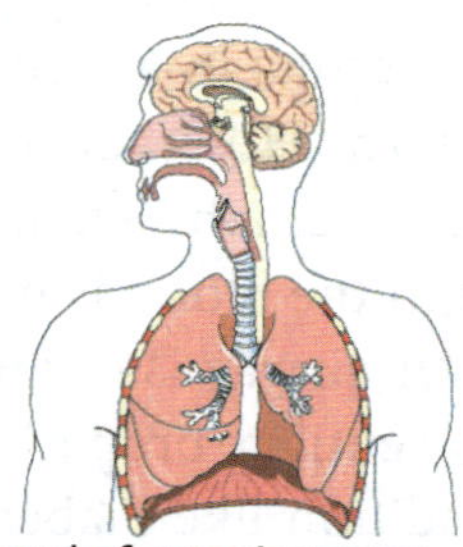

Upper Airway Obstruction

Obstruction is usually due to position, a piece of food, fluids, or swelling from trauma or infection. The obstruction may be partial or complete. With partial obstruction, the patient will have noisy and labored respiration characterized by wheezing, whistling, or stridor—the high-pitched raspy sound made by inhalation against an obstruction.

The ability to swallow saliva may be impaired, causing the patient to drool. Talking may be difficult or impossible.

With a partial obstruction, the first rule of treatment is: "Do no harm." If the patient is not yet in respiratory failure, they will be making their own efforts to dislodge an object or reposition the airway. Except for rolling a patient to drain fluids, any attempt by you to remove an obstruction carries the risk of making it worse. The ideal treatment is urgent evacuation to advanced life support and surgical care.

Upper Airway

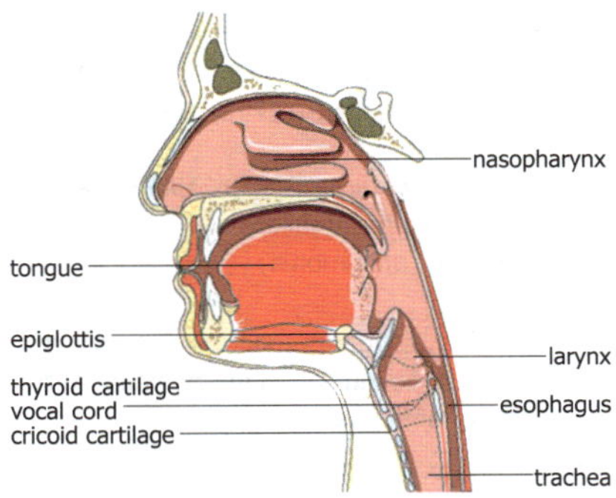

When the patient is in respiratory failure or arrest, immediate basic life support techniques are used to clear the airway (see the Basic and Advanced Life Support chapter). At this point, the benefit is obvious, and you have nothing to lose by trying. In cases where a foreign object is removed you may certainly take credit for the save. Remember, though, evacuation is prudent if swelling is anticipated, such as after a prolonged obstruction or a burn from hot food.

Airway obstruction due to swelling from burns, trauma, or infection is the most difficult to manage in the field. A partial obstruction carries the anticipated problem of complete obstruction, which can develop quickly in some cases. The patient will naturally find the best airway position, and there is little else you can do to improve on it. A patient with airway obstruction due to swelling is best evacuated urgently to advanced life support and surgical care. In a desperate situation with respiratory failure secondary to progressive airway obstruction, you may be able to improve symptoms temporarily with inhaled or injected epinephrine. The dose is the same as discussed in the protocol for anaphylaxis and asthma detailed later in this textbook.

Lower Airway Constriction

Spasm, swelling of the mucous membrane lining, or the accumulation of mucus or pus can cause narrowing of the bronchi and bronchioles, which are the tubes of the lower airway. This is what happens in asthma, bronchitis, and anaphylaxis. The constriction inhibits the movement of air in and out of the alveoli. In the initial stages of lower airway constriction, the patient may have a more difficult time exhaling than inhaling. This can render positive pressure ventilation ineffective, although the rest of the generic treatment for respiratory distress is certainly useful.

Lower Airway Constriction

MOI:
- Swelling (anaphylaxis)
- Spasm (asthma)
- Infection (bronchitis)

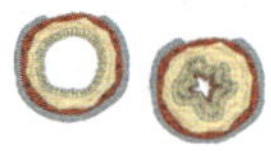

Assessment:
- Respiratory distress; forced expiration, wheeze, cough
- Exposure and Sx of anaphylaxis
- History of asthma or illness

Treatment:
- PROP
- Treat the cause (asthma, anaphylaxis)
- Evacuate to Advanced Life Support

In severe constriction, inspiration and expiration are often prolonged with pronounced wheezing and a cough. Sometimes the lower airway noise is loud enough to hear from a distance. Other times you may need a stethoscope or an ear to the patient's chest. Oxygen saturation will measure below normal.

Lower airway constriction by any mechanism is a serious problem when it causes respiratory distress. Your initial response should be PROP; but the ideal treatment is medication. Bronchodilators, such as nebulized albuterol, may be helpful in cases of bronchitis or smoke inhalation. Antibiotics may be added for infection. With a history of asthma or anaphylaxis, you can follow the Wilderness

Protocols for the emergency use of epinephrine detailed in the basic and advanced life support and the allergy and anaphylaxis chapters.

Alveoli

The usual problem in the alveoli is fluid accumulation blocking the exchange of oxygen and carbon dioxide between air and blood. The generic term for this is pulmonary edema. The source is usually capillary leakage within the lung as part of an inflammatory process caused by infection or inhalation injury.

Contusion of lung tissue can also result in pulmonary edema. You should anticipate this condition in patients with suspected rib fracture or any blow to the chest severe enough to "knock the wind out" of them. Capillary leakage can also be the result of congestive heart failure or the effect of reduced oxygen at high altitude. Contusion or laceration of the lung tissue may cause the alveoli to fill with blood.

Shortness of breath on exertion will reveal the reduced lung capacity in the early stages of fluid accumulation. The patient often develops a dry cough as the lung tries to clear itself. A low-grade fever may develop. In the presence of a mechanism of injury like submersion, high-altitude pulmonary edema, chest trauma, or infection, these early signs are reason to anticipate respiratory distress as the situation becomes worse.

As the problem progresses, crackles may be heard with a stethoscope or an ear to the chest as the patient inhales. Large amounts of fluid in the lungs will cause gurgling that can be heard at a distance. Fluid may froth from the mouth and may be tinged with pus or blood. At this point, respiratory distress will have become obvious, with imminent respiratory failure.

With alveolar fluid, PROP can make a significant difference. Positive pressure ventilation can help force alveolar fluid back into the circulatory system, restoring lung surface area for gas exchange and opening airways. You should not wait for the patient to stop breathing to apply positive pressure ventilation (PPV). This is a safe and effective basic life support treatment for respiratory distress. Do not worry about timing; a patient in trouble will adjust their respiratory effort to your efforts to assist.

The patient will prefer to sit up, even on a litter during evacuation. Supplemental oxygen will help and should be an early part of the plan for treatment and evacuation. Definitive care will require antibiotics for infection or medication to reduce edema from other causes. Access to advanced life support is high priority. For high-altitude pulmonary edema, the definitive treatment is immediate descent, but there are medications that can buy the patient some time (see the Altitude Illness chapter).

Fluid in the Alveoli
(pulmonary edema)

MOI:
- Swelling (water inhalation, HAPE, trauma)
- Congestive heart failure
- Infection (pneumonia)

Assessment:
- Crackles, cough, gurgling, respiratory distress
- Exposure to inhalation injury, altitude, trauma
- History of illness

Treatment:
- PROP, especially PPV
- Treat the cause (medication)
- Evacuate to Advanced Life Support

Chest Wall and Diaphragm

Trauma to the chest wall or diaphragm can interfere with the function of the respiratory system in several ways, but the most common cause of respiratory distress is pain from fractures or sprains. The effective application of PROP and pain relief will often significantly improve the respiratory status of the trauma patient. Sometimes a rib belt or wrap around the chest will make the patient more comfortable if walking or crawling is necessary. If you choose to apply a belt, monitor the patient carefully and be prepared to remove the belt if it seems to make breathing worse.

More serious structural damage to the chest, or pain that does not respond quickly to field treatment, deserves urgent evacuation. An unstable chest wall, also called a flail chest, indicates that the bellows system is damaged to the point that it is no longer rigid. Instead of the lungs expanding with inspiration, the chest wall collapses. Hemothorax and pneumothorax are terms used to describe the presence of blood and/or air in the chest cavity in the pleural space between the lungs and the chest wall preventing full expansion of the lungs.

A tension pneumothorax develops when air accumulates in the pleural space under pressure, shifting the heart and airways out of position and putting pressure on the great vessels of the circulatory system. It should be suspected with increasing respiratory distress, asymmetrical chest wall expansion, and deteriorating vital signs. In the rare case of an open pneumothorax, sometimes called a sucking chest wound, air may enter the chest cavity through a hole in the chest wall. The usual cause is a knife or gunshot wound.

The generic treatment for respiratory distress, like the field treatment for volume shock, is limited and only temporary. The patient with chest injury significant enough to cause respiratory distress needs a surgeon and a hospital. Assist the patient into whatever position allows for the best respiration and the least pain. Call for early advanced life support with pain medication, airway management and, in the case of suspected pneumothorax, emergency chest decompression.

Chest Wall Trauma

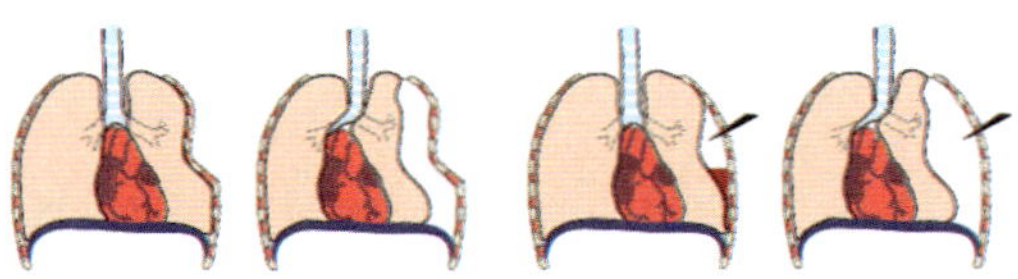

"Pain is the most common cause of respiratory distress in chest wall trauma. Treating the pain can improve respiration, even in the presence of significant injury."

Open chest wounds with air bubbling in and out of the defect should be covered with an airtight seal, like a piece of plastic bag or duct tape. You do not need to make a one-way valve or coordinate the patch placement with inspiration. Just put it on. If applying a patch improves the situation, leave it in place. If symptoms become worse during evacuation, remove it.

Nervous System Drive

The usual problem with nervous system drive is increased respiratory drive. Hyperventilation occurs with altitude, exercise, injury, and illness and is a normal response to physiological demands that require more oxygen and produce more carbon dioxide. Increased respiration also occurs with acute stress reaction (ASR), but not in response to an increased need. Fortunately, the condition is self-limiting.

The result of hyperventilation in ASR can be an abnormal decrease in the carbon dioxide concentration in the blood with the associated abnormal increase in pH. This out-of-balance blood chemistry can produce a variety of nervous system symptoms that are referred to as hyperventilation syndrome. The mechanism can be dramatic and emotional, or quite subtle. A slight increase in respiratory depth and rate over enough time will cause it.

Typically, the patient will complain of tingling of the hands and feet and numbness around the mouth. The patient may feel paralyzed, but their ability to move is not actually impaired. Vision may be affected with the patient seeing spots or experiencing a narrowed visual field. The symptoms may fuel further ASR and exacerbate the hyperventilation. The patient may ultimately faint, which will cure the problem.

It can be difficult to distinguish between hyperventilation syndrome and serious critical system problems, especially if there is a significant mechanism of injury. As with other components of acute stress reaction, however, it gets better with time, reassurance, and pain control. Telling the patient that hyperventilation is the cause of their symptoms almost always cures it.

Decreased Nervous Drive

MOI:

S – Sugar
T – Temperature
O – Oxygen
P – Pressure
E – Electricity
A – Altitude
T – Toxins
S – Salts

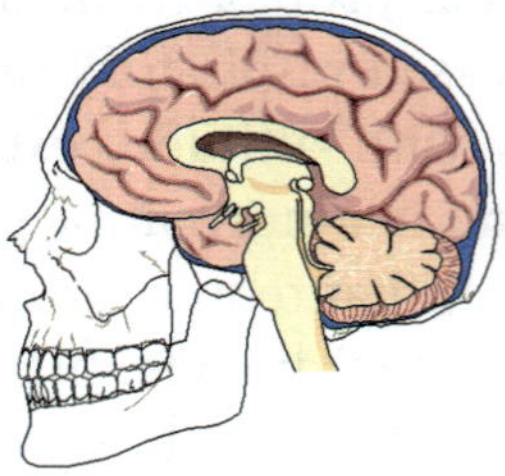

"If the brain is not functioning correctly, breathing may be irregular or very slow."

Decreased nervous system drive is less common, but more serious. If the brain is not functioning correctly, breathing may be irregular or slow. If the brain stops working, breathing will stop. The possible causes include low blood sugar, hypothermia, and toxins. The symptoms present in marked contrast to the other forms of respiratory distress.

Decreased nervous system drive is not noisy or fast. Because the patient is already V, P, or U on the AVPU scale, mental status is no longer a reliable indicator of oxygenation and perfusion. The patient is not awake enough to tell you that they are having trouble breathing. You won't see it unless you look for it. Observing skin color or measuring oxygen saturation may help.

Any injured or ill person with inadequate respiration and reduced level of consciousness needs PPV and oxygen. Do not be timid about this. PPV carries a very low risk of causing harm and provides great benefit.

Risk Versus Benefit

As with shock, the ideal treatment for respiratory distress is evacuation to definitive medical care. In the wilderness or offshore setting where evacuation may be impossible or involve a high level of risk, field treatment may be prolonged. In some situations, such as with asthma, anaphylaxis, or airway obstruction, field treatment may be definitive and there will be no emergency.

Your worry list includes situations in which you cannot reverse the progression of respiratory distress or signs and symptoms that indicate a poor response to treatment. These cases may be worth an emergency evacuation or an attempt to bring advanced-level care to the patient. The balance of risk versus benefit will depend on the situation and on the experience and skill of the practitioner making the judgment.

Respiratory Distress
Wilderness Perspective

High-Risk Problem:

- Cannot improve respiratory status
- Persistent altered mental status
- Coexisting major problems
- Cyanosis
- Cannot maintain body temperature
- Cannot maintain hydration and calories
- The patient is getting worse

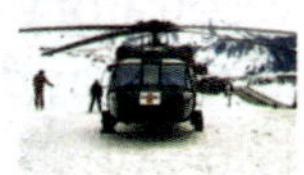

"These cases may be worth a high-risk evacuation or an attempt to bring advanced level care to the patient."

Chapter 5 Review:
The Respiratory System

- The respiratory system is responsible for bringing outside air into the alveoli of the lungs where the exchange of oxygen and carbon dioxide with the blood can occur.
- Problems with the respiratory system are described as respiratory distress, respiratory failure, and respiratory arrest. Distress is difficulty breathing. Failure is distress with inadequate oxygenation. Arrest is complete cessation of breathing.
- The generic treatment for respiratory system problems is abbreviated PROP: Position for best ventilation and airway control, Reassurance and coaching for efficient ventilation, Oxygen by mask or cannula if available, and Positive pressure ventilation if necessary.
- The five basic components of the respiratory system include the upper airway, lower airways, alveoli, chest wall and diaphragm, and nervous system drive. Identifying the component in which the problem lies will often identify the specific treatment for the problem.
- Respiratory distress is suspected or anticipated with mechanisms including upper airway obstruction, lower airway constriction, fluid in the alveoli, chest wall trauma, and brain failure.
- Respiratory distress that you cannot fix in the field is an emergency.

Chapter 6: The Nervous System

The central nervous system is one of the three critical systems and controls all essential life functions, both voluntary and involuntary. The brain receives stimuli directly from the eyes, nose, and facial nerves via the cranial nerves in the head, and indirectly from the rest of the body through peripheral nerves and the spinal cord. Impulses traveling from the brain in the other direction control most of the functions of our muscles, glands, and organs. Failure of the brain to adequately regulate and control body systems can result in failure of the circulatory and respiratory systems resulting in death. Brain failure is a serious critical system problem requiring immediate and aggressive treatment. Spinal cord failure is less likely to be immediately life threatening but is also an emergency (see the Spine Injury chapter).

Structure and Function

The soft tissue of the brain and spinal cord are enclosed and protected within the bony structure of the skull and vertebrae of the spine. From the gap between the individual vertebrae, unprotected peripheral nerves branch out from the spinal cord to reach all body tissues. Nerves controlling the most critical functions of the major body systems exit the cord at the base of the skull and the upper part of the cervical spine. Several serious problems can affect the central nervous system.

Brain Failure

Because nervous system tissue is exquisitely sensitive to oxygen deprivation, any significant problem with oxygenation and perfusion will affect mental status. A subtle change in brain function is often the first indication of a serious condition. This is the peeling of the evolutionary onion as discussed in the General Principles of Physiology and Pathology chapter. Inevitably, the level of consciousness will begin to decrease if the perfusion or oxygenation problem persists.

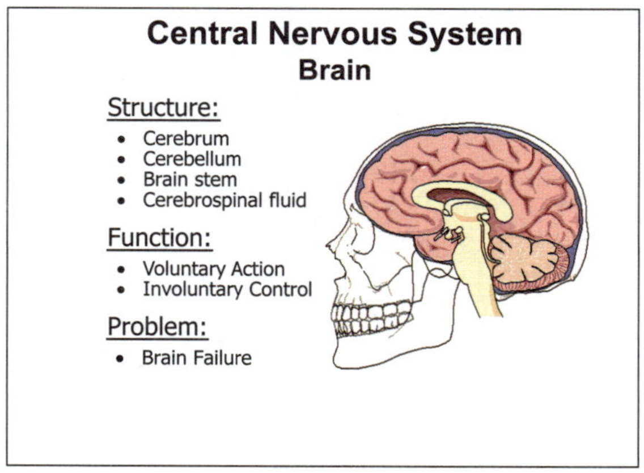

Assessing the Level of Consciousness

For field purposes, we describe brain function by using a scale abbreviated AVPU. This simple assessment tool is familiar to most emergency care providers. More complex evaluation tools, such as the Glasgow Coma Scale, are generally not necessary or useful in field medicine.

Describing Brain Function

AVPU:

A – Awake (describe mental status – oriented, confused, anxious, combative, lethargic, etc.)

V – Verbal

P – Pain

U – Unresponsive

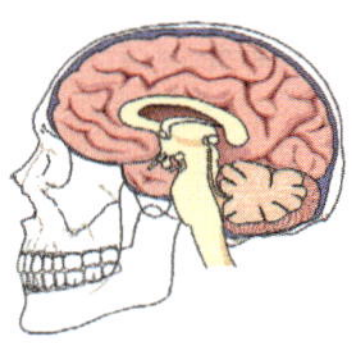

"In describing mental status, plain language is usually better…"

In the emergency medical services (EMS), normal mental status in the awake patient is often abbreviated A&O × 4. This means that the patient is Awake and Oriented to person, place, time, and event. Using this phrase to describe normal mental status is fine if everyone knows what this expression means. This description becomes confusing when the patient's mental status is not normal. Reporting a patient as A&O × 2 gives little useful information.

When describing mental status, plain language is usually better in a wilderness rescue or disaster settings that may involve multiple agencies and medical personnel at various levels of training.

Describing your patient as "awake, knows their name and where they are, but not sure how they got here or what day of the week it is," may seem cumbersome, but everyone involved in their care and transport will understand it. Furthermore, improvement or decay in mental status will be more easily detected.

Differential Diagnosis of Brain Failure

The term differential diagnosis describes a list of the possible causes of a condition or problem. The most common causes of impaired brain function can be summarized as a simple differential diagnosis with the acronym STOPEATS.

Brain Failure

Mechanisms:

S – Sugar

T – Temperature

O – Oxygen

P – Pressure

E – Electricity

A – Altitude

T – Toxins

S – Salts

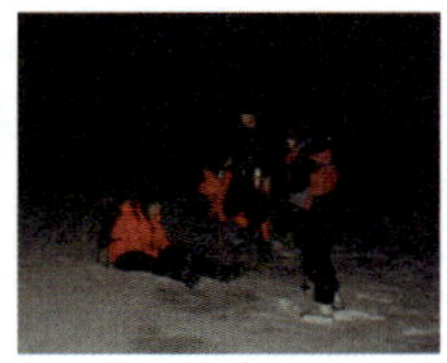

"The numerous causes of impaired brain function can be summarized … with the mnemonic *STOPEATS.*"

STOPEATS can be a handy diagnostic tool when you are evaluating mental status changes in the presence of a mixed or uncertain mechanism of injury. While reviewing the mnemonic, you will usually be able to eliminate some possible causes in your scene size-up and patient assessment. Other possibilities will have to remain on your problem list until they can be ruled out or confirmed over time.

Imagine caring for the subject of a successful 48-hour backcountry search. Your patient is found curled up under a spruce tree in a level area of forest at 950 meters in elevation. The weather is cool and wet without thunderstorm activity. The patient is V on the AVPU scale and shivering. There is no evidence of trauma.

Based on your survey of the scene and the patient, you can eliminate problems with pressure, electricity, oxygen, and altitude from your problem list. Even though you are fairly certain that their problem is hypothermia, the mnemonic reminds you to also consider blood sugar, toxins, and salts as possible contributing factors. Time and response to treatment may allow you to refine your problem list further in the field, or you may have to keep a potential problem on the list throughout an evacuation effort. This is an example of the generic to specific principle at work: Treat what you can and evacuate for what you can't.

Increased Intracranial Pressure

Increased Intracranial Pressure (ICP) is a swelling and pressure problem resulting in ischemia. The anticipated problem of increased ICP causes a lot of anxiety in wilderness and rescue medicine. This is part of the P in the STOPEATS mnemonic and the brain problem that is most likely to be fatal. We can worry about it and recognize it, but we cannot effectively treat it in the field. The one exception is increased ICP from high-altitude cerebral edema (HACE).

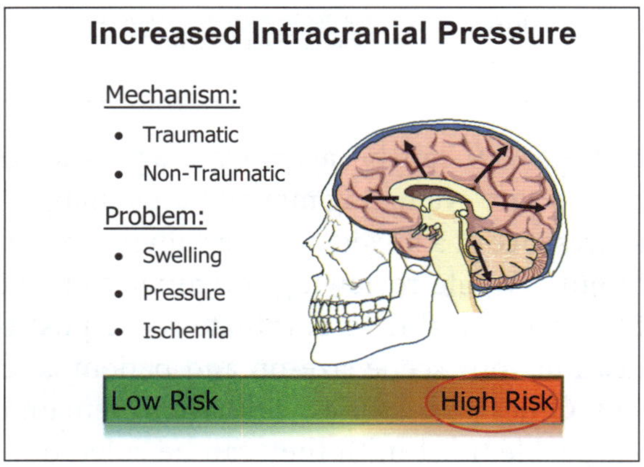

Like other body tissues, the brain will swell when injured. Unlike other tissues, the brain is confined within the rigid compartment of the cranium. Swelling from bleeding or edema within this confined space can raise ICP to the point there is not enough difference between intracranial pressure and systemic perfusion pressure to allow blood to flow into brain tissue. In effect, the brain becomes ischemic and begins to fail.

Like shock and respiratory failure, increased ICP has a typical pattern and spectrum of severity regardless of its cause or rate of onset. Altered mental status is often the earliest vital sign indicator of increasing ICP with the patient becoming more disoriented or restless. These signs are usually accompanied by headache, photophobia (discomfort with bright light), and nausea. If the pressure continues to increase, the deeper layers of the brain will begin to fail resulting in the patient becoming combative or somnolent with severe headache and persistent vomiting. This pattern of worsening mental status, headache, and vomiting indicates increased ICP until proven otherwise.

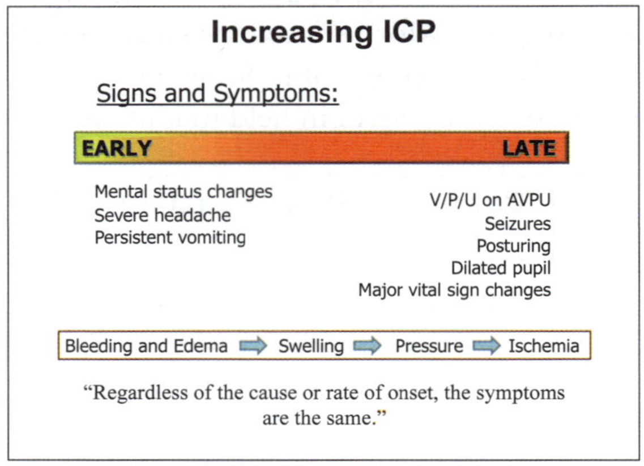

A severe increase in ICP will drive the patient through V, P, and U on the AVPU scale with seizures, posturing, and pupil dilation as the brain stem infarcts as it is squeezed through the base of the cranium. At this point, survival without neurosurgical intervention is very unlikely.

Field Treatment of Increased ICP

Although there is no definitive field treatment for ICP, your careful attention to BLS—airway control, ventilation, body core temperature, and hydration—can certainly improve the outcome. Swelling develops and swelling resolves. Most patients can live through a period of increased ICP if you can preserve systemic oxygenation and perfusion. Emergency evacuation to surgical care is certainly the ideal plan, but support of vital body functions is equally essential.

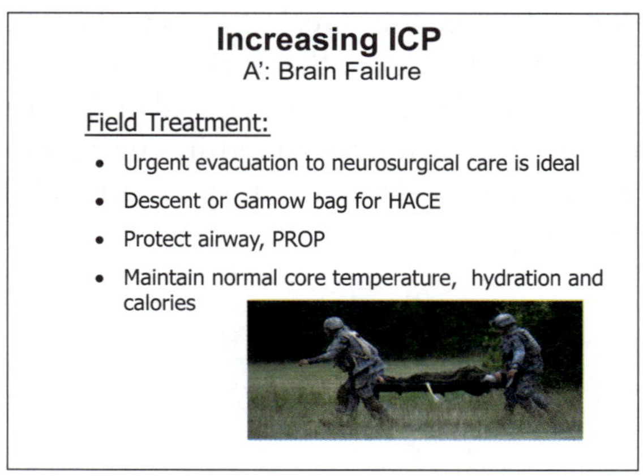

The rapid onset of increased ICP from severe illness or injury will be fatal in most backcountry or offshore situations. Cardiopulmonary arrest due to severe brain damage does not respond to CPR or defibrillation. It is the early recognition of slow-onset swelling from the accumulation of edema fluid or slow bleeding that can save lives.

Non-Traumatic Brain Injury

Non-traumatic mechanisms that can lead to increased ICP include HACE, hypoxia, stroke, infection, and hyperthermia. In essence, any problem that injures brain tissue can stimulate an inflammatory response and cause blood or exudate to accumulate inside the cranium.

Non-Traumatic Brain Injury
A': Increasing ICP

- Stroke
- Hyperthermia
- Hypoxia
- Electricity
- Infection
- Exercise-Associated Hyponatremia
- Altitude (HACE)
- Neuro Toxins

Sometimes, as with an ischemic stroke or electrical injury, altered mental status is just a symptom of the initial brain injury. There is no associated headache or vomiting unless the anticipated problem of elevated ICP actually develops. That is why persistent altered mental status carries the anticipated problem of elevated ICP, unless the cause is known to be unrelated (e.g. chronic dementia, alcohol intoxication).

Traumatic Brain Injury

Traumatic brain injury (TBI) is the common term for brain injury from trauma. The terms closed head injury and concussion are also used. The diagnosis of TBI is significant because it carries the anticipated problem (A') of increased ICP. Even if no serious problem exists yet, worrying about increased ICP can cause major safety and logistical issues in the remote setting. This is another case where a conscientious patient survey, careful monitoring, and good risk/benefit judgment will lead to the best plan.

Assessment of TBI

We cannot directly examine the brain in the field, at least in a living patient. Our assessment must be based on the mechanism of injury, estimating the force involved, and observing brain function. Generally, the less profound the signs and symptoms are, the less severe the injury is and the less likely the brain is to swell. Conversely, an impressive mechanism with a lot of force and profound changes in brain function indicates a high probability of significant brain injury.

The common sign of altered mental status immediately after a blow to the head is a symptom of the initial injury, not evidence of increased ICP. A rapid return to normal mental status, even after a period of unconsciousness, would suggest mild injury very unlikely to result in a significant increase in ICP. This patient may not remember the accident but will remember everything before and after, and remains oriented to person, place, purpose, and time. In the absence of other complications, this would be considered a low-risk TBI.

Traumatic Brain Injury

Field Assessment:

- Any degree of amnesia
- Any change in mental status
- A' is increased ICP and Brain Failure
- Other terms include:
  - Concussion
  - Brain Trauma
  - Closed Head Injury

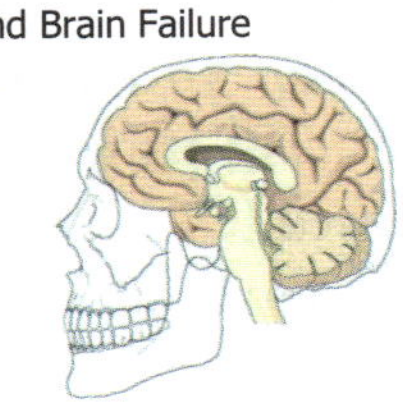

A more severe injury is evidenced by prolonged changes in mental status, loss of memory for the hours or days before the event, or persistent lapses of memory after the event. There may be bruising and swelling of the face and scalp or other

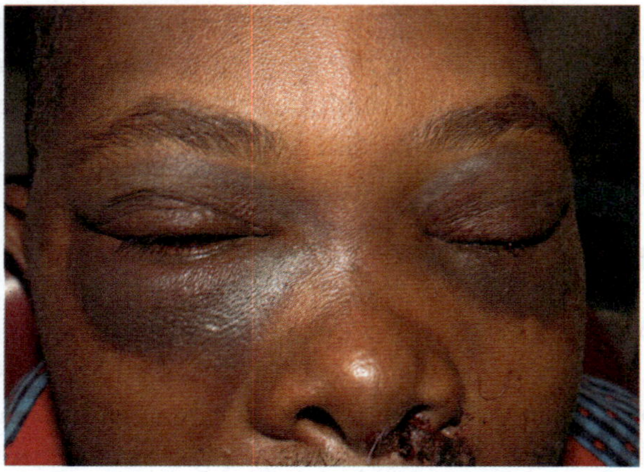

indication of high-velocity impact. A cracked helmet, damaged bicycle, or broken ski suggests a significant mechanism. A more severe injury carries a higher risk of increased ICP.

A history of previous brain injury with persistent symptoms, especially if recent, is an added concern. A patient taking blood thinning medication like warfarin or aspirin is at greater risk for persistent intracranial bleeding. Extremes of age are also worrisome considerations; infants and toddlers cannot give reliable information and older adults are more prone to intracranial bleeding. Elements of a patient's history like these can make the diagnosis of TBI more serious. All of this helps to answer the essential questions: How severe is the TBI? Are there other factors that increase risk? How worried am I about increased ICP?

Field Treatment of Traumatic Brain Injury

Generally, increased ICP from trauma will manifest within the first 24 hours or so if it is going to happen all. In a remote setting, it is ideal to evacuate a TBI patient early rather than waiting for increased ICP to develop, but this need not be an emergency. Simply moving your patient closer to medical care may be sufficient in low-risk cases.

If you choose to keep the patient in the field, it is important to monitor them closely during that first day. The patient should not use opioids or stimulant drugs or drink alcohol because this will confuse your assessment of mental status. Someone should always be with the patient, but it is not necessary to keep the patient awake. They will not sleep through the pain and vomiting of increasing ICP.

High-risk TBI should be evacuated directly to a Level I or II trauma center, if possible. Because vomiting is one of the signs you're watching for, you must include airway obstruction and dehydration on your anticipated problem list. The patient will not be moving around much and is at risk for hypothermia in all but the warmest of environments. BLS in long-term care includes positioning your patient for airway control, maintaining hydration and calories, and preserving body core temperature.

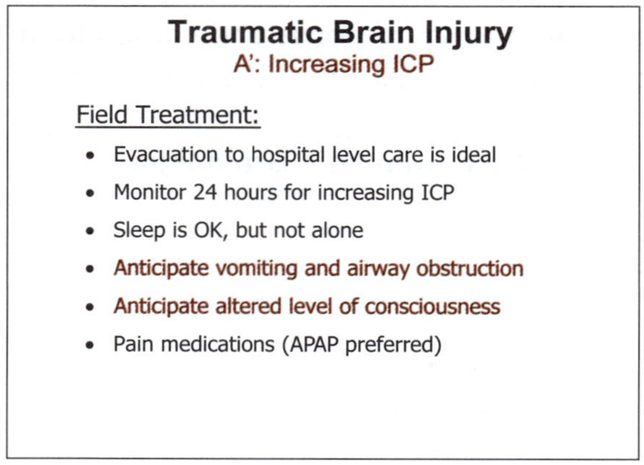

Risk Versus Benefit in TBI

Deciding what to do with an obvious high-risk TBI, especially where increased ICP is already developing, is easy. This is a serious critical system problem and the patient needs to be in a hospital right now. If evacuation is impossible or extremely dangerous, the plan is still straightforward: good basic life support and protection until evacuation can be safely accomplished.

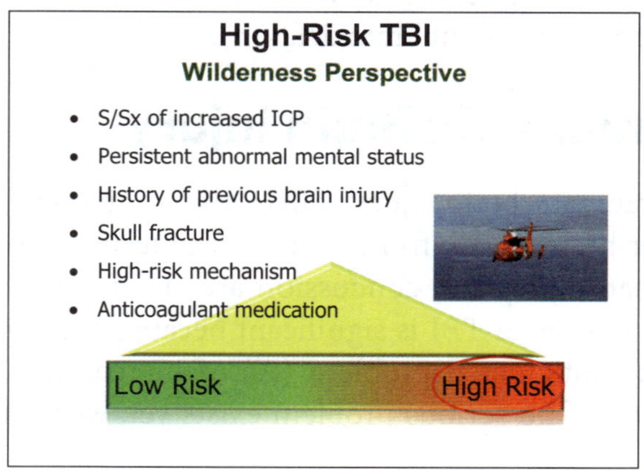

Lower-risk TBI creates more of a quandary when your evacuation options are less than ideal. Most of these will recover without serious problems and the risk and expense of emergency evacuation usually exceeds any real benefit. This creates the common backcountry medical dilemma: Evacuate now, or wait and watch?

There are no absolute rules to fit every situation, but there are some general guidelines to help with your risk/benefit assessment. As mentioned above, there is a low probability of increasing ICP when mental status returns to normal shortly after the event. By "normal," we mean awake, alert, and making sense. By "shortly," we mean within three hours or so. During this observation period, you should see steady improvement in memory and mental status. If so, there is no emergency and medical follow up can be delayed if necessary.

Sometimes, even more ominous signs like anterograde amnesia or loss of distant memory can quickly improve. Anterograde amnesia is the term for the inability to retain new memory and is a form of altered mental status. The patient may literally forget what has been happening from minute to minute as you talk to them. With loss of distant memory, the patient may not recall where they live, how they came to be where they are now, or even their age. In the absence of other serious signs or symptoms, improvement to normal mental status relieves the immediate emergency, but early evacuation to medical care is still advised.

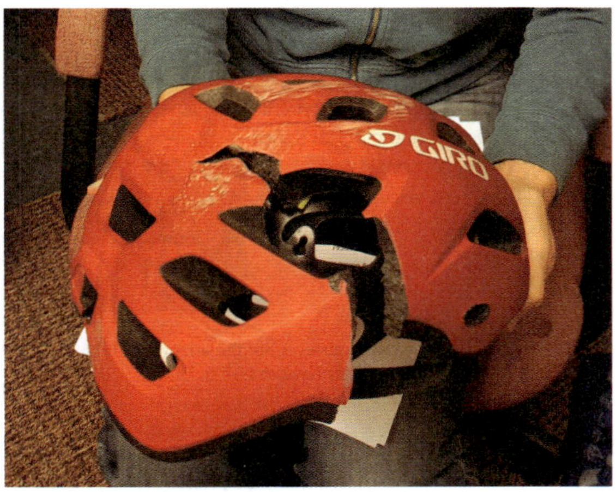

This helmet damage indicates a high-energy impact and an increased potential for brain swelling and increased intracranial pressure.

Finally, being able to diagnose a TBI means that you can also determine when the patient does not have a TBI. There may be an ugly scalp laceration or a broken nose, but if the patient has normal mental status and remembers everything that happened, there is no significant brain injury. Injuries to the face and scalp without a change in brain function do not carry the anticipated problem of increased ICP.

Post-Concussive Syndrome

Following a blow to the head, some patients experience symptoms including mild headache, photophobia, nausea, sleep disturbance, and dizziness developing a day or so after the injury. Some become depressed, angry, or tearful. This can develop with or without the field diagnosis of TBI. This post-concussive syndrome can last anywhere from hours to weeks, but 3–5 days is typical. Mental status remains near normal, but their discomfort alone may be a good enough reason to put the patient ashore or end a backcountry adventure early.

Post-Concussive Syndrome

- Can occur without measurable brain injury
- May develop quickly or > 24 hours after injury
- Normal mental status with:
  - mild to moderate headache
  - blurred vision, photophobia
  - disrupted sleep pattern
  - nausea, loss of appetite
  - dizziness
- Does not indicate elevated ICP
- Symptomatic treatment as needed
- Non-urgent medical follow-up

Field treatment is symptomatic: medicate for headache, allow for rest as possible, and avoid activities that require a lot of concentration. Generally, nonurgent medical follow-up is adequate. However, progressive worsening or the appearance of new symptoms, such as persistent vomiting, should motivate urgent evacuation.

Stroke

A sudden change in brain function without a history of trauma or intoxication should make you think of stroke. It may be as subtle as a little numbness in one hand or arm or a slight facial droop, or as dramatic as complete paralysis of one side of the body or the sudden loss of the ability to speak. In some cases, the symptoms are transient, resolving after a few minutes or hours as a clot forms and then dissolves. These transient ischemic attacks should be taken as a warning of serious and permanent problems to come if the patient is not treated soon.

Like a heart attack, a stroke is an example of ischemia leading to infarction in a critical body system. It is a serious problem with a critical system, and the patient needs a hospital. During evacuation, apply BLS and treat as you would any patient with existing or anticipated increased ICP. Do not give aspirin or ibuprofen in an effort to reduce clotting. The stroke may be caused by bleeding and you will have no way of knowing that in the field.

Seizure

Seizure is a symptom of brain malfunction, not a disease unto itself. In the wilderness context, seizure may occur with low blood sugar, heat stroke, hypoxia, increased ICP, lightning injury, HACE, toxins, or hyponatremia. You will recognize this list from the STOPEATS mnemonic. The problem may be relatively mild or very severe. Either way, the new onset of seizure activity indicates nervous system problems that may become significantly worse over time.

Of course, seizure can also be a relatively benign occurrence in a patient with a known seizure disorder such as epilepsy. The stress of backcountry travel or a voyage at sea can upset the blood levels of antiseizure medication allowing a breakthrough event. This is a surprisingly common problem in the backcountry. The medical practitioner should be alert to this possibility when a seizure occurs without an obvious mechanism of injury. With organized trips or outdoors schools it is possible that a patient with epilepsy will have chosen not to disclose this history on an intake medical form.

There are many types of seizures. The classic grand mal seizure is what you are most likely to notice easily and is characterized by generalized tensing of all body muscles and repetitive, purposeless movement. Although the patient's eyes may be open, they will be unresponsive during the seizure. They may be incontinent of feces and urine. There will usually be a period of drowsiness and disorientation after the seizure has ended.

Treatment of Seizure

Protection from injury is the most important treatment you can provide. Most seizures will resolve spontaneously in a short period of time. Protect the patient from injury when falling or thrashing. Also protect the patient from unnecessary treatments like chest compressions or rescuers trying to force objects between the patient's teeth.

Seizing patients will normally hold their breath briefly and become cyanotic (blue from lack of oxygenation). This is not a problem if it does not last more than a couple of minutes. Position the patient and ventilate if necessary after the seizure has resolved, or during the seizure if you feel that respirations are inadequate. The real worry is not the seizure itself but what may have caused it.

Seizure

Wilderness Perspective

High-Risk Problem:

- Result of trauma or environmental illness
- Persistent neurological deficit
- New onset seizure
- Recurrent seizure
- The patient is getting worse

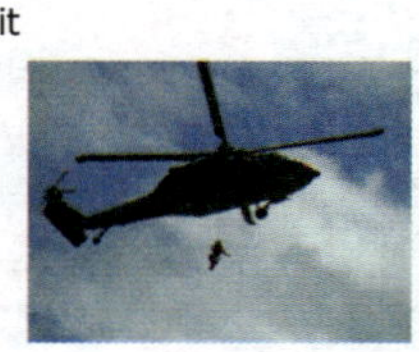

"The real worry, of course, is not the seizure itself but what may have caused it."

If the mechanism is not obvious, consider all the conditions on the STOPEATS mnemonic. In the field, you may be able to treat for problems like hyponatremia, hypoglycemia, heat stroke, and alcohol withdrawal. A careful survey of the scene may disclose problems like drug overdose, trauma, or hypoxia.

Sometimes, people will experience brief seizure activity with head injury at the time of impact. This seems to be more common in children and is not serious if it resolves quickly and there is an early return of normal mental status. However, seizure occurring later as part of a pattern of increasing ICP certainly is serious.

In the case of a known epileptic who improves spontaneously post seizure and seems otherwise okay, evacuation need not be an emergency. However, blood levels of medication will need to be checked and adjusted. The patient should not be allowed to perform risky activities or be left alone in dangerous situations. This is not a patient who can be trusted to belay a climbing partner or remain on the deck of a small boat alone.

Exercise Associated Hyponatremia

Exercise associated hyponatremia is most common with extreme athletes and others who have been working or playing hard and drinking too much water. This dilutes the salt content of the body to a point where function is impaired. The term hyponatremia means low sodium, one of the body's primary electrolytes. This is the Salts in the STOPEATS mnemonic.

Hyponatremia typically causes changes in mental status, particularly slow thinking, confusion, and tremors. Serious cases can cause loss of consciousness and seizures. The signs and symptoms can resemble heat exhaustion with weakness, nausea, and headache, but urine volume is near normal with relatively dilute urine. This can be a difficult diagnosis to make without a device to measure electrolytes.

Exercise-Associated Hyponatremia

Mechanism:

- Excessive fluid replacement dilutes sodium and other salts
- Some loss of salts through sweat, but primarily a problem of too much water

Signs and Symptoms:

- Altered mental state; slow mentation, lethargy, agitation
- Nausea, headache, weakness, seizures, tremors
- Urine output and core temperature near normal

The term dilutional hyponatremia describes the problem in patients who drink too much without significant sweating or vigorous activity. This is uncommon but can affect people using recreational drugs like MDMA or people on unconventional diets.

Treatment of Exertional Hyponatremia

Water restriction is the usual field treatment for hyponatremia. Salty food may help but is not definitive treatment. Evacuation to medical care is ideal. Fluid replacement with normal saline, as is often performed for dehydration, can actually make hyponatremia worse. Hydration should be initiated for hyponatremia only if signs and symptoms of dehydration are also present and when blood electrolytes can be measured. Worsening of mental status and level of consciousness suggests a serious problem requiring emergency evacuation. Giving an oral solution of 3% saline solution or the equivalent (e.g. ½ teaspoon of salt in 100 ml of water) and repeating in 10 minutes may help.

Exercise-Associated Hyponatremia

Treatment:

- Rest
- Fluid restriction unless there is evidence of volume depletion
- Evacuate if not improving, urgently if worse

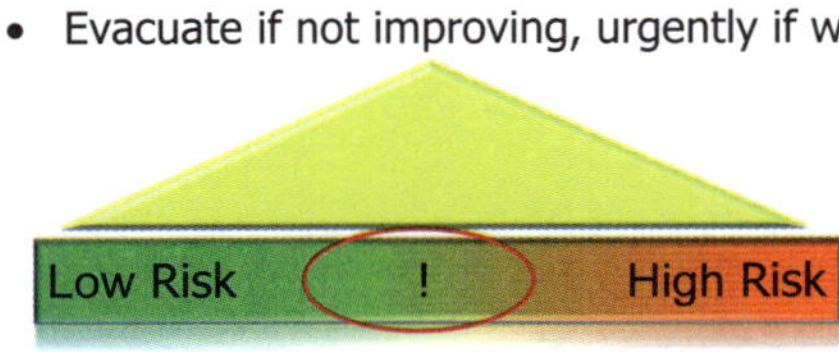

Chapter 6 Review: The Nervous System

- Brain failure can lead to loss of nervous system control over other critical systems. Possible causes are summarized by the mnemonic STOPEATS.
- Subtle changes in mental status are often the earliest indicators of a problem with brain perfusion and oxygenation and may indicate progression toward brain failure.
- Traumatic brain injury (TBI) is a common cause of temporary brain failure and carries the anticipated problem of increased intracranial pressure (ICP). Other causes of increased ICP include stroke, electrical injury, hyperthermia, and hypoxia.
- Increasing ICP produces a pattern of symptoms beginning with persistent vomiting, severe headache, and mental status changes. Late signs include seizure, unequal pupils, and posturing.
- The treatment for increased ICP includes urgent evacuation to neurosurgical care, airway protection, ventilation as needed, and maintaining body core temperature.
- Seizure is an emergency when it is caused by ICP or an undiagnosed problem. It is less of an emergency in a patient with a history of epilepsy who recovers to normal mental status following seizure.
- Exercise-associated hyponatremia is usually due to low blood salts from too much water intake and it is most common with extreme athletes.
- The signs and symptoms of hyponatremia include altered mental status, slow mentation, seizures, and nausea.
- Hyponatremia patients who do not begin to improve quickly with water restriction and salt intake should be evacuated to definitive care.
- Hydration should be initiated for hyponatremia only if signs and symptoms of dehydration are also present and blood electrolytes can be measured.
- Any condition of persistent altered mental status that cannot be corrected is an emergency.

Case Study 3: Snow Machine Accident

SCENE

Mountain Rescue responds to a snow machine accident 15 kilometers from the trailhead at 3300 meters elevation. The guide reports that a middle-aged male client was thrown from a machine, striking a tree. At 1500 hours the weather is partly cloudy with east winds at 12 knots and the temperature is -6°C. The forecast calls for increasing winds and blowing snow. The trail is rough. The team required 45 minutes to reach the scene. Ground evacuation to an ambulance will take an hour. The ambulance transport will take 30 minutes to a small community hospital. Air evacuation will require a 45-minute response to the scene and 45-minute return to a Level II trauma center.

S: A 42-year-old man is found awake and responsive lying on a tent fly and foam pad. There is a bandage around his head. The guide reports that the patient was "out" for a few minutes after striking the tree, then woke up and kept asking the same questions over and over for another 15 minutes.

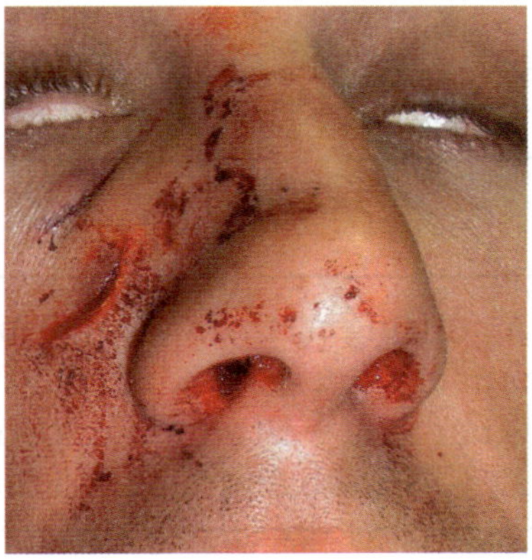

The patient now complains of a moderate headache and nausea, which seems to be getting worse. He denies neck or back pain and distal numbness or weakness. He is aware of being on a snow machine tour but does not remember who he is with or anything about the ride or the accident. He denies allergies. He takes one aspirin a day. He reports one previous TBI requiring hospitalization several years ago. His last meal was at 1200.

O: The patient is subdued but awake and cooperative. Moderate deformity of the face with superficial lacerations and abrasion. No skull deformity. Bleeding controlled by direct pressure. No spine tenderness. Distal CSM intact. Mild shivering. Vital Signs: Pulse: 80, Resp: 18, Temp: normal, Skin: cool, dry, pale, C: awake but subdued with significant memory loss, BP: 138/88.

A:

1. TBI with nausea and headache
   A': Elevated ICP
   A': Vomiting with airway obstruction and aspiration
2. Cold response
   A': Hypothermia
3. Facial lacerations and deformity
   A': Infection
   A': Bleeding
4. Decaying weather

P:

1. Recovery position in medic trailer. Oxygen. Suction device ready. Close monitoring.
2. Sugar and fluids as tolerated. Insulation.
3. Clean and dress scalp wound.
4. Evacuate to the trailhead while conditions permit.
5. Request helicopter response to the trail head.

Discussion:

This patient is worrisome because of the extent of memory loss and the delayed return to normal mental status. The diagnosis of TBI is clear and increased ICP is anticipated. Even if the team medic cannot do anything about the increasing ICP, she can improve oxygenation by maintaining a clear airway and giving supplemental oxygen by cannula. At this elevation it will help even if the patient's respiratory system is already working fine. The ability to maintain airway and oxygenation, along with body core temperature, while transporting is key to determining the evacuation method.

In this case, the medic felt comfortable managing the patient en route and chose to evacuate by ground. She also called an air medical helicopter to meet the team at the trailhead because the patient would be better served by evacuation to a trauma center rather than a small community hospital. At the same time, she is reducing the risk associated with possible cancellation of the helicopter due to weather by proceeding immediately to the trail head. If there is no helicopter and trauma center, at least there is an ambulance and hospital.

Case Study 4: Illness at Sea

SCENE
A cruising catamaran 250 nautical miles ESE of North Carolina bound for Saint Martin. One of the four crewmembers complains of shortness of breath upon returning from a sail change. The weather is fair with west winds at 20 knots and seas of 1 to 2 meters from the southwest. The temperature is 22°C. The boat is making 12 knots at 096 degrees true.

S: A 36-year-old woman is found awake and responsive sitting in the cockpit at 2300 hours. She is initially breathing hard and coughing but settles down after a few minutes. She complains of becoming short of breath and dizzy while raising the reefed mainsail and had to sit down on deck before recovering enough to return to the cockpit. She reports "coming down with a cold" 5 days ago before departure but has felt much worse over the past 5 hours with fevers and chills, persistent cough, and chest pain. The cough is occasionally productive of thick green sputum. She admits an allergy to penicillin. She has been taking over-the-counter cough medication with little success. She reports little appetite and has not been eating or drinking normally. She last produced a small amount of urine at 1700. She gives no history of asthma or other respiratory problems. She denies trauma. She denies any possibility of pregnancy with a last menstrual period (LMP) of one week ago.

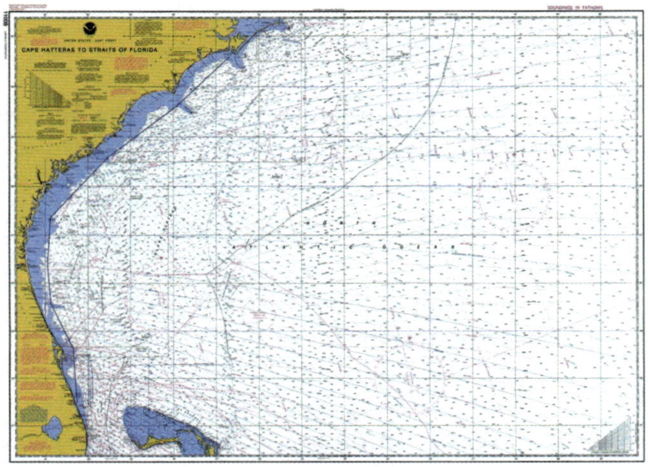

O: Subdued but awake, cooperative, occasional cough noted. Auscultation of the chest with a stethoscope reveals fine crackles and a slight wheezing in both lungs. The abdomen is soft and nontender with normal bowel sounds. Vital Signs: Pulse: 120, Resp: 24, Temp: 38°C, Skin: warm, moist, pink, C: awake and oriented but subdued, BP: 110/68.

A:

1. Respiratory distress due to infection with lower airway constriction and fluid in the alveoli.
   A': Respiratory failure
   A': Systemic infection
2. Compensated volume shock from dehydration
   A': Decompensated shock
   A': Hypoglycemia
3. Remote location, high-risk evacuation

P:

1. Non-penicillin antibiotics
2. Monitor respiratory status
3. Minimize activity
4. Encourage oral electrolyte drink. Monitor urine output. Consider hypodermoclysis.
5. Change course for land to improve access to evacuation. Advise Coast Guard of the situation and plan.

Discussion:

This patient's condition is serious but not yet an emergency in this remote setting. Shortness of breath on exertion is early respiratory distress and the problem seems to be progressing quickly. However, because the likely cause is infection, it is reasonable to start antibiotics and look for improvement while sailing toward land. Emergency evacuation could be initiated if the patient's condition worsens, with due consideration of the risks associated with a helicopter at the limits of its flight range.

The respiratory structures affected suggest pneumonia, which causes fluid to accumulate in the alveoli. The generic treatment for respiratory failure in this case would be PPV. The captain's plan is certainly contrary to the goal of the voyage. It would be very tempting to hope for the best and continue on course with fair wind and good boat speed. The presence of respiratory failure, decompensated shock, and systemic infection on the anticipated problem list, however, demand decreasing rather than increasing the distance to definitive care.

Section III: Critical System Problems and Treatment

Chapter 7: Basic and Advanced Life Support

Basic life support (BLS) is the immediate treatment of life-threatening critical system problems discovered during the primary assessment. Although BLS is outlined in a specific sequence, field treatment requires flexibility. The circulatory, respiratory, and nervous systems are equally important. It is often necessary to change the order in which things are done, or to manage several components at the same time. The primary goal is to support oxygenation and perfusion of the brain and other vital organs.

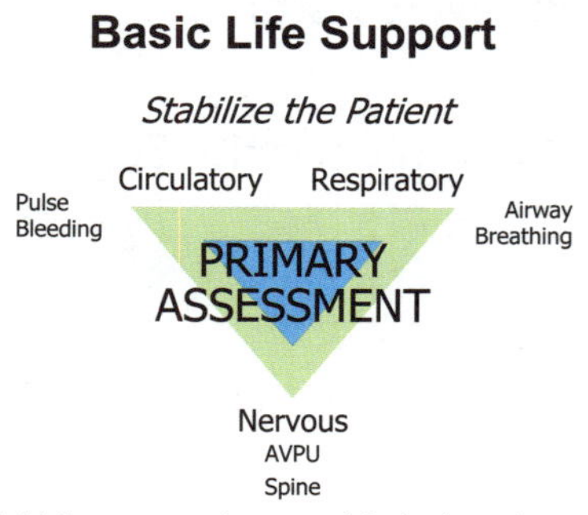

"The initial assessment is your quick check on the status of the patient's three critical body systems."

Where available, advanced life support (ALS) is also part of the immediate response to life-threatening critical system problems. ALS techniques are more invasive, using a range of medications, advanced airways, and some surgical techniques. However, the goals of BLS and ALS are the same: to preserve and enhance oxygenation and perfusion.

Some techniques that were previously reserved for advanced level practitioners have been added to the basic scope of practice. The time-critical treatments for anaphylaxis and asthma offered in the protocols for wilderness medicine are examples. The use of automated external defibrillators (AEDs) in the urban context is another.

At any level of medical expertise, it is important to understand what the next step along the chain of medical care should be. This allows for better referral and evacuation decisions. The BLS rescuer should know when ALS care may be beneficial, and, conversely, when it isn't. If you know what type of care the patient needs, you may refine evacuation decisions and routes based on services available at one hospital or another.

Respiratory Failure

Respiratory failure is presumed to exist whenever inadequate or difficult breathing is associated with an altered level of consciousness or severe changes in mental status. Your immediate response is to ensure an open and clear airway, begin positive pressure ventilation (PPV), and add supplemental oxygen if you have it. Your initial goal is to maintain oxygenation while you determine what specific treatment may be necessary. This will be easier if you are able to identify what part of the respiratory system seems to be affected. If the heart is still beating, PPV can help maintain oxygenation for many hours as assessment continues, and the patient is evacuated to definitive care.

You can apply PPV directly using mouth-to-mouth, as is still taught in some CPR courses, but a mask or other barrier device should be used whenever possible. This is part of standard precautions and serves to protect both you and your patient. A barrier device with a filter and one-way valve is an essential part of any emergency medical kit. These now come in two forms: the traditional face mask that covers the mouth and nose, and the newer intraoral mask that is placed inside the patient's lips and over the teeth like a snorkel mouthpiece. The latter has the advantage of being a much smaller unit unaffected by facial hair but has the disadvantage of requiring the rescuer to seal the nose or apply a nose clip.

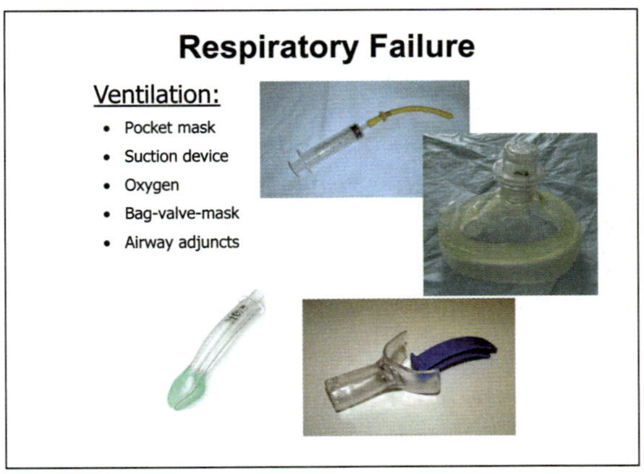

The rate of ventilation should be about 10 to 12 breaths per minute. If you are unable to keep count, just start the next breath as soon as the patient has finished exhaling. Blow in enough air to cause the chest to rise slightly. Each breath is done slowly over two to three seconds. Faster flow rates tend to blow air into the stomach, causing distension and vomiting.

Patients who are breathing on their own, but not deeply or frequently enough, can still be assisted with PPV. This is especially useful in treating inadequate respiration due to chest wall injury, fluid in the alveoli, or decreased nervous system drive. Timing your PPV to the patient's efforts is not critical; a patient in trouble will quickly adjust.

You may be able to apply more specific treatment for respiratory failure if you are able to identify which part of the system is affected. If you are unable to get air into the lungs, for example, the problem may be upper airway obstruction. You may have already found clues to the mechanism in your scene size-up, such as an unfinished meal. Other causes of obstruction include swelling, spasm, position, and deformity from trauma.

Airway obstruction may be complete or partial. Complete obstructions will be rapidly fatal if not corrected. Clearing a complete airway obstruction is a progression of actions from simple to desperate. Try to open the airway using a jaw thrust, chin lift, or direct pull on the tongue. Attempt to maintain in-line position of the head and neck to protect the spinal cord in trauma patients. If this type of positioning does not clear the airway, look inside the mouth. You may see a foreign body that can be pulled out with your fingers or a clamp.

If there is nothing to see, try using residual air to help clear the obstruction with chest compressions and abdominal thrusts. This can be done with the patient supine or sitting. Whether you are squeezing the abdomen or the chest, the effect is the same.

The sudden thrust can force out the air left in the patient's lungs under pressure, blowing out any obstruction with it. Current CPR training calls for the rescuer to begin chest compressions on any unresponsive patient, which will produce the same result. If chest compressions fail, try firm back blows between the shoulder blades. This also applies intrathoracic pressure and can help dislodge an obstruction.

Partial upper airway obstructions are indicated by choking, gasping, or coarse noise on inspiration (stridor). The patient may be unable to swallow their own saliva. These obstructions tend to become worse over time, especially if aggravated by treatment. Do not attempt to clear a partial obstruction in the field unless it is causing respiratory failure. Early access to ALS airway management skills and tools would be a priority in calling for assistance and evacuation.

BLS - Respiratory Failure

Position for easiest respiration:

- Clear airway, position for drainage
- Nasopharyngeal and oropharyngeal airway use, suction

Reassurance to improve respiration

Oxygen via mask or nasal cannula:

- Titrate to response
- Heat and humidify

Positive Pressure Ventilation:

- Can be effective for hours or days
- Can be used to assist inadequate respiratory effort

If the obstruction is caused by swelling of the airway, back blows and chest compressions will not help. The only BLS treatment is to continue PPV in an attempt to force air past the obstruction while repositioning the neck for the best air flow. These patients will need medication or a surgical airway.

If the cause of airway swelling is anaphylaxis, an injection of epinephrine can be lifesaving. This is part of the Wilderness Protocol for anaphylaxis, a technique taught to basic practitioners because it is a low-risk treatment for a high-risk problem (see the Allergy and Anaphylaxis chapter). Life-threatening lower airway constriction due to asthma can be treated with epinephrine and steroids. This procedure is part of the Wilderness Protocol for asthma, also taught to basic level practitioners for the same reason (see the Severe Asthma chapter).

Circulatory Failure

Cardiac Arrest

Chest compressions are used to temporarily support perfusion when the heart has stopped functioning. Unlike PPV, chest compressions are effective for only a few minutes. An early return of spontaneous circulation is necessary for the patient to have any chance of survival.

Current CPR standards call for 2 minutes of chest compressions, with or without PPV depending on the level of training, before checking a pulse on any patient who is unresponsive and not breathing effectively. This makes sense in the civilized setting where the most common cause of cardiac arrest is a heart attack and hospitals are nearby. The hope is that by circulating still-oxygenated blood through the heart and brain, the patient will be more likely to survive with early defibrillation and quick access to hospital care.

CPR

CPR 2020 Update:

- Begin compressions if unresponsive and in respiratory arrest.
- 30:2 ratio on adults and children (100 -120 per minute)
- 15:2 ratio for two rescuer CPR on infants and children
- Breaths given over 1 second, blow until chest rises
- One shock followed by 2 minutes of CPR before next attempt.

However, chest compressions are not the best immediate treatment for all unresponsive patients in the backcountry setting. If the primary cause is respiratory arrest, as in drowning, avalanche burial, or lightning strike, emphasis should be placed on ensuring an airway and ventilation. Chest compressions could be harmful to a patient in decompensated shock from internal bleeding or respiratory failure from chest wall injury. Chest compressions could cause cardiac arrest in a severely hypothermic patient. A quick but careful scene and primary survey, including a pulse check, should be used to determine if chest compressions are really indicated.

The pulse can be very difficult to find under adverse field conditions where you may be working with cold hands in dangerous places. The pulse can be weak or absent in the extremities of a person in shock, and very slow in cases of severe hypothermia. The carotid and temporal pulses are the easiest to access, and most likely to be felt if the heart is beating. The carotid is located on either side of the Adam's apple (larynx) in the neck. The temporal pulse is on the side of the head just in front of the ear.

Confirmed cardiac arrest in the field should be treated on scene with CPR, which is a combination of chest compressions and PPV that allows

Cardiac Arrest
WILDERNESS PROTOCOL

Do Not BEGIN CPR:

- Obviously dead from lethal injury
- Submerged under H_20 greater than 1 hour
- Trauma with no pulse

Start CPR and ALS otherwise*

* See Thermoregulation for recommendations specific to severe hypothermia.

some oxygenation and perfusion of the brain and vital organs. For CPR to be effective, the patient's critical systems must still be intact. CPR will not save or restore life in cases where the cardiac arrest was caused by massive trauma or shock.

The survivors of cardiac arrest are typically patients who have experienced ventricular fibrillation or other cardiac arrhythmia due to a heart attack. The lungs and brain are still intact and capable of resuming function if perfusion is restored. The application of electrical defibrillation within a few minutes of the arrest may be successful in reestablishing functional cardiac rhythm, at least temporarily.

Unfortunately, CPR and defibrillation are not very useful unless there is rapid access to hospital care. CPR by itself is unlikely to restore normal cardiac rhythm and defibrillation will not fix the cause of the cardiac arrest. The chance of a successful resuscitation without definitive medical care is extremely low. If your backcountry safety budget is limited in money, space, or weight, a defibrillator is not the best way to spend it.

The Wilderness Protocol for cardiac arrest reflects our current level of experience and understanding. We hold out some hope for cardiac arrest caused by respiratory failure due to events like drowning or lightning strike that could be reversed by prompt oxygenation of the lungs and chest compressions to boost perfusion. How often this might occur is left to speculation since there are simply not enough monitored cases to know.

Except under extraordinary circumstances not reproducible in the backcountry or offshore setting, normothermic patients do not recover after more than 30 minutes of CPR. Regardless of the cause of cardiac arrest, the minimal chance of a successful resuscitation does not justify any significant level of risk to survivors or rescuers.

Cardiac Arrest
WILDERNESS PROTOCOL

STOP CPR:

- Spontaneous pulse resumes
- Authorized medical professional pronounces the patient dead
- Rescuers are exhausted or at risk
- Fatal injuries are discovered
- After 30 minutes of sustained cardiac arrest*

* See Thermoregulation for recommendations specific to severe hypothermia.

Severe Bleeding and Shock

Controlling blood loss is the other essential element of circulatory support in the BLS process. Bleeding from an artery is the most immediately life threatening and can usually be controlled by wound packing and well-aimed direct pressure. The site must be exposed, and the bleeding source identified. Packing and direct pressure will be effective most of the time if applied firmly enough, in the right place, and long enough for the blood to clot.

A tourniquet may be used on an extremity to control severe bleeding temporarily while you deal with other critical system problems. It can also be used to stop bleeding long enough for you to expose and identify the source to better aim your direct pressure. A tourniquet can safely be left in place for up to an hour if necessary. Beyond that, the risk of significant tissue infarction due to ischemia will increase. In life-threatening circumstances, however, there may be no choice but to leave it in place.

Pressure points on proximal arteries, sometimes mentioned in first aid texts, are generally not effective for life-threatening bleeding. Hemostatic agents (bandages designed to facilitate blood clotting at the bleeding site) remain unproven in actual field use, and anecdotal experience is mixed. However, these products may offer the only viable alternative in treating severe bleeding that is difficult to access, such as axillary and groin injuries and gunshot wounds to the abdomen. To be effective, hemostatic agents must be properly applied or packed into the wound.

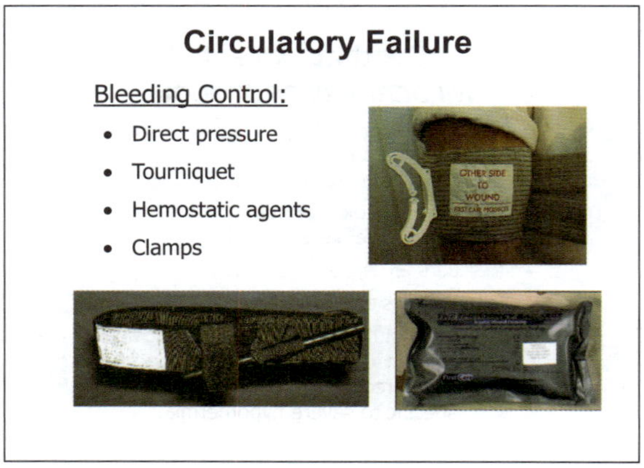

No technique for bleeding control will work if you don't find it. Even profuse external bleeding can be hidden by bulky clothing. This can be a real problem when the clothing is waterproof, and the weather is too extreme to permit undressing the patient. A thorough exploration with a gloved hand is a mandatory part of the primary assessment of a trauma patient.

Internal bleeding is difficult to control without surgery. Some BLS techniques, like binding a pelvic fracture or packing an abdominal wound with gauze (with or without hemostatic agents), may increase the pressure on the bleeding site or reduce the space available for blood to accumulate. This tamponade effect may occur naturally in other confined spaces such as around the kidneys or inside the capsule of the spleen or liver. This fortuitous condition may allow time to evacuate the patient to surgery before shock progresses.

There are no definitive ALS field techniques to control severe internal bleeding. In the presence of progressive shock, ALS providers may use IV crystalloids to increase blood volume and maintain minimal effective perfusion pressure during evacuation. This must be done cautiously because increased pressure can disrupt clot formation, and too much intravenous fluid can impair coagulation and contribute to hypothermia.

Another ALS option is a drug called tranexamic acid (TXA) which has been shown to reduce hemorrhage if given soon enough after the injury. It can be administered orally or by IV and works by inhibiting the breakdown of fibrin in clots. It is in use by some EMS systems in the U.S. and elsewhere, particularly where access to surgery and blood replacement products will be delayed. Nevertheless, for uncontrolled bleeding giving IV fluids and TXA in the field is less important than access to a hospital and a surgeon.

If the bleeding site is accessible and controlled, IV therapy may help to restore perfusion pressure and is less likely to be harmful. Shock stabilized like this, especially if patient protection and body core temperature is not an issue, becomes a lot less of an emergency. Evacuation can be slower and less hazardous.

Brain Failure

Changes in mental status or level of consciousness can be caused by direct trauma to the nervous system or by loss of brain oxygenation due to circulatory or respiratory system problems. There is no real way to treat brain failure other than to treat the cause. Examples include giving sugar to reverse hypoglycemia or naloxone to reverse opioid overdose. Otherwise, BLS is aimed at protecting the airway from fluids and vomit while assessment and treatment continue.

In trauma patients, the spine is also protected as part of BLS. This usually takes the form of restoring and maintaining normal spinal alignment while treatment of any life-threatening condition continues. However, spine management should not take precedence over patient protection, adequate ventilation, or circulatory support.

BLS – Brain Failure

Altered Mental Status:

- Treat the cause – STOPEATS
- Maintain normal body temperature
- Secure and monitor the airway
- Maintain ventilation
- Maintain hydration
- Protect the spine as needed

"There is no real way to treat this other than to treat the cause."

A major critical system problem carries a high risk of death and the benefit to the patient of almost any BLS/ALS treatment is obvious. What is less obvious, sometimes, is the risk to the rescuers performing the treatment.

Risk Versus Benefit in BLS

Any rescue effort, even the most desperate, must consider the overall probability and consequence of an adverse event. Performing CPR under a hang fire avalanche, for example, is a very low-yield procedure in a very high-risk environment. Discontinuing resuscitation under such a circumstance would certainly be appropriate but would be one of the most difficult decisions a medical officer would have to make.

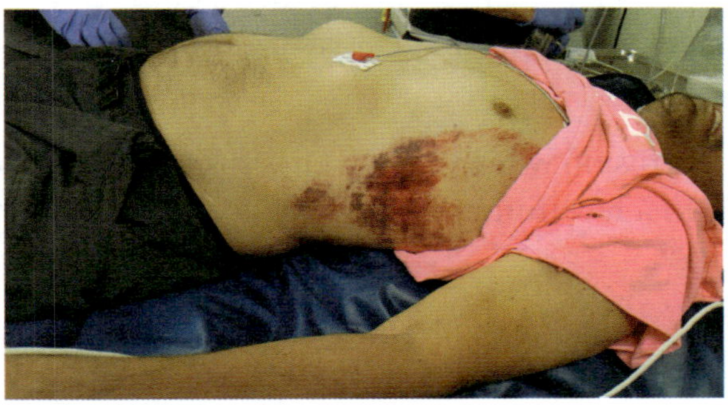

External injury highlights the anticipated problem of internal bleeding. However, significant blunt force trauma may leave no visible signs.

Even in the urban context, the global risks are often discounted in favor of low-yield procedures. Consider, for example, the AED-equipped police cruiser responding to a cardiac arrest call. The officer knows that a fast response is beneficial to the patient's chance for survival. But, at the same time, their code 3 race through town substantially increases the risk to drivers on the road, children and dogs in crosswalks, and bicyclists turning to watch the excitement. Add an ambulance, engine company, and helicopter to the response and the risks really start to pile up.

In the backcountry and offshore setting, the risk associated with rescue and evacuation is often extreme. It is incumbent on the medical officer to balance the chance of successful medical treatment against these risks to the rescuers as well as the patient. There will be situations where remaining on scene and performing good basic medical care while risks are mitigated and a safe rescue is organized will give everyone a better chance of survival. There will also be situations where rapid removal of the patient from the scene before initiating any medical care will be required.

And, of course, there are situations where access to the patient is impossible without exposing rescuers to unreasonable hazards and rescue efforts must be abandoned. Deciding which is which requires an objective, unemotional, concise valuation of probability and consequence and risk versus benefit.

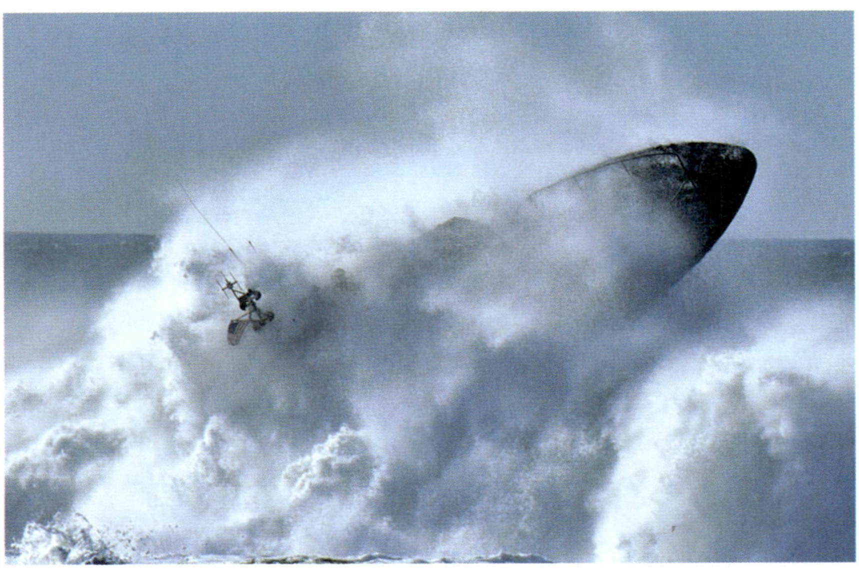

The risks are often extreme...

Chapter 7 Review:
Basic and Advanced Life Support

- Basic life support (BLS) is the immediate treatment of life-threatening critical system problems discovered during the primary assessment. BLS includes airway control, ventilation as needed, bleeding control, CPR as needed, spine protection, and protection from extreme heat or cold.
- BLS can also include the use of injectable epinephrine and a defibrillator, if available.
- Advanced life support (ALS) techniques use additional medications, advanced airways, and some surgical techniques. ALS should be accessed when such procedures would be a benefit to the patient and the rescue effort.
- The goals of BLS and ALS are the same: to preserve oxygenation and perfusion.
- Respiratory failure is evidenced by an altered level of consciousness and inadequate or difficult breathing. Your immediate response is to ensure a patent airway, begin positive pressure ventilation (PPV), and add supplemental oxygen if you have it.
- Chest compressions are used to temporarily support perfusion when the heart has stopped functioning. If functional cardiac activity is not restored within a few minutes, the patient will not survive. Early access to an AED and hospital is ideal.
- Bleeding from an artery is the most immediately life-threatening of bleeding types and can usually be controlled by well-aimed direct pressure or a tourniquet.
- Abnormal brain function indicated by reduced level of consciousness or mental status changes can be caused by direct trauma to the nervous system, loss of brain oxygenation due to circulatory or respiratory system problems, or other causes outlined by the STOPEATS mnemonic.

Chapter 8: Allergy and Anaphylaxis

The severe systemic allergic reaction known as anaphylaxis causes serious critical system problems that require immediate treatment in the field. The medications used are an important part of your basic life support (BLS)/advanced life support (ALS) tool kit. The emergency treatment for anaphylaxis should be memorized and rehearsed. This is a problem that will not wait for you to look it up in a book, or for an ambulance or helicopter to arrive.

Allergy and Anaphylaxis

Mechanism:

- Antigen injected, ingested, inhaled, or absorbed
- Antibody produced by the immune system marking the antigen for destruction by white blood cells
- Histamine and other inflammatory chemicals released by white blood cells (mast cells) during the process

Allergy and inflammation is a complicated process involving several chemical mediators and body responses. The actions of drugs used to treat it are equally complex and sometimes not well understood. Fortunately, a basic understanding of the important points is sufficient for field purposes.

Allergy

Allergy is an abnormally vigorous form of immune response resulting in the release of the chemical histamine and other inflammatory mediators into blood and body tissues from white blood cells called mast cells. These white blood cells are responding to signals from antibodies that have attached themselves to a foreign molecule, bacteria, or other allergen marking it for destruction.

The histamine and other chemicals mediate vasodilation and bronchoconstriction, causing swelling and lower airway constriction. These effects can be mild or severe, local or systemic. Onset can be nearly instantaneous or delayed by several hours.

When the response remains localized to the area of antigen contact, it is called a local allergic reaction. The patient experiences localized vasodilation. This allows fluid to leak from capillaries into the extracellular space causing localized swelling and itching. Hay fever is an example of a local reaction affecting the mucous membranes of the nose and eyes. These effects explain the familiar symptoms: swollen mucous membranes, itchy eyes, and a runny nose.

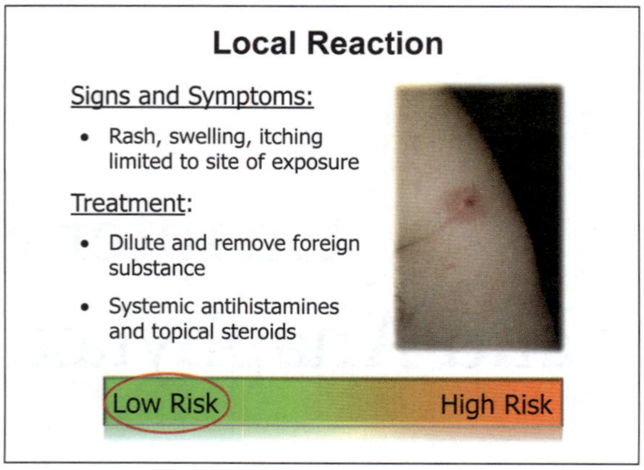

A systemic response to an allergen, by contrast, can produce generalized itching and hives all over the body surface. The patient may give a history of a specific allergy, or the history may be completely unrevealing. As long as there is no swelling, no facial involvement, no respiratory distress, and no signs of vascular shock, we call this a mild allergic reaction. It usually resolves on its own or responds well to treatment with oral antihistamines (e.g. diphenhydramine/Benadryl). Often, the patient will give a history of similar symptoms and successful treatment with oral medications. This is reassuring for field treatment, but still requires careful monitoring because any reaction can be more severe than expected.

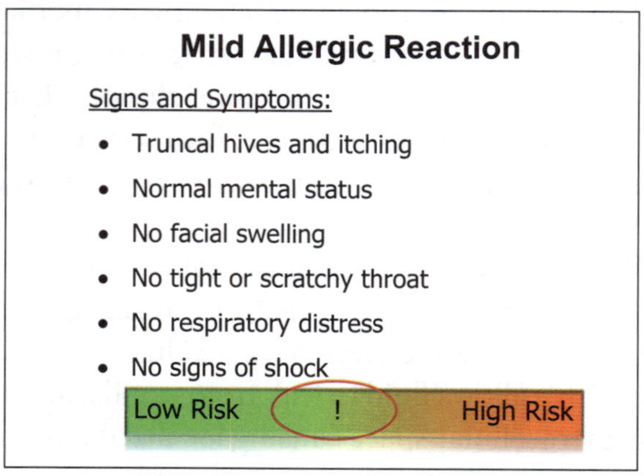

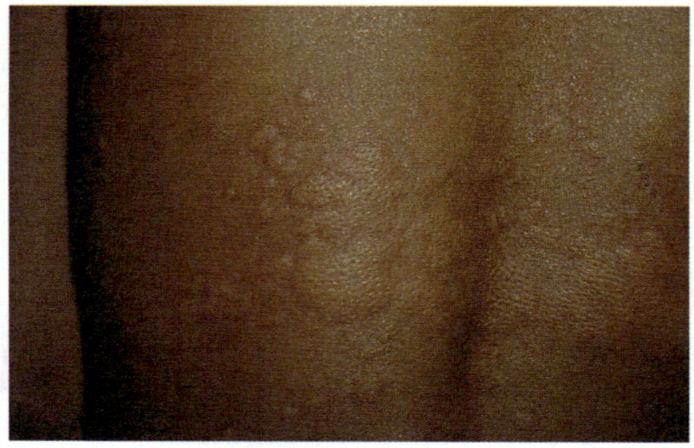

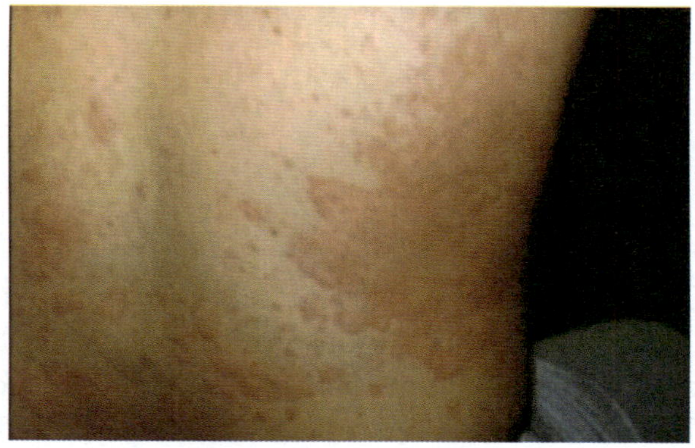

Hives tend to appear and disappear from various areas of the skin surface, sometimes within minutes.

Anaphylaxis

Anaphylaxis is a severe form of systemic allergy that results in critical system problems. Widespread vasodilation and fluid shift into the interstitial space can cause vascular and volume shock, upper airway swelling, vomiting, and diarrhea. Lower airway constriction results in wheezing and respiratory distress. The patient can die within a matter of minutes.

Symptoms can progress quickly from an initial complaint of itchy skin and hives with a scratchy or constricted feeling in the throat. Patients often report feeling a sense of impending doom. As the reaction becomes more severe, signs and symptoms including wheezing, stridor, facial swelling, nausea, vomiting, or diarrhea may develop. There will be weakness and mental status changes with the onset of vascular and volume shock.

Anaphylaxis

Signs and Symptoms:

- Generalized and facial hives
- Tight or scratchy throat
- Vascular and volume shock
- Respiratory distress
- Nausea, vomiting, diarrhea
- Altered mental status

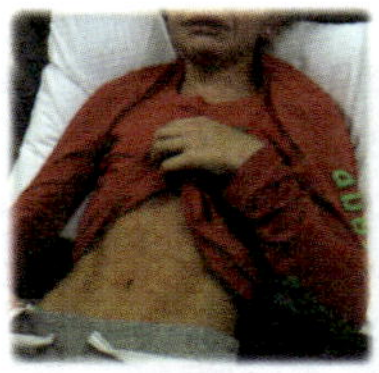

Low Risk — High Risk

A previous history of anaphylaxis is not necessary to make the diagnosis. A significant percentage of patients presenting with anaphylaxis will have no known history of allergy. In the remote setting, early and aggressive treatment for evolving anaphylaxis is always warranted.

Treatment of Anaphylaxis

BLS and PROP is appropriate, but not definitive. Specific treatment with epinephrine is required to immediately reverse the systemic response. The Wilderness Protocol for anaphylaxis adds the use of oral antihistamines and prednisone which may help prevent the reoccurrence of the problem. The recognition of anaphylaxis and the use of these medications are important skills for the wilderness medical practitioner.

Epinephrine (adrenaline) is a potent vasoconstrictor and bronchodilator that also helps to stabilize the activated mast cells, reducing the release of histamine and other mediators. It is most effective when injected into the muscle of the lateral aspect of the thigh at a dose of 0.3 to 0.5 mg. The patient's symptoms usually improve within 90 seconds. Repeat doses may be necessary if symptoms do not improve or if a rebound (biphasic) reaction occurs.

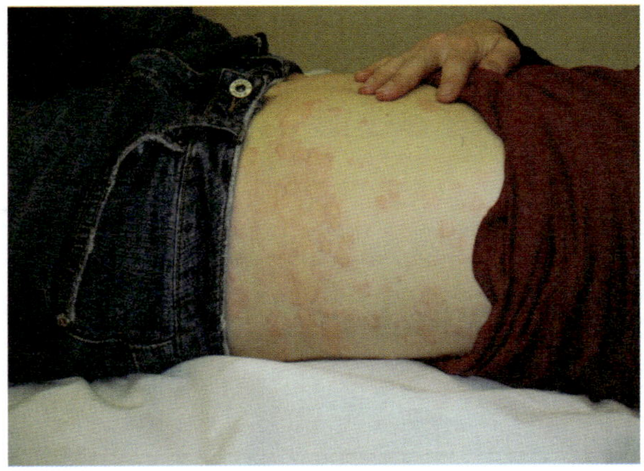

Hives on the abdomen of a patient with anaphylaxis, prior to the administration of epinephrine.

Epinephrine is supplied as a liquid specifically for the treatment of anaphylaxis in the form of a pre-loaded autoinjector such as an EpiPen that automatically injects the specified dose when pressed firmly against the skin. In the United States, these devices are available only by prescription. Patients known to have severe allergies often carry one. Many other countries like Canada and Mexico allow autoinjector sales without prescription.

Anaphylaxis Treatment

WILDERNESS PROTOCOL

Epinephrine:

- 0.01 mg/kg up to 0.5 mg by intramuscular injection. Average adult dose is 0.3 – 0.5 mg.
- Repeat as soon as 5 minutes if needed
- Action: bronchodilation, vasoconstriction, stabilizes mast cells

Antihistamine

- Action: blocks histamine at receptor sites
- eg: diphenhydramine 25 – 50 mg or cetirizine 5 – 10 mg by mouth

Prednisone:

- 40 to 60 mg by mouth
- Action: anti-inflammatory, may help prevent biphasic reaction

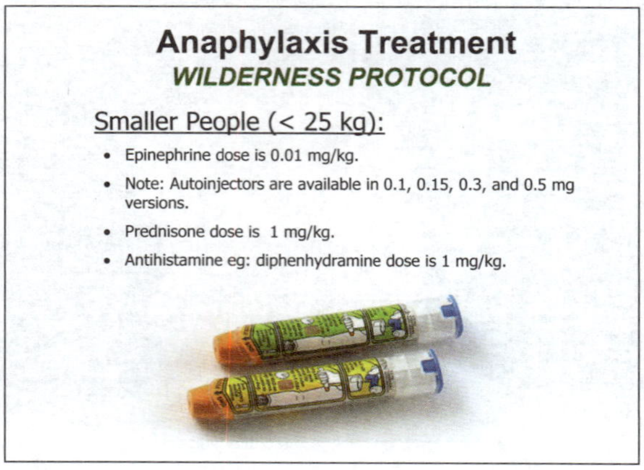

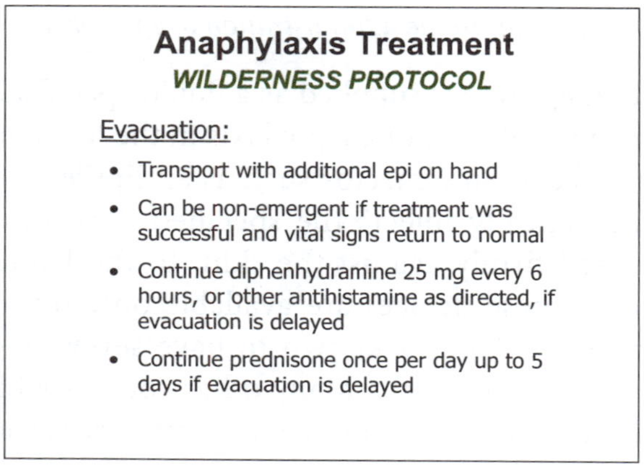

In the backcountry setting, it is advisable to carry at least three doses of epinephrine to cover biphasic reactions during evaluation and evacuation. Practitioners trained and comfortable with syringes and ampoules or vials may choose to carry epinephrine in that more economical and compact form. Epinephrine should be protected from light, freezing, and excessive heat.

The epinephrine injection is often followed by an antihistamine, a type of drug that is believed to directly block the attachment of the histamine molecule to receptor sites on body tissues. Diphenhydramine is a common example. It takes effect in about 15–20 minutes.

Neither epinephrine nor diphenhydramine will remove the antigen or the histamine. It is possible to see a biphasic reaction with the reappearance of symptoms minutes to hours later. Because the effects of epinephrine are temporary, evacuation and medical follow-up should be planned.

For offshore situations or long evacuations, adding prednisone at a dose of 40–60 mg once a day may suppress the inflammatory response associated with the reaction. This will make a biphasic reaction less likely. Prednisone can be used at this dose for up to 5 days.

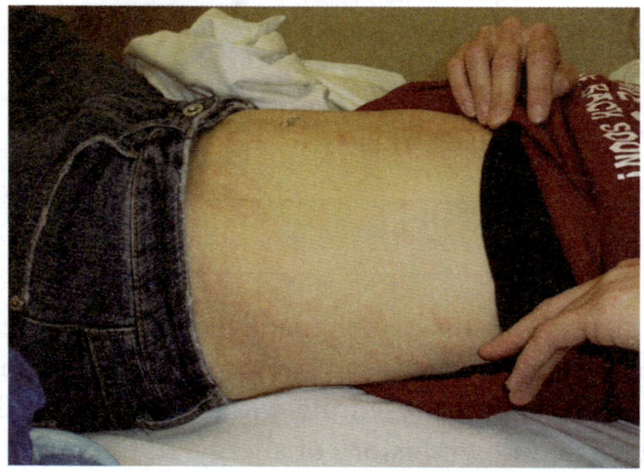

The patient in the photograph on the previous page approximately 12 minutes after the administration of epinephrine and diphenhydramine.

Risk Versus Benefit

The field treatment of anaphylaxis is a low-risk solution to a high-risk problem. You have a much better chance of saving a life with an injection of epinephrine than almost any other piece of medical equipment you can carry. Furthermore, the drugs and dosages specified in the protocol are highly unlikely to produce an adverse outcome, even if the problem is misdiagnosed and the treatment turns out to be unnecessary.

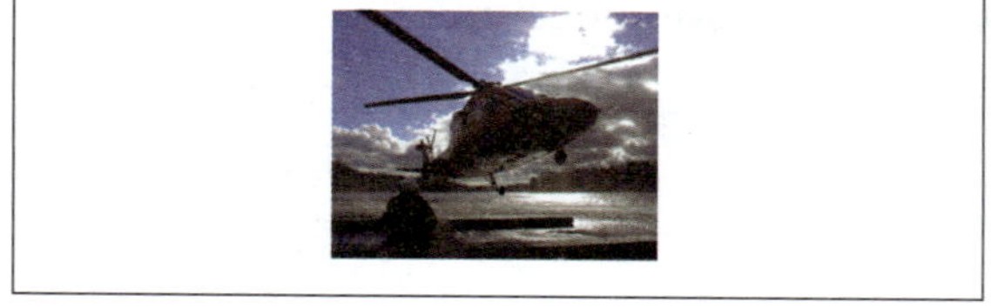
Anaphylaxis
Wilderness Perspective
High-Risk Problem:
• Persistent abnormal mental status
• Incomplete response to treatment
• The patient is getting worse
• Second injection of epi is needed

The greatest direct risk would be in giving epinephrine to a patient who is suffering a heart attack. Fortunately, the signs, symptoms, and mechanism are markedly different and unlikely to be confused with anaphylaxis. The most common problem to be mistaken for anaphylaxis in the field is acute stress reaction following multiple wasp or bee stings.

In any case, once you have initiated field treatment with epinephrine, evacuation for medical follow-up is considered ideal. If the patient has recovered from the event, it need not be an emergency. However, a history of previous hospitalization for anaphylaxis or failure to improve to normal after the first injection indicates a higher risk patient.

In remote or dangerous circumstances where evacuation is not safe or practical, continued use of the diphenhydramine every 4 to 6 hours may be advisable for several days. Continuing the prednisone once a day may also help prevent biphasic reactions and is safe for treatment up to 5 days. Careful monitoring is crucial.

Chapter 8 Review: Allergy and Anaphylaxis

- Allergy and anaphylaxis are mediated by histamine, a chemical causing vasodilation and lower airway constriction.
- Vasodilation results in fluid shift and soft tissue swelling capable of causing shock and respiratory failure.
- The Wilderness Protocol for anaphylaxis calls for 0.3–0.5 mg of epinephrine by intramuscular injection, 25–50 mg of diphenhydramine orally, and 40–60 mg of prednisone orally.
- Epinephrine reverses the effects of histamine, diphenhydramine blocks the effects of histamine, and prednisone reduces the immune and inflammatory response.
- Following treatment, evacuation for medical follow-up is ideal. In high-risk and remote settings, continued monitoring and use of diphenhydramine, and prednisone for several days may be indicated.

Chapter 9: Severe Asthma

Asthma is a chronic inflammatory disease that causes lower airway constriction. The mechanism involves both spasm of the smooth muscle walls and swelling of the mucous membrane lining of the bronchial tubes. Acute asthma attacks are sometimes triggered by infection, cold air, exercise, or other stressors. Sometimes asthma flares without apparent reason. Some patients need to use medications daily to keep their asthma under control.

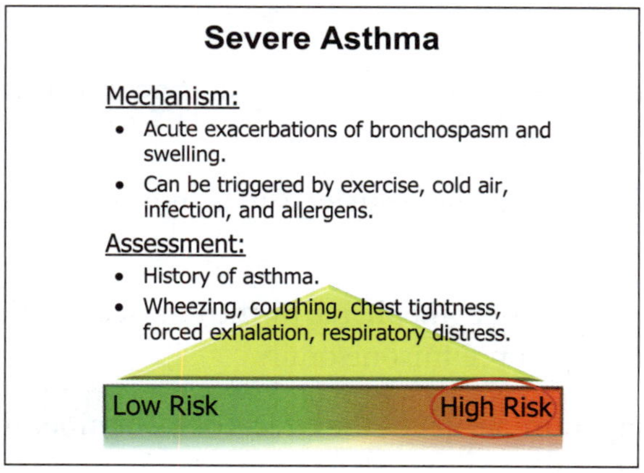

An acute asthma attack can be mild or severe. It can be a major critical system problem when it causes respiratory distress. If bronchospasm is allowed to persist, the lower airway constriction will be exacerbated by secondary swelling.

Early signs and symptoms include respiratory distress, chest tightness, wheezing, and a non-productive cough. Fortunately, most people with asthma are aware of their condition and are familiar with its presentation. Acute symptoms are usually relieved with self-administered medication, such as inhaled albuterol, that reverses the characteristic bronchospasm.

Occasionally, an asthma attack will not respond to inhaled medication. This is usually due to the patient waiting too long to administer it or not having it available at all. When early treatment is delayed or ineffective, the initial bronchospasm in the lower airways is made worse by secondary swelling. At this point, it will be difficult or impossible for the patient to inhale medication deep into the bronchioles where it can exert its effect.

Severe respiratory distress can rapidly progress to respiratory failure, at which stage respiration will be labored and the patient will be able to speak only one or two words between breaths. Immediate treatment is required, and it should not wait for evacuation or for ALS to be brought to the scene.

You should first assist your patient in the proper use of their HFA inhaler. Be sure that you are using the fast-acting bronchodilator. The patient may recognize this as their "rescue inhaler" which is usually red in color. The distinction is important because some patients also use an inhaled steroid or other medication as an adjunct to therapy.

These do not act fast enough to help in an acute attack.

Encourage the patient to inhale as deeply as possible while the inhaler is discharged into the mouth. The efficiency of the inhaler can be improved using a spacer to contain the vapors while the patient inhales. This is simply a plastic tube with the inhaler on one end and the patient on the other. You can improvise a spacer by using a plastic water bottle with the end cut off.

Asthma

Treatment:

- PROP
- Rescue inhaler (albuterol, salbutamol)
- Emergency evacuation or ALS support if not responding to the inhaler

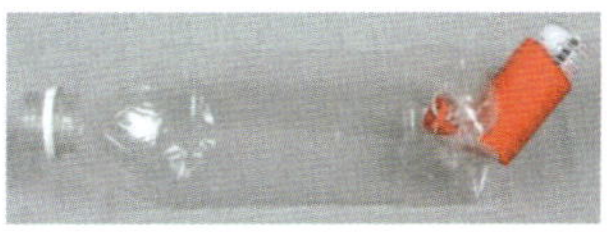

Rescue inhaler with water bottle spacer

It is safe to make several attempts to abort the asthma attack with an inhaler. However, do not delay moving to the next step if it is apparent that the patient cannot effectively inhale the medication. If use of the inhaler fails to reduce symptoms within a few minutes, the patient will need an injection of epinephrine.

Before medications like albuterol became available, epinephrine was a first-line treatment for an asthma attack. It is the same medication used for the emergency treatment of anaphylaxis. It is given in the same concentration and dose by intramuscular injection (see the allergy and anaphylaxis chapter).

The Wilderness Protocol for severe asthma calls for 0.3–0.5 mg injected into the lateral aspect of the thigh. For children, the dose is 0.01 mg per kilogram up to 0.3 mg. The patient will usually feel better within a few minutes. One dose of epinephrine may completely abort the asthma attack, but a second dose may be given within as little as 5 minutes if needed. Once symptoms improve, the patient should self-administer their own inhaler at a dose of 6 to 10 puffs up to three times over the next hour. Each 6 to 10 puff dose is roughly equivalent to a nebulizer treatment in a clinic or hospital.

If evacuation is likely to take more than 3 hours, add a dose of prednisone at 1 mg/kg given by mouth (40–60 mg for an adult, 20 mg for a child). As with anaphylaxis, this will reduce lower airway inflammation and the chance of another attack.

Asthma Treatment

WILDERNESS PROTOCOL

Respiratory distress not responding to the inhaler:

- PROP
- Epinephrine 0.3 mg IM.
- β-agonist rescue inhaler (6–10 puffs up to 3x over the next hour), then as prescribed.
- Prednisone 1–2 mg/kg up to 60 mg PO.
- Evacuation

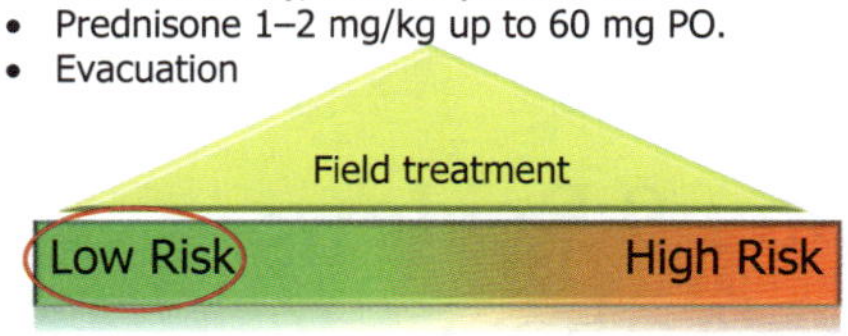

Risk Versus Benefit

This protocol is for use in severe respiratory distress leading to respiratory failure caused by lower airway constriction in a known asthmatic. It is safe, effective, and carries little risk compared to the problems associated with inadequate oxygenation. It is an important life-saving skill for both basic and advanced practitioners operating in remote areas.

Severe Asthma

Wilderness Perspective

High-Risk Problem:

- Persistent abnormal mental status
- Incomplete response to treatment
- HFA/MDI continues to be ineffective
- The patient is getting worse

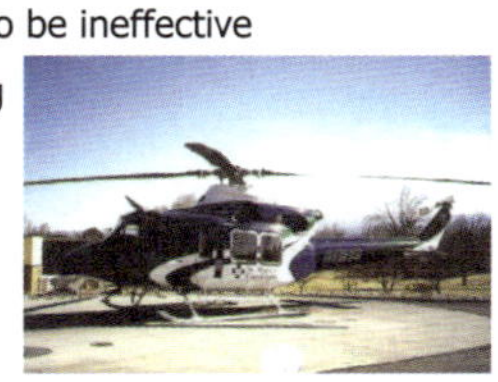

The disease itself can become a significant problem when the triggers cannot be avoided. Asthma can also generate significant lower airway inflammation and continued wheezing with exacerbations that may continue for several hours or days. Even if the initial attack is completely aborted, the risk of further exacerbations may warrant evacuation from the field.

Ideally, anyone whose life you have just saved with epinephrine should receive early follow-up medical care. If the symptoms are under control, the evacuation need not be an emergency one. In settings where evacuation is unreasonably dangerous or impractical, prednisone can be continued daily for up to 5 days. The patient should continue to use their albuterol inhaler as needed.

Chapter 9 Review: Severe Asthma

- Asthma causes lower airway constriction and, if severe, respiratory distress and failure.
- The Wilderness Protocol for severe asthma calls for 0.3–0.5 mg of epinephrine by intramuscular injection followed by albuterol by inhalation and 40 to 60 mg of prednisone orally.
- Following treatment, evacuation for medical follow-up is ideal. In high-risk and remote settings, continued monitoring and use of albuterol and prednisone for several days may be indicated.

Chapter 10: Problems with Sugar

Diabetes has become a common chronic medical problem so practitioners in any environment are likely to see a diabetic patient at some point. Fortunately, most diabetics are well-informed and do a good job of managing their disease. It is very likely that your diabetic client or traveling partner will know much more about it than you do. It is worth having a pre-trip discussion with the patient about anticipated problems and the appropriate treatment. It is also worth reviewing the patient's experience with managing their disease in similar situations.

Monitoring Blood Sugar

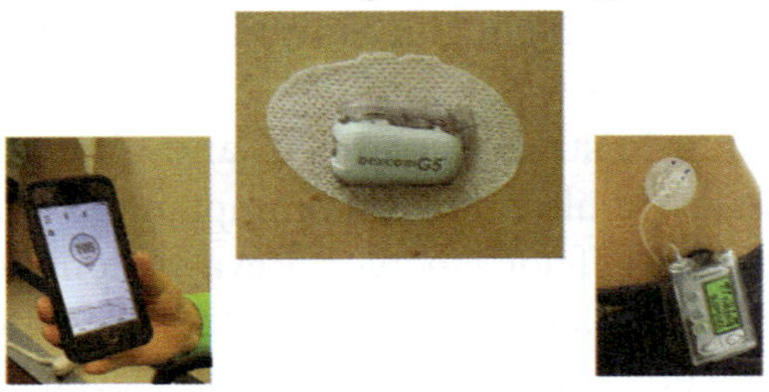

"Many diabetic patients can monitor blood sugar regularly, and adjust diet and insulin dosage accordingly."

Some diabetics manage their disease with oral medication in the form of pills. More significant cases use insulin by injection, infusion pump, or oral spray. The latter group is more likely to have problems in a new environment.

Diabetic Emergencies

Diabetes is, in basic terms, the inability to produce the appropriate amount of insulin in response to rising blood glucose levels. Insulin is a hormone produced in the pancreas. One of its primary jobs is to help facilitate glucose uptake into body cells where it is processed and stored for use as fuel. When the diabetic patient eats, blood glucose levels rise as they do in everyone, but insulin levels do not rise enough to meet the need. Supplemental insulin is usually injected or inhaled in a prescribed amount to match the glucose content of the meal.

Patients often adjust the amount of insulin and sugar intake in response to changing environmental conditions and activity. Most can monitor blood glucose at any time with a portable glucometer. It is rare for a conscientious patient to have a diabetic emergency while living within a well-established routine.

Hypoglycemia

Unfortunately, many backcountry and marine situations are far from well-established routine. Even a well-controlled diabetic can have trouble adjusting to a new environment. The problem is almost always low blood glucose, also known as hypoglycemia.

The symptoms of hypoglycemia can develop rapidly and result in brain failure, usually starting with easily observable mental status changes. Your patient may be behaving normally one minute and then become irritable, forgetful, or otherwise inappropriate the next. If hypoglycemia is not corrected, the patient can become combative, completely disoriented, or unconscious. Tachycardia and profound sweating are also commonly seen. Hypoglycemia is sometimes mistaken for intoxication or traumatic brain injury, delaying treatment until it is too late.

You are much less likely to see the opposite problem: hyperglycemia. The problem of too much sugar in the blood develops slowly over hours or days. Signs and symptoms include frequent urination, extreme thirst, weakness, and a fruity odor on the patient's breath. Most diabetics are aware that it is happening, and will adjust their insulin dose accordingly, or seek medical care before serious problems develop. Field treatment, when needed, is limited to aggressive hydration and emergency evacuation.

Treatment of Hypoglycemia

A diabetic with altered mental status is considered to be hypoglycemic until proven otherwise. The treatment is to administer easily absorbed sugar. For the patient who is still awake, the easiest route is orally in the form of a glucose gel kept in a first aid kit for that purpose. One dose is 15 grams of sugar. It is also fine to give granulated sugar, honey, candy, juice, or any other sweet food. Sugar substitutes like saccharin will not work.

If the patient's level of consciousness has decreased to the point that airway protection is a concern, intravenous sugar is preferred. If IV therapy is not available, glucose, honey, or granulated sugar can be rubbed on the mucous membranes under the tongue or inside the mouth where some will be directly absorbed into the blood. Sugar, diluted in warm water or D50, can also be given rectally in the form of an enema.

Your unconscious patient may be carrying a glucagon injector. This is a kit (available by prescription) containing a vial of powdered glucagon that is mixed with a solution, drawn up into a syringe, and injected into the upper arm, thigh, or buttocks. Glucagon can also be administered as a nasal spray, and autoinjectors are under development. Glucagon is a hormone that increases blood glucose levels by releasing glycogen, a concentrated form of glucose, from the liver. Improvement should be seen within 10 minutes. As the patient regains consciousness, sugar should be given orally.

Glucagon Injector

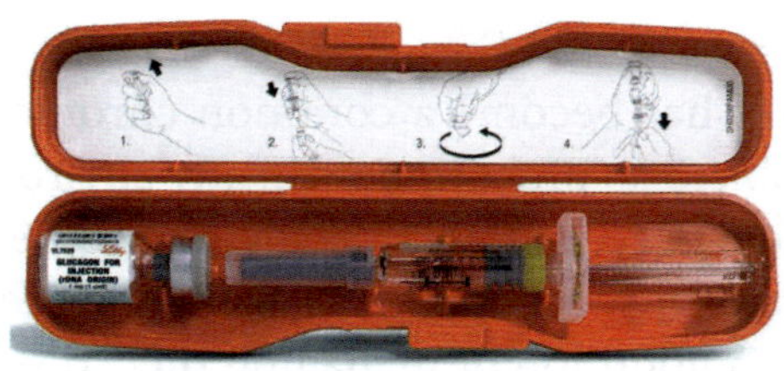

This glucagon injector contains a syringe of sterile water that is manually infused into the vial of powder to reconstitute the drug.

If your client is carrying a glucagon injector or atomizer, be sure that you examine it before you need it. Know where it is kept and consider instructing someone else in the group in its use. Like epinephrine, a glucagon kit should not be allowed to freeze.

The administration of sugar, and glucagon if necessary, should result in a prompt improvement of symptoms. If not, emergency evacuation should be initiated. Never give insulin to a diabetic, or trigger a bolus on their insulin pump, even if you have reason to believe that the problem is high blood glucose (hyperglycemia). The primary field treatment for that is aggressive hydration. You should also remind yourself of the STOPEATS mnemonic; low blood sugar may not be the only cause of the patient's condition.

Risk Versus Benefit

Complete recovery from an episode of hypoglycemia ends the immediate problem, but the practitioner must consider the patient's future safety. Can the patient reasonably expect to prevent another episode, and to treat it effectively if it does reoccur? As with other chronic conditions like asthma and angina, definitive treatment is a long way off if the emergency field treatment is not effective. Continued participation in a remote expedition may represent an unacceptable risk to the patient and the rest of the participants.

Pre-trip screening can be a useful preventive measure. Diabetics who are poorly controlled in a civilized setting are going to be at considerable risk in the backcountry or offshore. Although well-controlled diabetics will likely fare better in a new situation, lack of experience with the type of trip planned is a serious cause for concern for both the patient and the guide. The diabetic patient's first backcountry experience should probably be less remote with careful consideration given to treatment and evacuation options.

Chapter 10 Review: Problems with Sugar

- Hypoglycemia is inadequate blood glucose levels resulting in brain failure.
- Altered mental status in a diabetic is considered hypoglycemia until proven otherwise.
- The immediate field treatment is glucose, orally or via an IV. Glucose can be administered rectally if it is the only available alternative.
- A glucagon injector carried by the patient may be used if the patient is unresponsive.
- Emergency evacuation is indicated if the patient does not respond fully to treatment.
- Discontinuation of the trip may be advisable if blood glucose levels cannot be controlled.

Case Study 5: Incomplete Medical Screening

SCENE
Maine Island base camp, 8 kilometers offshore, 1930 hours. Weather 15°C, winds ENE 30 knots, visibility 0.5 nautical miles in fog and rain.

S: A 16-year-old girl is carried into the staff hut with the report of difficulty breathing for the past 2 hours and getting worse. She is no longer able to speak. Friends reported that she had complained of chest tightness and dizziness and had been asking around for an asthma inhaler with no success. No allergies or other medication use was listed on her medical screening form. No one had observed any recent trauma or respiratory illness. Her friends denied seeing any recreational drug use or smoking. Her last meal was lunch at 1300.

O: Awake, but subdued and incoherent. Unable to sit upright without help. VS: Pulse: 138, Resp: 24, shallow and labored with an audible wheeze, Skin: pale, lips blue, Temp: feels cool. No obvious severe injury noted on primary assessment.

A:

1. Respiratory failure due to lower airway constriction
   A': Respiratory arrest
2. Cold patient
   A': Hypothermia
3. Hazardous evacuation

P:

1. Oxygen by mask at 12 liters/minute. Wilderness Protocol for severe asthma initiated with 0.3 mg epinephrine IM by autoinjector.
2. Bag-valve mask readied for positive pressure ventilation if necessary. Albuterol and prednisone available.
3. Patient wrapped in sleeping bag, and the hut stove is fired up for heat.
4. Staff member tasked to initiate contact with the Coast Guard for a possible emergency evacuation by larger vessel.

Discussion:

Respiratory failure is a primary assessment problem requiring immediate treatment. The secondary assessment can wait. Wheezing suggests lower airway constriction as the generic problem meaning that epinephrine will be required. Based on a limited history, asthma was presumed, but anaphylaxis is also a possibility. The problem list was compounded by the weather, resulting in a cold patient at risk for hypothermia. Warming was therefore an important part of the primary treatment.

In this case, field treatment was successful, and an emergency evacuation was not necessary, but the staff had been wise to initiate the process early. It is usually safer to call off an evacuation in progress than to rush an evacuation started too late. In this case, the availability of a warm hut, oxygen, and medical supplies allowed for good basic medical care on scene. It was later determined that the patient has a history of asthma and normally carries medication. This significant element was omitted from her screening form for fear that it would have disqualified her from participating in the program.

Case Study 6: River Trip Disaster

SCENE

River kayak day trip, Quebec, 12 kilometers from the nearest road. Weather: 5°C, overcast and windy with snow flurries. A group of three kayakers encounters a second group on the riverbank with one guide performing CPR on another. There were five other kayakers lying and sitting around, apparently unconcerned. The exhausted guide reports that he has been doing CPR on his unresponsive assistant for 15 minutes and asks for help. His group of six clients had also been in the water helping with the rescue. He did not know if any of them were injured. He has been unable to call for help because there is no cell phone service.

S: The patient was pulled from the water after a 40-minute entrapment fully submerged. He was last seen upright just before dropping into a large hydraulic. No other history is obtained. Five other people were noted in various stages of altered mental status and reduced level of consciousness. One was apparently missing.

O: A male in his 30s, unresponsive. CPR in progress. VS: Pulse: undetectable, Resp: absent, Skin: pale, Temp: cold. Helmet cracked. Deformity noted above right eye.

A:

1. Multiple casualty incident with one fatality
2. Multiple people in mild to severe hypothermia
3. Missing person
4. Cold, no shelter, high-risk evacuation

P:

1. Discontinue CPR
2. Push sugar and fluids for the other patients and build a fire; improvise shelter
3. Initiate a hasty search of the nearby riverbank for the missing person
4. Activate your personal locator beacon

Discussion:

The most serious medical problem in this scene was not the unresponsive subject of CPR. His chance of survival after a 40-minute submersion and 15 minutes of CPR is extremely low, whereas the risk of severe hypothermia in the other six is quite high. And, there is still one person missing. This was a clear case for recognizing the limits of CPR in the wilderness context and for focusing on the people who need immediate care and protection.

Activating a beacon or employing other means of declaring an emergency was justified in this case even though you have stopped CPR. Your ability to treat six exhausted and cold people with inadequate equipment and supplies, while searching for a seventh, is severely limited. You are dealing with high-risk problems in a high-risk environment.

Section IV: Trauma

Chapter 11: General Principles of Trauma

Energy can be neither created nor destroyed. It can change form, but it must go somewhere. The faster an object is moving and the more massive a moving object is, the more energy there is to be transformed and dissipated as the object is slowed or stopped. The faster this transformation takes place, the higher the risk of damage to the object or person gaining or losing the energy.

The more you can dissipate energy over time and area, the less energy any structure must contend with at any point in time. This is the principle behind crumple zones in cars, helmets on skiers, and body armor on bull riders. It also explains why some impacts are just annoying and others produce significant trauma.

The problems associated with trauma tend to be cumulative, especially in the backcountry. Patients are often cold or hot, dehydrated, calorie depleted, and dirty as well as injured. This explains an important part of the Generic to Specific Principle discussed in the chapter on general principles of wilderness rescue, and the reasons that you need to look well beyond the immediate event and specific complaint to consider the whole patient and all the influences on their health.

Energy and Injury

Kinetic energy is the energy of motion. When a moving object stops moving, its kinetic energy must be converted into another form or absorbed by the object and whatever stops it. The brakes on your truck, for example, slowly transform the vehicle's kinetic energy into heat as you slow down.

Potential energy is possessed by an object waiting to fall. When the frost finally dislodges the rock above you, its potential energy is converted into kinetic energy. When the rock strikes you, the foam lining in your helmet absorbs the energy as it deforms, reducing the amount of energy transmitted to your head. Trauma happens when the human body absorbs too much kinetic energy too quickly, resulting in damage to its structure, just like the foam in your helmet.

$$\mathbf{K = 1/2\ mv^2}$$

Kinetic energy is equal to mass times velocity squared, divided by two. This formula tells us that velocity contributes substantially more than mass to the kinetic energy possessed by a moving object. This explains how a very small high-velocity bullet can do so much damage. It also tells us that a fast-moving skier stopped by a large maple tree will dissipate a lot more energy than a skier moving at half the speed. It explains why a fall from two meters in height may be no big deal, but four meters can be fatal.

Deceleration

The rate of change in speed is called acceleration. Because injuries are usually caused by a sudden decrease in speed, or negative acceleration, we use the term deceleration. Deceleration requires the transformation or dissipation of energy over time.

When you step on the brakes, your truck does not decelerate instantly. There must be time for the brakes to absorb and diffuse the truck's kinetic energy without damage to the vehicle or its occupants. If your truck were to decelerate instantly, against a bridge abutment, for example, massive deformation would result as the kinetic energy was absorbed instantly by the vehicle and the occupants. The difference between braking and crashing is the rate of deceleration.

Deceleration causes injury due to inertia, the tendency of a moving body to keep moving until acted on by an outside force. If a skier's head is suddenly stopped by a maple tree, their brain will continue to move forward until it strikes the inside of the skull. This causes direct injury to the front of the brain from the impact, and indirect injury to the back of the brain as suspended arteries and veins tear away from the brain tissue (known as a contra-coup injury). The heart and great vessels in the chest can experience the same forces, resulting in a torn aorta.

Rapid deceleration concentrates energy and magnifies its effect. High kinetic energy with rapid deceleration causes the most damage. A good helmet and body armor can reduce trauma by decreasing the rate of deceleration, but if your patient was moving fast and stopped quickly you still have a lot to worry about. This would be a good time to use the Generic to Specific Principle in assessment.

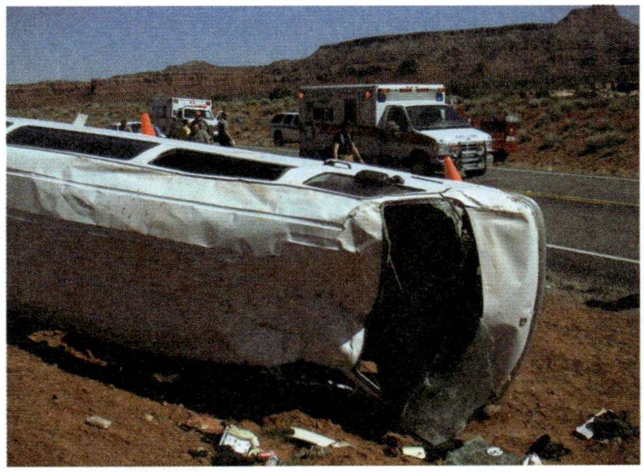

Rapid deceleration offers a high probability of multi-system trauma. Be sure to examine the whole patient, not just the most obvious injuries.

By contrast, slow deceleration can dissipate the same amount of energy without deforming structure. The high-speed skier who falls on a steep, open slope can dissipate their kinetic energy while sliding several hundred meters to a stop. They might even emerge uninjured. Ski patrollers call this a yard sale because ski equipment and clothing tend to dissipate as well. The skier's kinetic energy is absorbed by the snow as the skier slides along, and by the flexion and compression of body tissues and clothing at the points of contact. If the energy of each impact is low enough, the skier's body can accept the momentary deformations without lasting damage.

Cavitation

High-velocity trauma can cause injuries remote from the point of impact due to an effect called cavitation. This is the sudden displacement of internal organs creating a shock wave that can distribute energy throughout the body. Low-density organs like the gut and lungs are elastic, like foam rubber, and they can move and compress as they absorb the energy transmitted by cavitation. It is unusual to see rupture of hollow organs from blunt trauma.

High-density solid organs and bones are less elastic; they are more like watermelon and tend to split and fracture as energy is absorbed. This is how the spleen is ruptured by blunt trauma.

There may be no visible external injury, but the solid organs inside can be shattered.

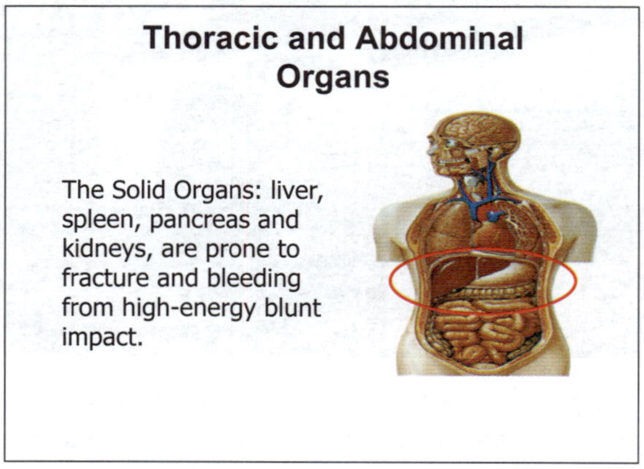

Pay Attention to the History

Attention to the mechanism of injury and how kinetic energy was absorbed often gives you more information than the secondary assessment does. For example, a patient who reports having the wind knocked out of them has just told you that their body absorbed enough energy fast enough to disrupt nerve function and possibly rupture internal organs. A sport climber whose fall was caught by a stretchable dynamic rope will have experienced substantially less deceleration than a rescue worker unfortunate enough to drop several meters and be stopped suddenly by a static rope.

If your scene size-up or history reveals a high-velocity and rapid deceleration mechanism you have good reason to suspect serious injury, perhaps remote from the site of impact. Trauma like this is more likely to involve shattered bone, ruptured organs, traumatic brain injury, and/or cardiac contusion. A thorough exam and careful monitoring is prudent, regardless of the chief complaint and outward appearance.

Conversely, low-velocity trauma tends not to cause injury elsewhere. It does not cause cavitation, and deceleration is minimal. The initial damage is restricted to the point energy is applied or is transferred by leverage or torque. In essence, what you see is what you get. In the patient with a complaint of knee pain following a slow twisting fall, you need not anticipate shock from solid organ rupture. In this case, the mechanism and history are reassuring.

Even when kinetic energy is high from a large mass, low-velocity trauma remains localized. The patient with a foot crushed by a ship rolling against the pier was exposed to massive kinetic energy because of the size of the ship. But this is still a low-velocity injury with slow deceleration and no cavitation; the damage is limited to the foot.

Problems Are Cumulative

An isolated injury to an otherwise healthy and safe individual is a rare delight in emergency medicine, especially in the backcountry. Unfortunately, it is common for trauma to be complicated by multisystem involvement, environmental extremes, and preexisting injury or illness. A patient who is already in compensated volume shock from dehydration is not in a good position to survive blood loss from a fractured femur. Mild hypothermia by itself can be cured in the field, but it vastly reduces the chance of survival for a patient in shock. Fractured bones might well be combined with skin abrasions, lacerations, and the risk of infection. Cold weather and ischemia is a setup for frostbite. The immediate traumatic event can be combined with everything that has developed before, leaving you with a long and complicated problem list.

Extremes of age and chronic illness also elevate your level of concern. Elderly people are less able to compensate for volume loss due to less elasticity in the vascular system and reduced cardiac output. Small children lose heat much faster due to a larger surface area-to-weight ratio. Diabetics have more difficulty maintaining perfusion of the extremities. A careful history, exam, and application of the Generic to Specific Principle can alert you to greater risk or provide some degree of reassurance.

Critical Systems Come First

Major multi-system trauma can present a confusing picture. Assessment is complicated by acute stress reaction and the distractions caused by deformed fractures and pain. It is important to remember that musculoskeletal injuries and lacerations are never, by themselves, life-threatening problems.

The severe bleeding associated with a femur or pelvis fracture is a circulatory system problem. Difficulty breathing in the presence of a rib fracture is a respiratory system problem. Altered mental status with a skull fracture represents a nervous system problem. Your primary assessment and basic life support (BLS) should recognize and treat the critical system problems without being distracted by broken bones, pain, and superficial wounds. Trauma patients do not die of fractures, sprains, strains, and contusions. They die from shock, respiratory failure, and brain injury.

The Golden Hour

The emergency medical services (EMS) subscribe to the golden hour in trauma management as the ideal time within which the patient should access surgical care and stabilization. This is rarely possible in wilderness and offshore situations but speed can still save lives. It is time to move fast if your scene size-up or primary assessment reveals existing or anticipated critical system problems. Multiple-trauma patients need a hospital. In some situations, the secondary assessment will have to wait, perhaps even until the patient is out of the operating room.

Hold the Fluid

Experience in combat medicine from the beginning of the 20th century through the Vietnam War demonstrated that aggressive fluid resuscitation of trauma patients in the field can often be deadly rather than helpful. The intent in giving intravenous (IV) fluid to patients in shock is to maintain perfusion pressure and cellular oxygenation. Unfortunately, higher pressure within the circulatory system can also disrupt clot formation, dilute clotting factors, and exacerbate bleeding.

During more recent conflicts in the Persian Gulf, American medics have been instructed to withhold IV fluid from bleeding casualties who were still producing enough perfusion pressure to maintain A on the AVPU scale. If fluid is deemed necessary it is titrated to maintain peripheral pulses, not necessarily to restore normal blood pressure. Volume is not fully restored until operative control of bleeding is established in the hospital. Fatalities from major battlefield injuries have fallen to 12% from a century-long constant of 22%.

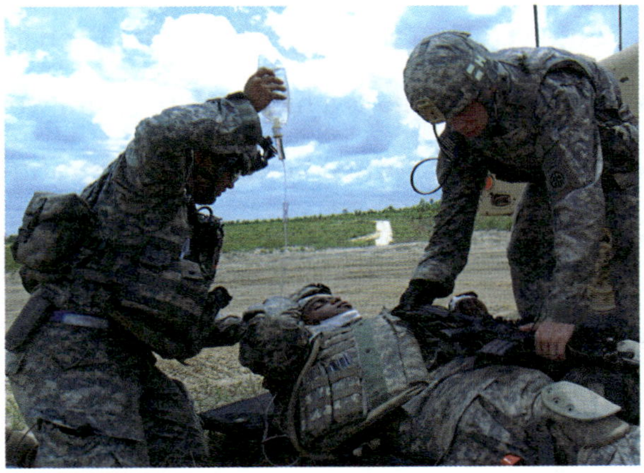

Use caution in trauma; rapid IV fluid administration can exacerbate uncontrolled bleeding and contribute to hypothermia.

The implications for wilderness rescue are clear: for the trauma patient in shock from internal bleeding IV fluid replacement is less of a priority than finding a surgeon and a hospital. If fluid replacement is performed, care should be exercised to avoid diluting blood and clotting factors with IV solutions. Maintaining body core temperature to preserve clotting function, ensuring oxygenation, and evacuating rapidly are more likely to save a life than reading blood pressure and starting an IV.

Chapter 11 Review: General Principles of Trauma

- High-velocity rapid deceleration events are most likely to cause multi-system trauma.
- Low-velocity, high-mass events are likely to cause only local injury.
- Multiple trauma is a high-risk problem worthy of conscientious BLS and evacuation to a hospital.
- Maintaining normal body core temperature is a critical part of BLS for multiple trauma patients.
- Multiple trauma complicated by environmental issues and preexisting problems can be confusing; remember the generic to specific principle, and that critical systems come first.
- Be cautious with fluid resuscitation if bleeding is not controlled.

Chapter 12: Pain Management

Pain has a purpose: to keep us from damaging ourselves. Once the damage is done, however, pain becomes a management problem. It is a natural and appropriate reaction for you to want to relieve someone's suffering, especially if you are the caregiver.

The most effective form of pain relief is to correct the cause. Reduce the dislocation, loosen the splint, drain the abscess, or rehydrate the dried-out hiker with the headache. Secondary swelling can be reduced with elevation and cooling. Unstable injuries are less painful when effectively stabilized. Acute partial-thickness burns are less painful when occlusive dressings are applied. Ask the patient what feels better and help them achieve it.

Sometimes, however, definitive field treatment is not possible or does not completely fix the problem. The pain remains, and you are left to treat the pain as a symptom, being fully aware that the original problem may remain. Nevertheless, pain by itself is not a true emergency.

Pain Medication

Medications for pain come in two basic forms: analgesics and anesthetics. Analgesics work systemically to reduce the production of pain impulses, or the perception of pain by the brain. Anesthetics work by inactivating nerve cells, causing temporary numbness. The two forms are often used concurrently, and both have a place in pain management in the backcountry setting.

Analgesics can be divided into three classes: nonsteroidal anti-inflammatory drugs (NSAIDs), other non-opioid analgesics, and opioids. NSAIDs include such medications as aspirin, ibuprofen, and naproxen sodium. These medications work by inhibiting the action of some of the chemical mediators of inflammation and pain at the site of injury. The result is fewer pain impulses being transmitted from the injury to the brain. The various NSAIDs work in slightly different ways, but all work to reduce pain, fever, and inflammation. Ibuprofen is a good example, and very effective in therapeutic doses of 400–600 mg every 8 hours for an adult.

Pain Medication

Non-steroidal anti-inflammatory drugs:

ibuprofen, naproxen sodium, aspirin, ketorolac...

Non-opioid analgesics:

acetaminophen, paracetamol

Opioids:

morphine, hydrocodone, oxycodone, fentanyl...

Combinations:

Vicodin, Percocet, Vicoprofen, Lortabs...

NSAIDs like ibuprofen do not significantly affect brain function. The patient remains awake and functional, which is a distinct advantage in a hazardous setting. Another advantage is that the best NSAIDs are widely available without prescription. For these reasons, NSAIDs are the first-line medication for the treatment of pain, inflammation, and fever in most backcountry situations. Just be sure to maintain adequate hydration to prevent kidney damage when using NSAIDs.

The primary side effects of NSAIDs include stomach irritation and increased bleeding. These drugs may not be a good choice for someone with nausea from sea sickness, or for a patient where life-threatening bleeding is an anticipated problem. A better non-opioid analgesic for these patients would be acetaminophen (paracetamol). Like NSAIDs, acetaminophen provides good pain relief and fever reduction. Unlike NSAIDs, it tends not to cause stomach upset or increased bleeding. Acetaminophen, however, does not have significant anti-inflammatory effects and will not help reduce swelling or tissue damage caused by inflammation.

Carrying both an NSAID like ibuprofen, and acetaminophen, offers the opportunity to combine the two. The effect is synergistic and is a very good way to manage moderate pain with minimal side effects. The dose can be alternated to keep the blood level of at least one of the medications above therapeutic levels at all times.

Alternating Dose
For Moderate Pain

Time	Dose
1200 hours:	ibuprofen 400mg
1500 hours:	acetaminophen 500mg
1800 hours:	ibuprofen 400mg
2100 hours:	acetaminophen 500mg
0000 hours:	ibuprofen 400mg
0300 hours:	acetaminophen 500 mg

Continue as needed...

Unlike NSAIDS and acetaminophen, opioids relieve pain by reducing the brain's ability to respond to pain impulses from the site of injury. Unfortunately, opioids depress other brain function as well. Side effects include increased reaction time, drowsiness, and depressed respiratory drive. Opioids also reduce gut motility causing constipation and suppress shivering which can make it difficult to maintain body core temperature in cold weather. In some wilderness and rescue situations these side effects may be unacceptable.

Despite these disadvantages opioids are often the best choice for severe pain if the patient can be monitored and protected. In most of the world opioids are controlled substances and should be used only under the guidance of a medical practitioner. This would be a good reason for basic level personnel to call for advanced life support (ALS) help on scene or to meet an evacuation underway.

For backcountry use, opioids are most easily administered orally and usually combined with an NSAIDs or acetaminophen in a single tablet. Vicodin, for example, is a brand name for a combination of hydrocodone and acetaminophen. Vicoprofen is hydrocodone combined with ibuprofen. Percocet is oxycodone combined with acetaminophen. If basic level practitioners are authorized to use opioids in the field, it will likely be this type of medication.

To avoid an overdose be sure that you know what you are dispensing, and what medications your patient is already using. Many cold and flu preparations also contain acetaminophen or an NSAID. To avoid liver damage, do not exceed a total acetaminophen dose of 3000 mg per day for an adult. Many other drugs like alcohol and antihistamines are also respiratory depressants, so beware of the effects when combined with an opioid.

Anesthetics, or "numbing agents" (like lidocaine and bupivacaine), relieve pain by blocking the function of nerve cells. They are injected into joints, fracture sites, and wounds to block the pain of local injury or for doing procedures. Hematoma block (injection into a fracture site) and wound infiltration are relatively safe and easy for trained personnel to perform and can make a big difference in the comfort and effectiveness of treatment. Even topical preparations such as viscous lidocaine or spray benzocaine can be very effective when combined with systemic analgesics to decrease the discomfort of wound debridement and irrigation.

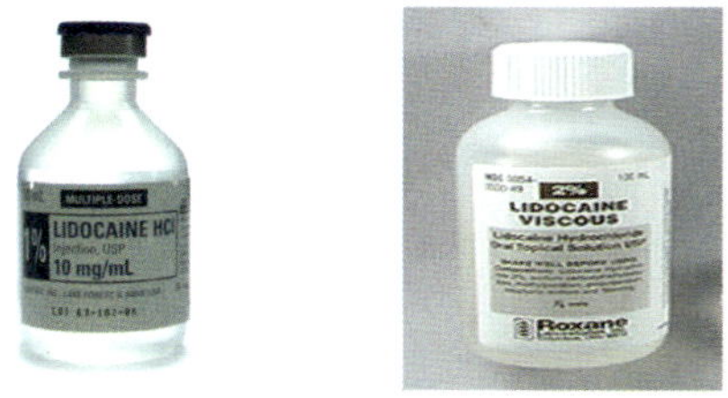

Anesthetics like lidocaine can be injected into wounds to block the pain of exploration and cleaning. Lidocaine is also available in a viscous solution for topical use when injection is not feasible.

Injectible Anesthetics

Injectable Anesthesia:

- lidocaine, bupivacaine, diphenhydramine
- intradermal infiltration
- intraarticular
- digital block
- hematoma block

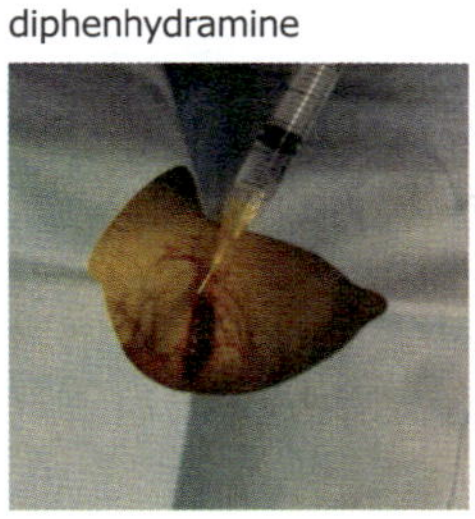

Ketamine is another anesthetic that may be used by advance practitioners in the field. It is systemic rather than local, and can be given orally or by intramuscular or IV injection. At lower dosages it is a good pain reliever when used alone, and even better when combined with a low dose of an opioid.

A separate class of drugs worthy of mention for pain management is benzodiazepines, such as diazepam and lorazepam. These are anxiolytics (anti-anxiety), not analgesics, but can substantially enhance the pain-relieving effect of opioids and NSAIDs. An opioid at the lower end of its dose range combined with a low dose of benzodiazepine may have a better effect than a larger dose of either drug alone.

In a well-controlled setting, opioids, benzodiazepines, and ketamine are typically administered by injection. Some of these can also be given by intranasal atomizer, as can the opioid antagonist (antidote) naloxone. Use of these medications and routes is generally restricted to advanced level providers.

As any practitioner using these medications should be aware, opioids and benzodiazepines are central nervous system depressants and can depress respiration, mental status, and level of consciousness. When used in combination, the effects are cumulative. Care must be taken to use the lowest effective dose and to monitor the patient carefully.

Risk Versus Benefit

The goal of pain management in the wilderness and rescue setting is an awake patient with tolerable pain. When using opioids and benzodiazepines, titrate the dose gradually to achieve the desired effect. Avoid the temptation or pressure to give a large dose initially or to increase the dose quickly. Putting your patient to sleep will run the risk of respiratory depression, aspiration, airway obstruction, and the development of ischemia or other problems that may go undetected.

An awake patient will tell you when the leg goes numb or the splint is beginning to cause an abrasion. An awake patient will provide feedback on the success or failure of your treatment. An awake patient, even with analgesics on board, will not hurt themself by overusing an injured body part.

This reassurance, however, does not extend to local anesthetic agents. These medications can eliminate pain perception, even if the patient is wide awake. Injecting a joint with lidocaine, for example, can allow the patient to cause significant self-inflicted injury without feeling anything. A patient given anesthetic eye drops could tear or abrade the cornea just by rubbing the eye without the benefit of painful feedback.

The use of injected and ophthalmic anesthetics should include a plan for minimizing these risks, such as not allowing a patient to return to normal activity until the anesthetic has worn off.

Dispensing or administering any medication carries considerable responsibility, requires informed patient consent, and usually requires legal authorization. The medical officer should know the legal implications, indications, contraindications, precautions, dosage, route, side effects, and drug interactions of any medication carried. Practitioners typically get to know the medications they frequently administer or prescribe. When an unfamiliar medication is considered, they look it up. Basic level practitioners should do the same, even if the medications are common nonprescription types.

Chapter 12 Review:
Pain Management

- Pain is both a symptom of a problem and a problem to be treated.
- Pain management includes treating the cause of the pain and reducing the perception of pain with the use of medication.
- Medications commonly used in pain management include analgesics and anesthetics.
- Analgesic classes include NSAIDs like ibuprofen, non-opioid analgesics like acetaminophen, and opioids like morphine.
- Benzodiazepines like lorazepam may be used as adjuncts.
- Anesthetics like lidocaine inactivate nerve cells, causing temporary numbness.
- The goal of pain management in the wilderness and rescue setting is an awake patient with tolerable pain.
- Most pain can be managed with NSAIDs or acetaminophen. More severe pain may require the addition of opioids and benzodiazepines. Localized or procedural pain may be managed with anesthetics.
- The risks associated with opioid and benzodiazepine use include excessive sedation with respiratory depression, airway obstruction, aspiration, and undetected ischemia.
- The risks associated with the use of anesthetics include self-inflicted injury due to loss of pain feedback.
- Practitioners should know the legal implications, indications, contraindications, precautions, dosage, route, side effects, and interactions of any medication carried.

The goal of pain management in the wilderness and rescue setting is an awake patient with tolerable pain.

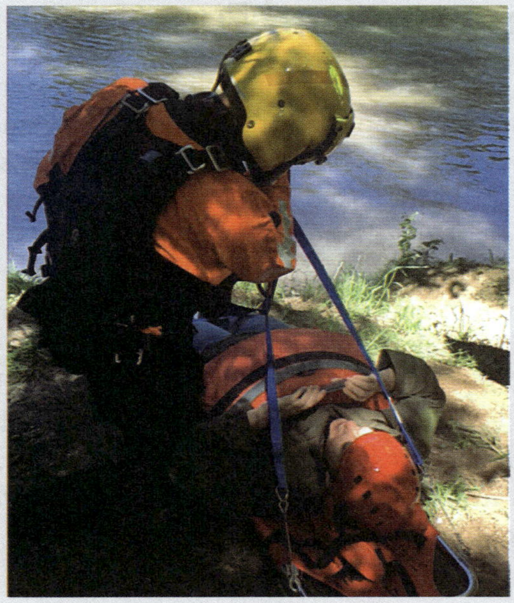

Chapter 13: Musculoskeletal Injury

Like most backcountry medical problems, musculoskeletal injuries are more often a logistical dilemma than any kind of emergency. It is the potential for serious associated circulatory, respiratory, and nervous system problems that should demand your immediate attention. If your scene size-up and primary assessment reveal no existing or anticipated critical system problems, you have the luxury of time to perform a secondary assessment to find and catalog the not so serious bumps, bruises, and breaks. You can develop a problem list and plan, and safely evacuate your patient to medical care hours or days later.

Structure and Function

The structure of the musculoskeletal system is composed of bone, cartilage, tendon, ligament, muscle, and synovial fluid. Its function is support, protection, and mobility. The problems can be described generically as stable injury, unstable injury, and associated neurovascular injury.

Bone provides structural support and protection for soft tissue, and leverage for mobility. It is living tissue with a rich blood supply and an overlying membrane called the periosteum, which is abundantly supplied with sensory nerves. As with any other tissue, bones bleed and hurt when injured.

Bones meet at joints and are held together by ligaments. Some joints are highly mobile and some do not move much. Cartilage provides the smooth surface and padding for bones to slide or pivot against each other. The synovial fluid contained inside the ligamentous joint capsule lubricates the surfaces.

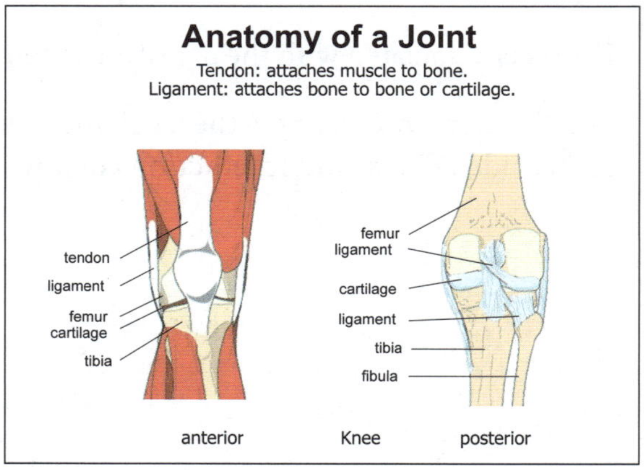

Tendons are cord-like connective tissue that join muscle to bone, crossing joints in the cable and pulley system that effects movement. The muscle tissue itself is encased in connective tissue compartments called fascia. This structure in cross section is well illustrated by a typical rib-eye steak: the muscle is the steak's soft red tissue, and the fascia is the tough white gristle that you don't eat.

Because muscle contraction is active and elongation is strictly passive, muscle groups must work in balanced opposition. One group is responsible for pulling a bone one direction, and the opposite group is responsible for pulling the bone back. For example, the contraction of your biceps flexes your elbow and the contraction of your triceps extends it. Balanced opposition is an important concept to remember when splinting an injured joint or reducing a dislocation.

There are many types of bones and joints, and many forms of injury. The mechanism can be direct or indirect force, overuse, infection, or even frostbite. Chronic conditions such as arthritis also affect structure and function. Knowing all types of injury in detail is interesting, but not required for effective field treatment.

The medical practitioner's primary concern is whether an injured bone or joint can still safely perform its function or must be stabilized and protected. This explains our generic and very practical assessment for the wilderness context: stable or unstable.

When the structure and function of the system are compromised, surrounding soft tissue is also at risk. Of primary concern in extremity injuries are the arteries, veins, and peripheral nerves that run adjacent to bones and joints. They tend to be grouped in a neurovascular bundle, much the way electrical wires and plumbing are fixed together as they run through a ship. These unprotected structures can be damaged during the initial injury or pinched by misalignment or swelling after the injury.

Neurovascular Bundle

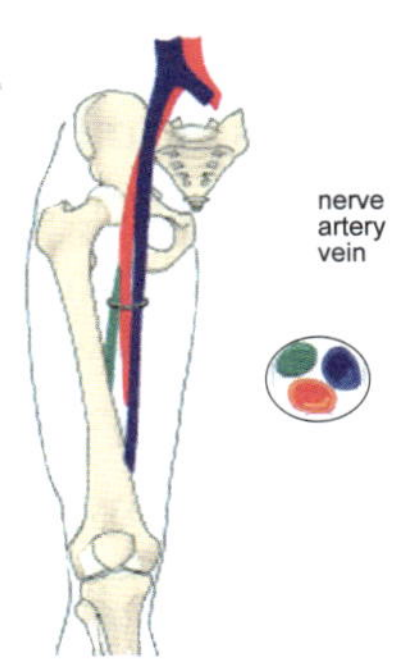

Structure:
- Peripheral nerves
- Blood vessels

Function:
- Motor/sensory function
- Perfusion and oxygenation

Problem:
- Ischemia
- Bleeding

Unstable Injury

Fractures, sprains, strains, and dislocations in extremities can be caused by a variety of mechanisms reflecting the different ways force can be applied to bones and joints. The injury may be caused by leverage, twisting, direct impact, or a piece of bone being pulled away at the site of attachment of a tendon or ligament.

High-velocity injuries, dissipating tremendous kinetic energy in a short period of time, tend to cause ligament and tendon rupture and bone fractures. Low-velocity injuries are more prone to cause partial tears of ligament and tendon and are less likely to fracture bones. For field purposes, defining the mechanism of injury can be generalized to a yes-or-no question: Was there sufficient force to cause a fracture or to rupture a ligament or tendon?

Unstable Injury

Specific signs and symptoms:
- Deformity, crepitus, instability on exam
- Impaired circulation (ischemia)
- Inability to use, feels unstable.

Non-specific signs and symptoms:
- Pain, tenderness
- Swelling
- Bruising
- Pain out of proportion to the apparent injury

The signs and symptoms of an unstable musculoskeletal injury are sometimes obvious. Deformity, crepitus, and instability on exam make the assessment rather clear. Also, the patient may report the instability by telling you that their knee gives out every time they try to walk. These criteria are very specific and indicate an injury that is unstable.

Sometimes you will have to rely on nonspecific signs and symptoms. Rapid swelling, for example, indicates significant bleeding at the injury site. The inability to use a joint or extremity after trauma indicates a more serious injury. Impairment of circulation, sensation, and movement (CSM) distal to the injury implies damage to the neurovascular bundle. The patient may report a snap or pop at the time of injury. Although these nonspecific criteria are less definitive, you might choose to treat the injury as unstable pending more information or response to treatment.

Ischemia

Mechanisms:

- Deformity
- Swelling (compartment syndrome)
- Tight splints, boots, jewelry
- Vasoconstriction from cold exposure
- Tight litter straps, pressure points

Low Risk — High Risk

It is worth noting that the amount of pain is not a reliable indicator of the severity of the injury. For example, a minor grade I ligament sprain will hurt much more than an unstable grade III ligament rupture. The primary pain receptors in ligaments are stretch receptors. Because the ruptured ligament is no longer being stretched, pain is minimal. The primary complaint is often instability rather than discomfort.

Manipulation or use of extremities with fractured bones and loose or dislocated joints can cause further damage to surrounding soft tissue like the organs, muscles, and neurovascular bundle. This potential for damage is especially important to evaluate whenever the associated soft tissue is part of a critical system, such as the spinal cord running through damaged vertebrae, or the femoral artery lying adjacent to a fractured femur.

Assessment for neurovascular bundle injury involves checking distal CSM. Problems with circulation are found by observing for signs of ischemia such as cool and pale skin or a weak or absent pulse in the distal extremity. Problems with sensation are usually reported by the patient as numbness and tingling. Because nervous system tissue is exquisitely sensitive to oxygen deprivation, these are usually the first symptoms noted. The examiner can further evaluate the problem by checking the patient's ability to distinguish sharp from dull touch on the distal extremity. Often sharp and dull sensation is fully intact even with the complaint of numbness and tingling. Ultimately, ischemic injuries can become very painful, with loss of motor control developing later in the process.

Extremity tissue can usually survive up to two hours of ischemia with minimal damage. Beyond this, the risk of tissue death and permanent damage increases quickly with time. Ischemia also increases the risk of frostbite in freezing weather and makes infection more likely in open wounds. If your treatment efforts do not succeed in restoring CSM, you have a limb-threatening emergency. Immediate evacuation is indicated if conditions permit.

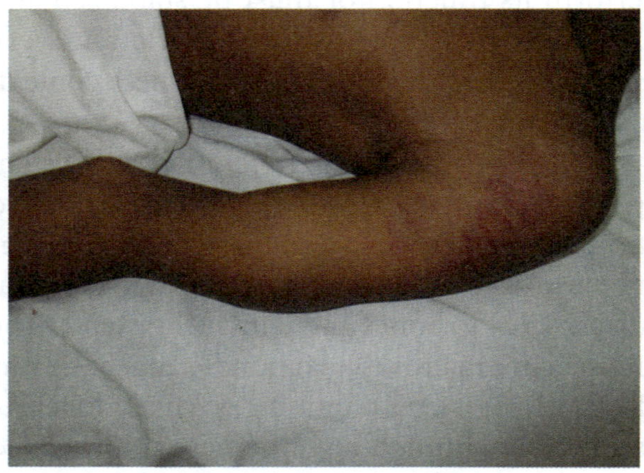

Before you begin, check and document the status of the neurovascular bundle (check CSM). You will want to know that your treatment has improved the situation, or at least not made it worse. Most of the time, CSM will remain normal throughout the process.

Sometimes, an extremity feels numb or cold immediately following trauma, especially if a fracture or dislocation results in deformity, pain, and acute stress reaction. Your treatment should result in a significant improvement in CSM status as circulation is restored. Beware, however, that distal CSM may become impaired later as swelling develops under a splint or bandage. Detecting and correcting ischemia is an important function of continued care throughout your treatment and evacuation.

Traction into Position

Injured bones and joints, and the soft tissues around them, are much more comfortable and much less likely to be damaged further and cause ischemia if splinted in normal anatomic position. Although many injured extremities remain in good position or return there spontaneously, some will require manual realignment. Like everything else we do, the fundamental goal is the preservation of oxygenation and perfusion.

To restore anatomic position, the first step is to apply traction. This separates bone ends and reduces pain. Then, while traction is maintained, position is restored. Shaft fractures of long bones are returned to the "in-line" position so that the effect of opposing muscles is most balanced, and the neurovascular bundle is least likely to be compressed.

Unstable Injury
Long Bones

Treatment:

1. Check Circulation
2. Gentle Traction into Position
3. Hand Stable
4. Splint Stable
5. Re-check Circulation

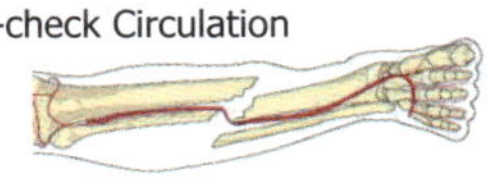

TIP →

"Your patient will be reassured to hear that traction into position is intended to be a slow and gentle process."

The amount of force necessary depends on the structure being realigned. Forearm and lower leg fractures usually require only gentle traction. Femur fractures, with the large surrounding muscle mass, may require significant traction to restore alignment. Deformed wrist fractures may also require significant traction and manipulation because the bone ends tend to lock against each other.

Open shaft fractures with bone ends protruding through the skin are still managed with traction and repositioning following thorough cleaning of the exposed bone ends and surrounding skin (see the chapter on soft-tissue injury). Be aware that the bone may not slide easily back under the skin with traction alone. To keep skin from becoming trapped under the bone as you realign the fracture, you may have to pull it free with forceps or a gloved finger as the bone is manipulated back into the wound.

Injured joints without dislocation usually do not need to be repositioned. If the patient is conscious and mobile, they will have already found the most comfortable position for the injured joint. If not, stabilize it in place unless there is impaired CSM or the position prevents safe packaging. If manipulation is necessary, move toward the mid-range of the joints normal motion.

Unstable Injury
Joints

Treatment:

Splint in position found unless

- Persistent ischemia (photo)
- Position or pain impedes effective splinting or evacuation
- Simple dislocation of shoulder, patella, digits in wilderness context (dislocation protocol)

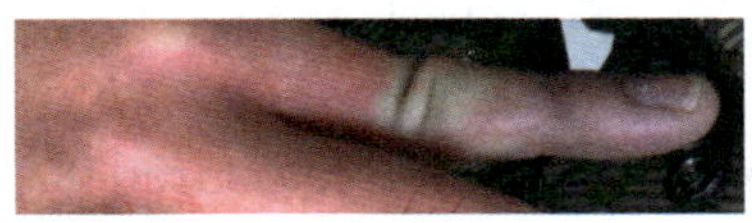

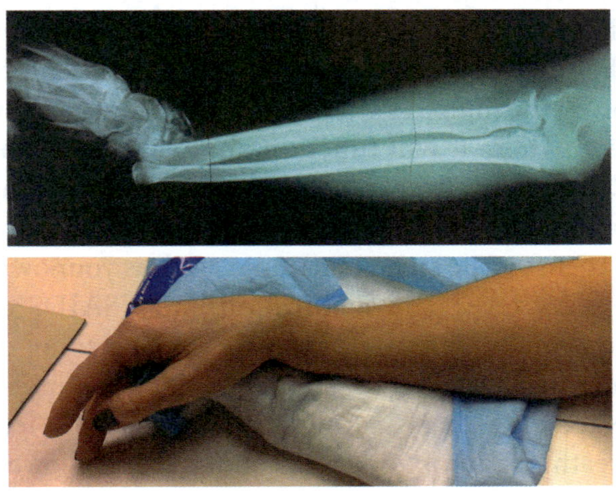

Complex joint injuries like this fracture dislocation of the wrist are manipulated in the field only when necessary to restore perfusion or enable a safe evacuation.

In joint dislocations, there is likely to be some loss of CSM distal to the injury. Under these conditions, traction and repositioning are used until circulation is reestablished. In specific cases, covered in the Simple Dislocations chapter, repositioning can be used to completely reduce dislocations of the shoulder, digits, and patella with a significant improvement in comfort and circulation. The use of traction on more complex dislocations, such as the elbow, wrist, or ankle, is indicated only for restoration and preservation of perfusion.

Spine injuries are also realigned by considering the stacked vertebrae of the spine to be a single long bone with a joint at the pelvis and the skull. However, traction should not be used. Spine alignment and protection are discussed in more detail in the spine injury chapter.

Traction and repositioning is a safe procedure if done properly, but it is not pain free. To be successful at reducing pain and restoring position, it is critical to have the cooperation and confidence of the injured person. Muscle groups in spasm, or a patient fighting your efforts, will vastly complicate the procedure. If possible, realignment should be accomplished as soon after the accident as possible.

Your patient will be reassured to hear that repositioning is intended to be a slow and gentle process. It will also help to let the patient know that they are in control, and that you will stop the process if asked. Explain that you intend to bring the injured extremity into the normal position where it will function and feel better. The therapeutic effect of a calm voice and reassuring manner is truly amazing. What this treats is the patient's acute stress reaction, as well as your own.

Basic level pain medication like NSAIDS or acetaminophen, or sedatives such as alcohol or marijuana, can be a valuable adjunct if the anticipated side effects can be safely managed. Field treatment, combining reassurance with the lowest effective dose of medication, can offer less risk with equal benefit.

Advanced practitioners are reminded that it can be dangerous to use opioids, anxiolytics, or general anesthetics in the backcountry setting at the dosage necessary to completely relax a scared and uncomfortable patient. Make your patient feel better but keep them awake. That way, you won't have to worry about airway compromise, inadequate ventilation, or doing a lot of damage without hearing about it.

Occasionally it will be impossible to restore position comfortably and safely. You should discontinue traction and stabilize the injury in the position found if traction causes a significant increase in pain or resistance. These rare situations represent a limb-threatening emergency if deformity is significant or ischemia is detected.

Hand Stabilization

Once you have repositioned an extremity injury, stability must be maintained until the splint can take over. This may mean having someone hold gentle traction on the extremity while you prepare for splinting. If you are alone, you can use snow, rocks, or pieces of equipment to hold the limb in place.

This simple step may seem blindingly obvious, but you do need to plan for it. You may find yourself holding stabilization on a beautifully realigned wrist only to find your first aid kit and splint just out of reach. Think ahead; this is an entirely avoidable personal embarrassment. Whether you use a commercially manufactured product, or something improvised from your equipment, a splint should be complete, comfortable, and compact.

Splint Stabilization

Complete. Long bones should be splinted in the in-line position, and the ideal splint should immobilize the injured bone as well as the joint above and below the injury. To splint a lower leg fracture effectively, the ankle and knee should be immobilized. Joint injuries are splinted in the mid-range position, including the bones above and below the injury. To splint the elbow, for example, the forearm and upper arm are included in the splint.

For splinting purposes, the stacked vertebrae of the spine may be viewed as a long bone with joints at the pelvis and base of the skull. Splinting an unstable spine injury would require stabilizing the pelvis, shoulders, and head. Unstable pelvis injuries require stabilization of the spine and femur. Femur fractures require stabilization of the pelvis and knee. For these spine, pelvis, and femur injuries, the ideal treatment is whole-body stabilization in a litter or vacuum mattress.

Comfortable. Splints should be well-padded, strong, and snug. There should be minimal movement of the injured bones and no pressure points or loose spots. A splint should allow you to monitor distal CSM and should be easily adjustable if ischemia or pain develops. A good splint decreases pain and preserves CSM; attention to this principle is critical to prevent pressure sores and infection during long-term care and transport.

Compact. For wilderness use, a splint should be no larger or more complex than necessary. It should not inhibit the evacuation you have in mind. A simple sling and swathe, for example, splints everything from the clavicle to the elbow. This simple structure can be created with a safety pin and the patient's shirt. No additional material is necessary.

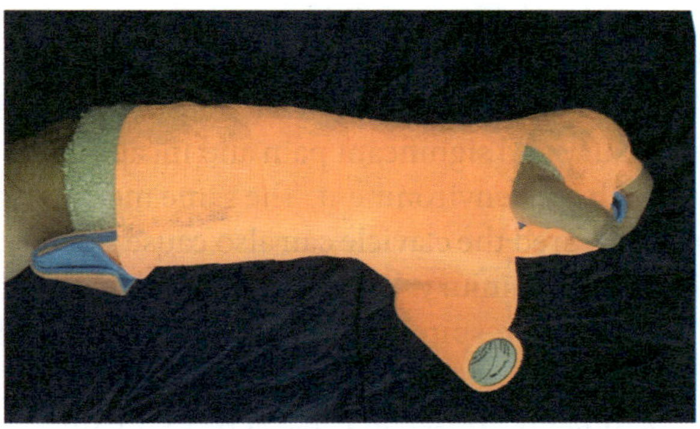

A wrist splint of malleable aluminum secured with vet wrap; complete, comfortable, and compact in the position of comfort.

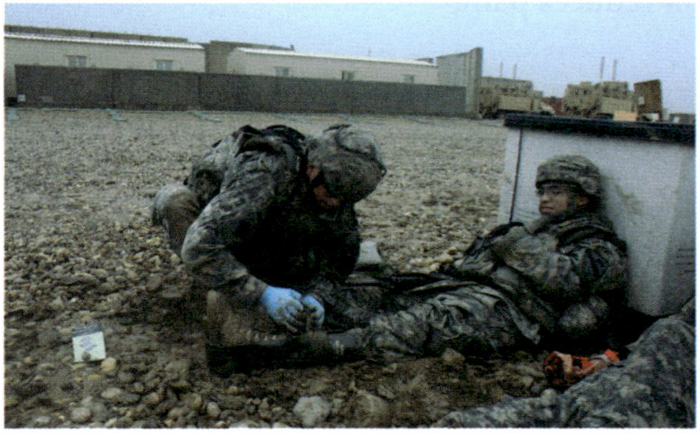

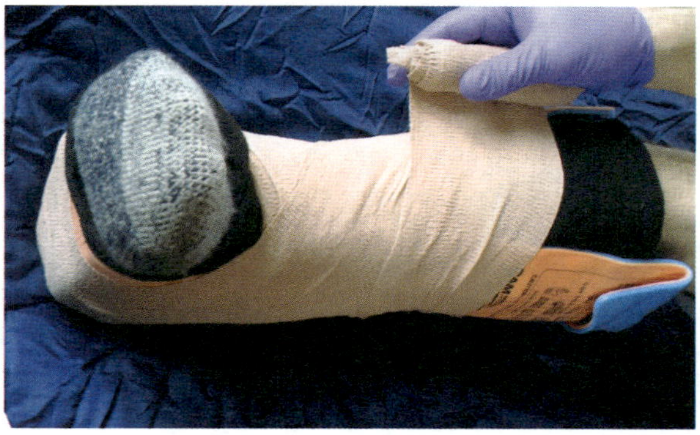

A quick splinting job is OK for extrication from a dangerous spot, but it needs to be fitted and padded later for long term use.

Once an injury is stabilized, the most important anticipated problem for long-term care becomes distal ischemia caused by compression of the neurovascular bundle as swelling develops inside splints or bandages. Treatment should include medication, rest, and elevation to reduce swelling and pressure. This is essentially the same as the generic treatment for stable injuries. If distal CSM remains normal or continues to improve, you can take your time planning a safe and comfortable evacuation.

Special Wilderness Considerations

Femur Fracture

Shock and distal ischemia are anticipated problems due to the proximity of the neurovascular bundle to the femoral shaft. The usual treatment for a femoral shaft fracture in the EMS setting has been the application of a traction splint and rapid evacuation to a hospital. This may be appropriate for short-term care, but the risks outweigh the benefits in long or difficult evacuations.

In many backcountry situations, it can be impossible to distinguish a femoral shaft fracture from a femoral neck or pelvis fracture that might be further deformed by the application of traction. Even when properly applied, traction splints are notoriously difficult to monitor and package.

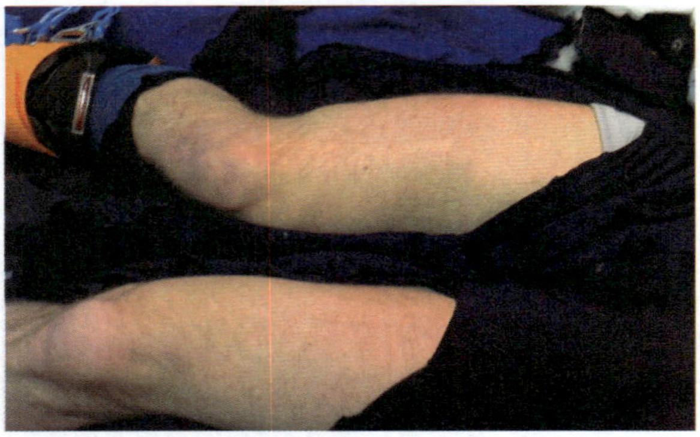

Traction into Position should be used to restore alignment and reduce soft tissue injury in this femur fracture.

When the recommended amount of traction is applied with a traction splint, the pressure at the anchor points will inevitably cause skin and soft tissue ischemia. For these reasons, the use of a traction splint is not appropriate for backcountry rescue or long-term care. In this setting femur fractures are best stabilized in a well-padded litter or vacuum mattress. Many EMS and ski patrol systems have adopted this practice as well.

Pelvic Fracture

Shock and distal ischemia are anticipated problems due to the proximity of the iliac arteries and veins. The assessment is made by feeling pelvic instability as motion or crepitus on gentle exam, or by noting obvious deformity. There is the potential for catastrophic internal bleeding, so the patient should be handled gently and the exam should not be repeated.

Pelvic binding with a padded strap or wide compression bandage may be useful to help stabilize a pelvic fracture and reduce the space available for internal blood loss. This can be accomplished by wrapping a tarp or backpack hip belt around the pelvis and tightening gently to restore anatomy. The patient is then further stabilized by a litter, vacuum mattress, or well-padded backboard. Emergency evacuation is indicated with the anticipated problem of volume shock.

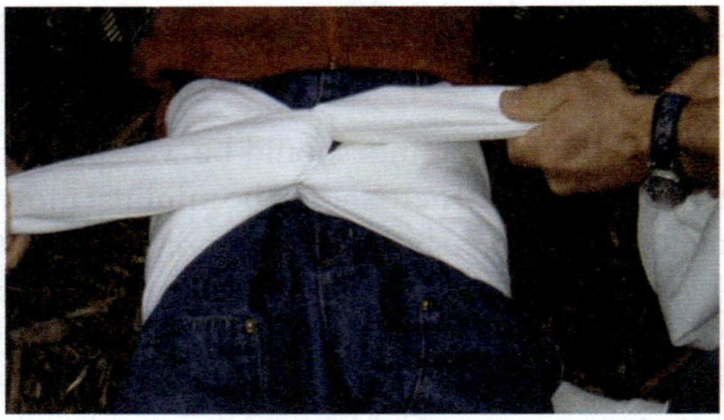

Effective pelvic binding can be accomplished by wrapping a tarp, sheet, tent fly or backpack hip belt around the pelvis and tightening gently to restore anatomy and reduce pain and instability.

Clavicle Fracture

We mention this here because the clavicle is the most frequently fractured bone in childhood, right up to about age 70. If your work or play involves falls at speed you will probably experience or see one eventually.

As with other bones, it is not the fracture itself that presents much of a problem. We worry more about the possibility of associated respiratory system injury and significant pain and incapacitation in a high-risk environment. The same mechanism that fractured the clavicle can also cause fractured ribs and lung injury. Your primary survey should focus on the respiratory system, not the clavicle or the pain.

Fortunately, most clavicle fractures are uncomplicated. They hurt, sometimes a lot, and the patient may feel the bone ends grinding together with movement of the arm or torso. Use a sling if it reduces pain.

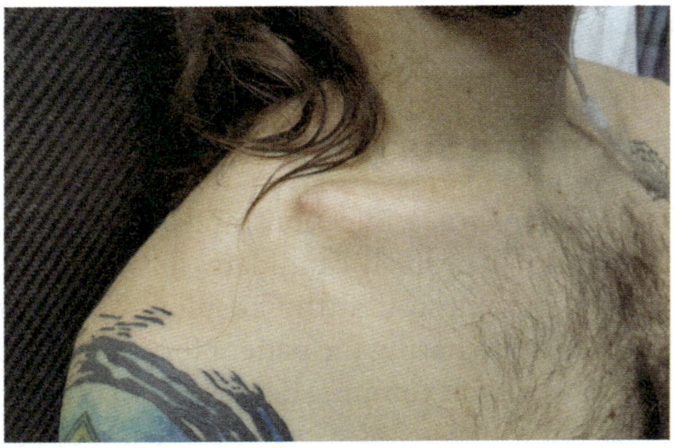

Tenting or trapping of the skin by clavicle fragments can cause problems with ischemia. Prolonged deformity can result in skin breakdown if not corrected.

In rare cases, a clavicle fracture will be complicated by tenting or trapping of the skin by fracture fragments causing skin ischemia. While this is not a critical system problem it will result in infarction and skin breakdown if not corrected. Usually the problem can be relieved by the patient changing position, moving the arm, or the rescuer pressing the fragments into better position. If the ischemia cannot be relieved, early surgical intervention is ideal. In the absence of a serious respiratory or circulatory problem, there is no emergency and the patient remains ambulatory and otherwise functional.

Compartment Syndrome

Swelling due to bleeding or edema inside a muscle compartment can increase intra-compartment pressure to the point that perfusion is impaired. The mechanism is usually blunt trauma or collateral damage from a fracture. It is also possible to see compartment syndrome develop from repetitive motion injury. Ischemia develops, with necrosis of muscle and nerve tissue as the anticipated problem. Typical symptoms include severe pain out of proportion to the apparent injury, distal numbness, and pain on passive stretching of the affected muscle group.

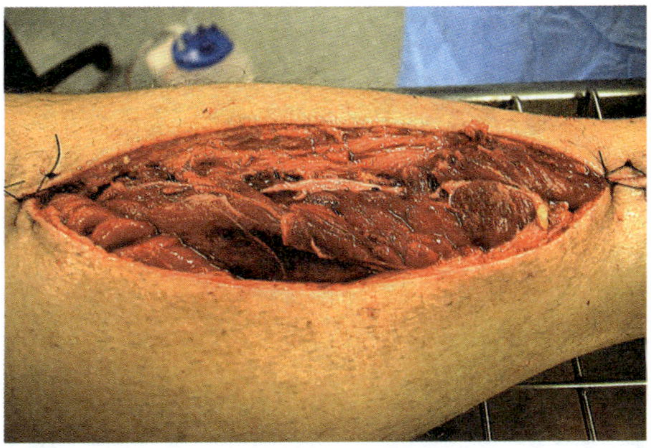

This fasciotomy was performed to relieve pressure and restore perfusion to muscle tissue affected by compartment syndrome. This is not a field procedure. It is shown here to better illustrate the problem.

With the right training and equipment, it is possible to measure intracompartmental pressures and this is sometimes performed in the hospital. However, it is more often the same signs and symptoms seen in the field that motivates an urgent trip to the operating room; pain out of proportion, pain on passive motion, and distal numbness. The compartment is decompressed (fasciotomy) to relieve the pressure and allow blood to flow into the injured muscle.

Compartment syndrome can develop hours to days after the initial injury. Field treatment includes anti-inflammatory medication, rest, elevation, and cooling of the extremity. Emergency evacuation is indicated if immediate improvement is not noted. A field fasciotomy would be a high-risk procedure, and become a significant wound management challenge.

Open Fracture

In an open fracture, the site is exposed to the outside environment through a wound in the skin. This opening can be produced from inside by sharp bone ends, or from outside by the same object that caused the fracture (such as a bullet). Unfortunately, this adds serious infection to the anticipated problem list.

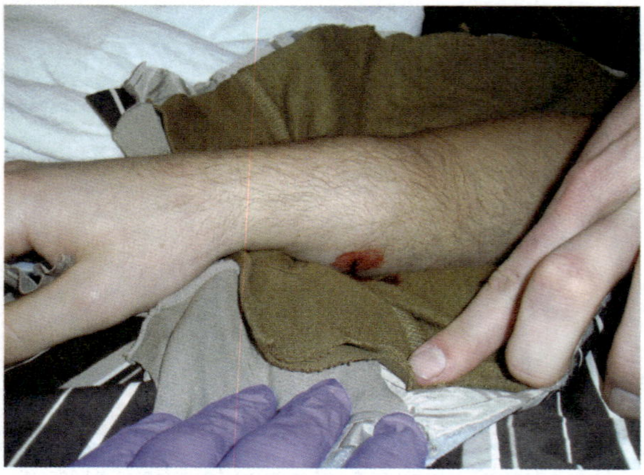

An open fracture is a high-risk problem that can be hidden by layers of clothing.

Aggressive debridement (removal of foreign material and dead tissue) and irrigation with clean water are necessary before bone ends are pulled under the skin. The early use of prophylactic antibiotics should be considered as part of the ideal field treatment. In cases such as crush injuries where bones remain exposed, moist dressings over the wound will help preserve tissue. Urgent evacuation is indicated.

Open Fracture
Wilderness Perspective

- A' is ischemia, bleeding, infection, and systemic infection.
- Free skin entrapments.
- Aggressive irrigation and debridement.
- Immediate treatment with antibiotics.
- Evac for surgical debridement.

Low Risk — High Risk

Joint Infection

The symptoms of joint infection (also called septic arthritis) include swelling, redness, pain, and warmth. The patient may develop a fever. Joint infection usually develops shortly after a laceration or puncture wound that penetrates the joint space, but it may develop after a minor abrasion or without any skin defect being visible. These infections have the potential to become systemic, and result in life-threatening vascular shock.

Impending Surgery

Deformed fractures, infections, and compartment syndrome will be likely candidates for immediate surgery upon arrival at the hospital. The anesthesiologist preparing the patient for surgery will anticipate patient vomiting because it is a problem associated with general anesthesia and intubation. For that reason, EMS personnel in the ambulance context do not give any fluids, food, or medications by mouth to such patients. This is referred to as keeping the patient NPO, an abbreviation for the Latin nil per os. Intravenous (IV) fluids and IV or intramuscular (IM) medications are used instead.

However, during a long evacuation in the backcountry, priority must be given to maintaining hydration, perfusion, and body core temperature. Fluid replacement by IV line is ideal, but oral intake of fluids will be necessary if the IV route is not available or is impractical. Food is important in maintaining calories for heat production. You can help the anesthesiologist by giving your patient easily digested and absorbed simple sugars and carbohydrates and avoiding protein and fat when possible. NPO is not an option in most prolonged evacuations.

Stable Injury

Stable musculoskeletal injuries have none of the specific signs and symptoms associated with instability. Often, the patient will be able to move, use, or bear weight with the extremity within a short time after injury, and there will be no history of instability. Any swelling will develop slowly over several hours. You will find no deformity, crepitus on movement, or instability on exam.

Treatment is designed to reduce and control swelling and pain and includes using anti-inflammatory medication as well as rest, ice if available, compression, and elevation (RICE). Because a stable injury is safe to use within the limits of discomfort and the patient is allowed pain-free activity; anything that does not increase pain is OK.

Elevation and rest are the most effective elements of RICE and most useful early on when the swelling is likely to be the worst. Ice can also be helpful if it is available, but not so much that it is worth carrying chemical cold packs in a backcountry medical kit.

Compression of an injured extremity with an elastic bandage is intended to limit the space available for swelling or to force accumulated fluid out of the extracellular space. Sometimes this is helpful, but it can also contribute to compartment syndrome and increase swelling of the distal extremity. Compression bandages may also be employed to provide some support to a sore joint. Frequent monitoring of the distal CSM is important when using a compression bandage.

Medication such as ibuprofen or acetaminophen can help reduce discomfort. A regular dose over several days will raise an appreciable level of the drug in the body and will work better than just taking it occasionally in response to pain. Because NSAIDS like ibuprofen inhibit blood clotting and increase swelling from bleeding, acetaminophen may be preferred in the immediate post-injury period.

Pain-free activity is allowed after the first 24 hours, or when most of the pain and swelling has resolved. The patient may perform whatever activity is possible if pain is not increased. This may include skiing, or it may require very limited use around camp for several days.

Stable Injuries

S/Sx:

- No deformity, no instability on exam
- No sense of instability reported by patient
- Able to move and bear weight after accident
- Distal circulation intact
- Slow onset of swelling
- Pain proportional to apparent injury

Low Risk — High Risk

Stable Injuries

Treatment:

- Rest, ice, compression, elevation
- Pain-free activity
- Splint or sling for comfort
- NSAIDs for pain and swelling
- Monitor circulation
- Follow-up as needed

Following these treatment guidelines, all stable injuries should show steady improvement. If not, your patient is being too active, or your assessment may be wrong. It is possible to have a stable injury with a small fracture causing prolonged discomfort. Medical follow-up is indicated if rapid improvement is not noted or if symptoms persist at the end of the trip.

Overuse Syndromes

Bursitis, tendonitis, and traumatic arthritis can be symptoms of overuse. These injuries develop over time without an obvious precipitating traumatic event other than repetitive motion. A long hike or bike ride can bring on pain and near-complete disability. You should be able to rule out unstable injury by history, but that may not make the patient any more functional.

You will note pain, swelling, and sometimes redness over an inflamed muscle, tendon, or joint structure. Moving it will hurt, and you may be able to feel crepitus as a damaged tendon slides roughly through an irritated tendon sheath. Resting it will bring relief. These symptoms are typical of all kinds of repetitive motion injury. Bikers get it in the knee, hikers in the foot, and rowers in the wrists.

To treat an overuse syndrome effectively, you must break the cycle of injury and inflammation. Treatment includes RICE and anti-inflammatory medication. If travel is required, functional splinting for support and mobility will be necessary. As pain subsides, remove the splint two or three times a day and do gentle exercises, taking the part through its normal range of motion as pain allows. Apply heat after the initial inflammation has settled down. Use warm soaks four times a day for 15 minutes at a time. This is good to do just before range of motion exercises.

Overuse Syndromes

S/Sx:

- MOI is repetitive motion, not isolated event
- Pain, swelling, tendon or joint crepitis
- Exacerbated by use, relieved by rest

Treatment:

- RICE
- NSAIDs
- Functional splinting
- Modify activity

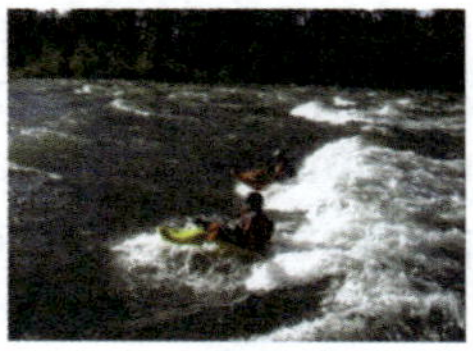

Change the way your patient performs the repetitive motion. This will put the stress on different muscle/tendon groups. For example, using a short loop of webbing as a handle on a kayak paddle can allow the paddler to pull with the wrist held vertically instead of horizontally. This may not be ideal, but it may allow the group to continue its travel.

The patient should take the maximum dose of anti-inflammatory medication if tolerated, at least for a short time. For ibuprofen, this is 2400–3200 mg a day. Gastrointestinal and kidney problems can be minimized by taking these drugs with ample water and food. The stomach may allow a couple of days of this, which can suppress the inflammation enough to prevent complete disability. Reduce the dose as soon as improvement is noted.

Using tape and padding, you can create a soft splint that will help reduce the stress on the irritated structure. Joint taping is another technique for providing support and limited mobility. Encourage the patient to rest frequently, letting pain be the signal to stop. Continue only after the pain is under control.

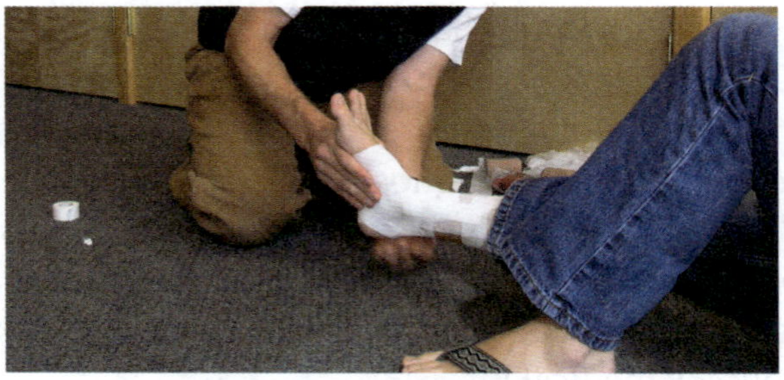

Joint tape can provide support, reduce pain, and improve mobility. This can be useful for the ankle and the wrist where continued use of the extremity is necessary for travel and survival.

Risk Versus Benefit

Traction into Position to restore alignment in significantly deformed fractures and dislocations can be painful for the patient and intimidating for a practitioner inexperienced in the procedure. It is worth remembering that significant deformity represents a high risk of ischemia to infarction and increased bleeding and tissue damage. It is also more painful and difficult to stabilize and evacuate safely. Gentle repositioning is a low-risk procedure for a high-risk problem.

Procedures that seem to cause intolerable pain or require a lot of force are more dangerous. When you meet significant resistance, you should stop and reassess. Wait a few minutes or modify the technique and try again. If you are still unsuccessful, consider the persistent deformity and severe pain to indicate a high-risk problem and the need for evacuation.

Even stable injuries, with continued use, run the risk of becoming worse. This must be balanced against the benefit of continued mobility and self-sufficiency. Moderating activity with splinting or wrapping to minimize the increase in pain and swelling is a reasonable goal for early treatment in a difficult situation.

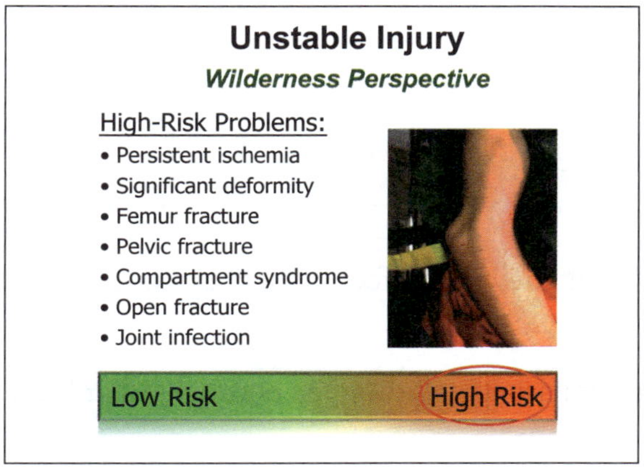

Splints and wraps are applied where necessary to reduce the risk of further soft-tissue trauma in unstable musculoskeletal injury. At the same time, they can create an increased threat to the patient's safety and survival. A sling and swathe, for example, can inhibit a skier's ability to negotiate a cliff band safely. Backboard or litter stabilization can drown a patient on an overturned boat. Sometimes the benefit of a stabilized injury does not match the overall risk to the patient and the plan must be modified.

Chapter 13 Review: Musculoskeletal Injury

- Musculoskeletal injuries alone are not emergencies, but they can affect critical system function, causing ischemia, respiratory distress, and shock.
- Unstable injuries present risk of injury to surrounding soft tissue, including the neurovascular bundle, and should be protected and stabilized.
- Deformed long bone fractures should be restored to normal alignment using Traction into Position.
- Open fracture represents a high risk for serious infection.
- Unstable joint injuries should be splinted as found unless circulation is impaired, or the position will inhibit safe evacuation.
- Splints, if needed, should be complete, comfortable, and compact.
- Stable injuries are safe to use and move within the limits of pain-free activity.
- High-risk musculoskeletal injury should be evacuated to definitive medical care.

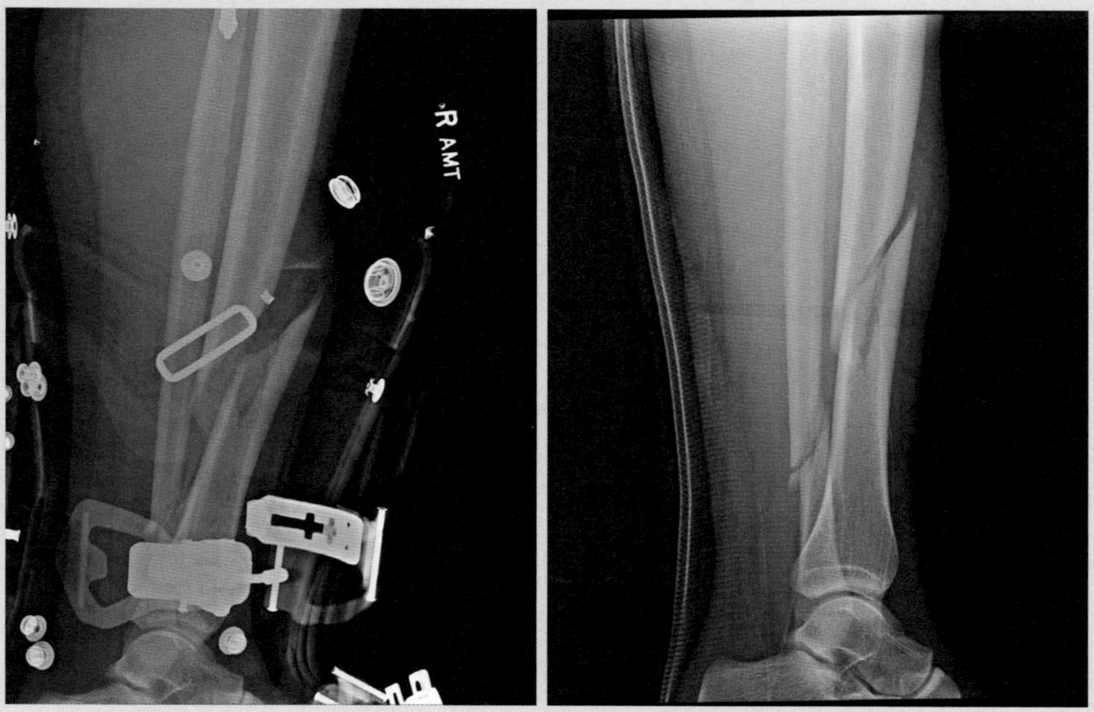

A displaced tibia and fibula fracture inside a ski boot (left). The process of removing the boot applies Traction into Position. The alignment of the extremity is significantly improved (right).

Chapter 14: Dislocations

A joint is a complex assembly of bones, ligaments, cartilage, tendon, muscle, and synovial fluid. These structures can be injured in a wide variety of combinations and levels of severity. A dislocation occurs when enough force is applied to the bone to stretch or tear the restraining ligaments and allow the joint to come apart. The process of restoring a joint to its normal anatomical position is called reduction.

Dislocations

Joint Structure:
- Bone, cartilage, tendon, muscle, ligament, fluid

Function:
- Support, mobility

Problem:
- Disability
- Pain
- Ischemia

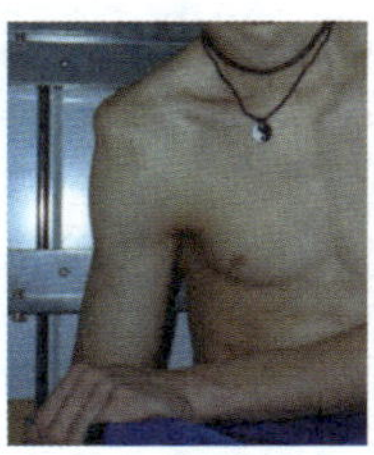

"Early reduction of a simple dislocation is a low-risk treatment for a high-risk problem."

There are three simple dislocations that are easy and safe to reduce in the field: the shoulder, patella (kneecap), and digits (fingers and toes). The Wilderness Protocol for joint reduction is for use in situations wherein the mechanism involves low-energy and indirect force. With proper technique, the medical officer can transform a gruesome and painful medical emergency into a minor logistical dilemma.

In cases where the deformity is the result of a direct impact, such as a fall while climbing or skiing into a tree, a dislocation is more likely to be complicated by fractured bone and cartilage. Reducing a dislocation under these circumstances involves more risk. Splinting in place and urgent evacuation is best when definitive care can be accessed quickly.

Dislocations

Mechanism:
- Indirect
  - leverage
  - torque
- Direct
  - impact
  - crush

S/Sx:
- Pain
- No active ROM
- Deformity
- Distal CSM often impaired

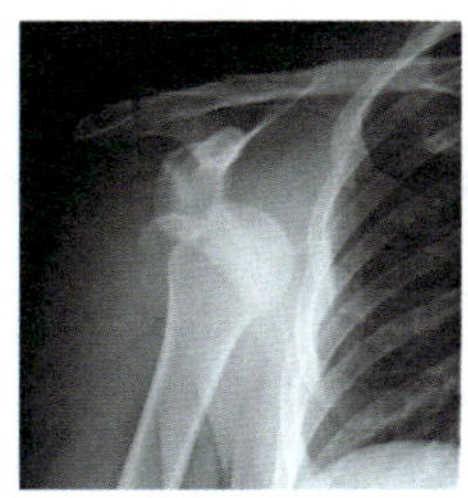

Dislocations
WILDERNESS PROTOCOL

Treatment:

Immediate field reduction if:

- Simple dislocation from indirect force
- Shoulder, patella, digits
- Wilderness context
- Patient consents

"The damage to the joint and surrounding soft tissue due to ischemia will increase significantly after a couple of hours."

Shoulder Dislocations

Shoulder dislocations can be extremely painful and acute stress reaction is common, leading to unwarranted high-speed and high-risk rescue efforts. However, this is one emergency that you can often fix in the field. The usual mechanism is external rotation and abduction by indirect force, such as high-bracing with a kayak paddle or catching a fall on an outstretched arm while skiing. The velocity is usually low, and the mass is restricted to the weight of the patient. Fractures are uncommon, and generally do not interfere with treatment.

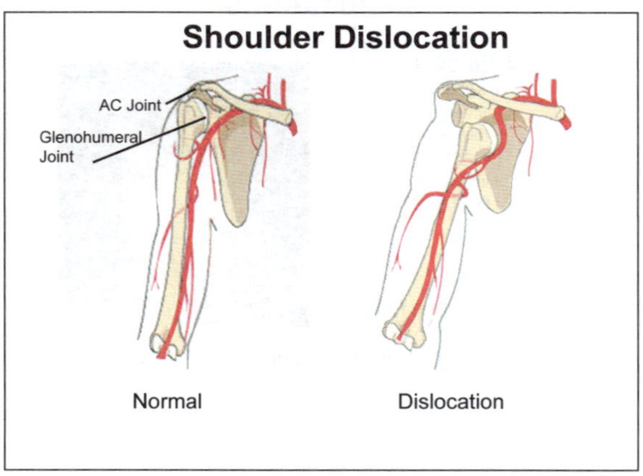

The shoulder itself loses the contour of the deltoid muscle and becomes a step-off deformity, with a hollow area where the shoulder is normally full and rounded. The patient will lose active range of motion (i.e., be unwilling to move the shoulder joint without help). There is often some degree of impaired circulation to the arm as part of an evolving ischemia to infarction problem: the main reason for early reduction in the field.

Occasionally, a shoulder dislocation can be confused with a shoulder separation. In a shoulder dislocation, the proximal end of the upper arm (humerus) is displaced from its socket (glenoid) in the shoulder blade (scapula). This glenohumeral dislocation results in gross deformity and complete loss of active range of motion of the arm.

A shoulder separation is a disruption of the joint between the distal end of the clavicle (collar bone) and the acromion process of the scapula (shoulder blade). The usual mechanism of injury is a direct blow to the top of the shoulder during a forward fall. This is a common skiing and over the handlebars bike accident.

This acromioclavicular joint lies directly above the shoulder joint and, when unstable, can have a similar step-off appearance caused by the displaced and elevated distal end of the clavicle. However, the shoulder joint itself remains intact with the rounded deltoid contour, and the arm retains active internal and external rotation. An acromioclavicular separation does not require field treatment other than pain management and a sling for comfort. If there are no other problems, non-urgent medical follow-up is sufficient.

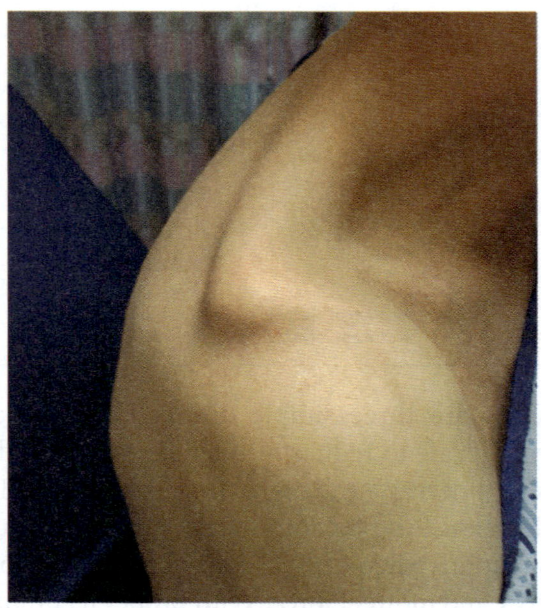

Acromioclavicular separation (shoulder separation)

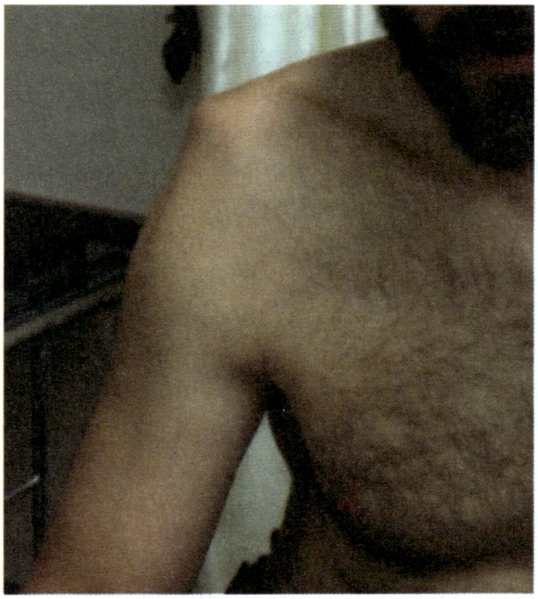

The shoulder dislocation seen here can be difficult to distinguish from the AC separation seen on the previous page. The diagnosis can be confirmed by assessing the mobility of the shoulder joint.

Treatment of Shoulder Dislocation

Ischemia to infarction is an anticipated problem, as is increasing pain and disability. A shoulder dislocation from indirect force should be reduced in the field if the evacuation time to definitive care is greater than two hours, or if the evacuation will be difficult, dangerous, or unreasonably painful to perform. It is safe to say that these criteria are met by most backcountry and marine situations.

There are many techniques that are effective in reducing dislocated shoulders. The best for field use are performed gently and slowly and there is low risk of causing further injury. The patient's cooperation and relaxation are essential to the process. Three example techniques are described here.

The Cunningham Technique

The Cunningham technique and its variations takes advantage of the fact that the joint is most balanced and stable in its normal position and, given a chance, will sometimes return there on its own. The idea is to put the dislocated joint at rest, encourage the muscles and the patient to relax and allow the humeral head to slip back into place against the glenoid. It is the most benign shoulder reduction technique and is worth a few minutes of trial before moving on to manipulation.

This principle can be applied in almost any position, but sitting is best. The practitioner sits facing the patient on the injured side and places the patient's hand on their own shoulder. The practitioner then gently massages the muscles around the patient's shoulder while encouraging the patient to relax and allow the joint to reduce. As with any of the techniques described here, patient relaxation is the key.

Shoulder Reduction

Cunningham:

- Patient sitting up straight, shoulders back, arm adducted, hand on practitioner's shoulder, relaxed as possible.
- Practitioner massages shoulder muscles until reduction occurs.

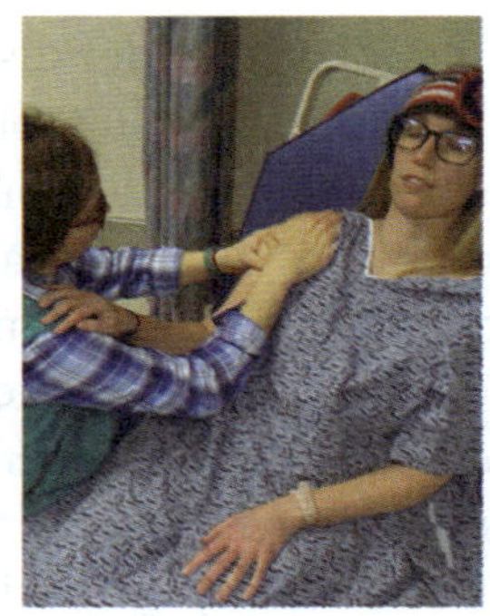

Simple External Rotation

Simple external rotation can be used when the patient presents with the arm down with the elbow near the chest. Reduction is usually performed with the patient sitting up straight with shoulders back and relaxed.

Shoulder Reduction

Simple External Rotation:

- Patient sitting or lying down.
- Practitioner externally rotates humerus with slight traction.
- Assistant or practitioner massages shoulder muscles.

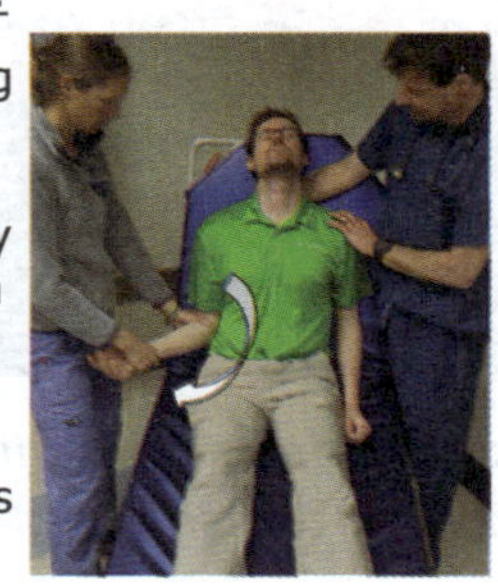

While you stabilize the patient's elbow against the body, slowly externally rotate the arm while massaging the muscles around the shoulder and encouraging the patient to remain relaxed. Slight downward traction at the elbow will allow the humerus to slide rather than snap back into place.

Usually, the shoulder will reduce before the limit of normal external rotation is reached. If not, hold the external rotation and continue to massage the shoulder muscles for several minutes. If reduction still does not occur, consider adding scapular manipulation or laying your patient back and trying the baseball position (both described in this chapter).

The Baseball Position

To reduce a shoulder dislocation using the baseball position, first support the patient's arm while you help them into a supine position. Apply gentle traction on the upper arm to help relieve pain during movement. Laying the patient down may take some time. Once the patient is supine, slowly externally rotate the arm while abducting into a position about 90° from the body, with the elbow bent. It is exactly the position in which the patient would have their arm if they were about to pitch a baseball. Once the arm is in position, make yourself comfortable and begin to apply steady traction. Reduction may take up to 15 minutes.

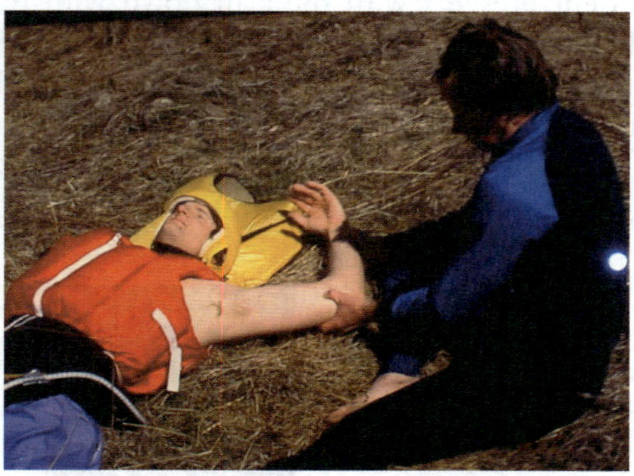

Peter Goth demonstrating the baseball position for shoulder reduction.

Traction should be firm, but there should be no need for counter-traction unless you are working on ice or snow. Gently and repeatedly encourage the patient to relax their shoulder muscles. Usually, within a few minutes, the muscles fatigue, allowing the joint to slip back into place.

If the joint has not slipped back into place after about 5–10 minutes, try a move called throwing the baseball. This movement involves exactly what it sounds like. Watch the patient's shoulder and pick a moment when you see the muscles really relax. Gently rotate the arm and hand forward as if the patient were throwing a ball. This is almost always successful in encouraging the shoulder to pop back into its socket.

Scapular Manipulation

Another safe reduction technique for field use is scapular manipulation. Instead of rotating the humeral head into place in the socket, slide the socket (glenoid) into place behind the humeral head. Have an assistant apply traction or externally rotate the humerus while you push the lower portion of the scapula medially. This rotates the scapula to drop the socket into place behind the humerus. If you do not have an assistant, the patient may be positioned face down on anything that allows the dislocated humerus to hang off the edge. This could be lying on a picnic table, downed tree, large rock, or the deck of a boat.

As with any reduction technique, slow and gentle manipulation with a relaxed patient will have the best chance for success. Scapular manipulation can also be used simultaneously with most other reduction techniques, including simple external rotation and the baseball position. Whatever technique you use, the goal is to find the right position in which the humeral head will drop back into its socket.

You will recognize a successful reduction by the dramatic relief of pain and return of mobility. You can sometimes feel and see a sudden shift of the upper arm as it relocates in the socket. A successful reduction can be confirmed by the patient's ability to reach across and touch the opposite shoulder. If CSM impairment was present before reduction, it will rapidly improve afterward.

Scapular Manipulation

- Rotate the bottom of the scapula medially and the top laterally
- Assistant applies traction to the arm or uses external rotation technique
- Scapular manipulation may be added to any other shoulder reduction technique

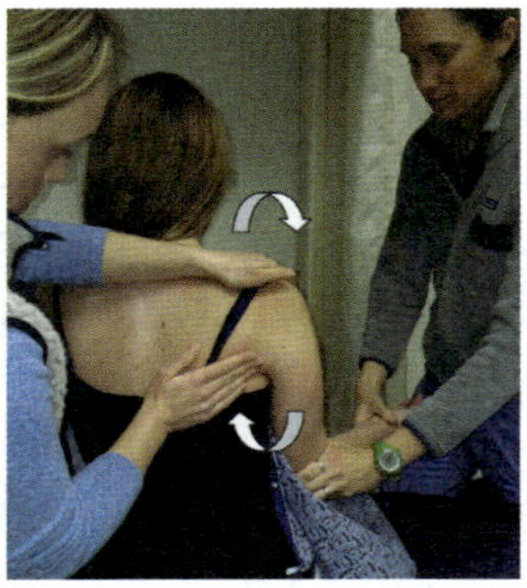

Remember to check and document CSM both before and after reduction. Use a simple sling to splint the shoulder, adding a swathe if it makes the patient more comfortable. The patient should plan for medical follow-up within a week, if possible. Pain-free activity is safe as long as the patient avoids abduction and external rotation.

Some shoulders may remain quite painful immediately after reduction. This sometimes indicates that a small piece of bone is chipped from the head of the humerus. This should not be a cause for urgent evacuation if distal CSM (particularly circulation) is intact.

Dislocations that result from direct force or are part of multiple trauma are more complicated and are best cared for in a medical facility with x-ray capabilities. Manipulation in the field is directed only at restoring CSM, if necessary and at positioning the patient for safe evacuation. If the patient is to be walked out, a sling with a swathe or pinned to the patient's shirt or jacket is effective immobilization. If field reduction must be attempted, use the same techniques discussed above. Pain medication may be required.

Patella Dislocation

The patella is a sesamoid bone imbedded as a fulcrum in the quadriceps tendon. This large structure transmits the force of the contracting quadriceps muscle in the front of the thigh to the front of the lower leg to allow you to extend your knee. The tendon passes over a groove in the femur like a cable through a pulley. In patellar dislocation, the tendon and patella slip off the femoral groove, making it impossible for the knee to function.

Like the shoulder, the patella can dislocate with a direct blow or an indirect mechanism—typically a sudden extension of the knee while twisting or turning with the foot fixed in position by a crampon or ski. The patient often has a history of recurrent dislocation. An indirect dislocation always leaves the patella pinned against the outside of the knee by the pull of the quadriceps (a lateral dislocation). The appearance can be deceiving. Shifting the patella laterally will make the end of the femur on the inside of the knee stand out and look like the missing patella.

Like the shoulder, these dislocations are extremely uncomfortable and there is little or no active range of motion. Because the neurovascular bundle is not nearby, distal circulation and sensation are usually unaffected. Damage to other surrounding soft tissue will increase with time, as will the difficulty of reduction.

Treatment of Patella Dislocation

As with shoulder dislocation, a dislocated patella should be reduced if access to medical care will be delayed by more than two hours, or if the evacuation will be unreasonably difficult. Take the tension off the structure by sitting the patient up to flex the hip. Then slowly straighten the knee. If the patella does not reduce on its own by the time the knee is in full extension, push it gently into place with your thumbs. Like the shoulder, relief of pain and return of mobility will indicate success. Also like the shoulder, these injuries are likely to result in swelling and significant pain later.

Patella Dislocation

Reduction:

- Have the patient sit up and lean forward
- Slowly straighten the knee, manually shift the patella medially when leg is straight
- Usually there is no impairment of distal CSM

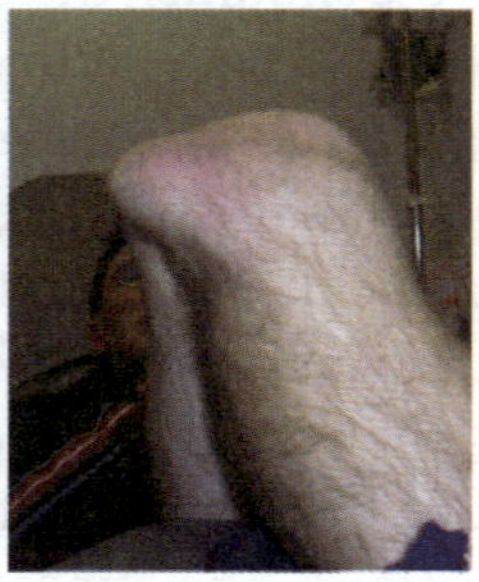

Ideally, a reduced patella dislocation should be splinted as an unstable injury and the patient carried out. In more common and less than ideal situations the knee could be wrapped or braced, and the patient walked out if pain and terrain permits. Taping the patella to prevent lateral displacement is often effective. It is important to avoid repeating the mechanism of injury. If CSM is intact there is no emergency, but medical follow-up is important.

Patella Post Reduction

Long-Term Care:

- Ice, NSAIDs. Swelling and pain are anticipated problems
- Splint or tape to limit ROM and keep patella in mid-line
- Carry-out evacuation is ideal, but walk-out is OK if patella is stabilized

"As long as pain and swelling can be controlled there is no emergency, but medical follow-up is important."

Dislocations of Finger and Toes

Joints in the digits usually dislocate due to an indirect force that levers the bone ends apart. Active range of motion is impossible, and there is often some degree of CSM impairment. These dislocations often have an associated small avulsion fracture that does not inhibit treatment. Like all dislocations, ischemia to infarction is an existing or anticipated problem.

Treatment of Digit Dislocation

Digits usually dislocate at the proximal and distal interphalangeal joints (PIP and DIP). Reduction is relatively easy and should be performed in the field. Dislocations of the metacarpal-phalangeal joints (MCP), where the fingers join the hand, can be more difficult. Sometimes the base of the phalanx pokes through the joint capsule and becomes trapped there, preventing field reduction. If several attempts fail, splinting and evacuation for surgical reduction are indicated.

Digit Dislocation

Reduction:

- TIP to normal anatomy
- Check ROM and distal CSM

Long-Term care:

- RICE and splint or buddy tape to next digit
- Medical follow-up, non-emergent if CSM is OK

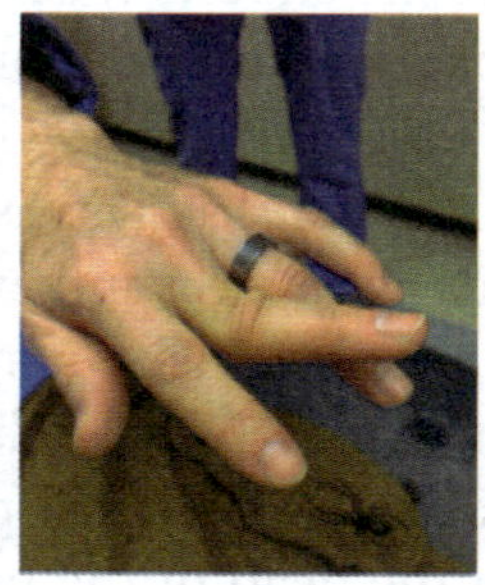

Reduction will be easiest right after the injury has occurred, before swelling and pain inhibit it. Grasp the end of the dislocated finger with one hand, and the rest of the finger in the other. Slowly but firmly pull the end of the finger in the direction it is pointing and then, while maintaining traction, swing it back into normal position.

You will probably need to wrap the end of your patient's finger in gauze or a bandanna to help keep your grip. Some crepitus will be felt during manipulation.

Digit Dislocation Treatment

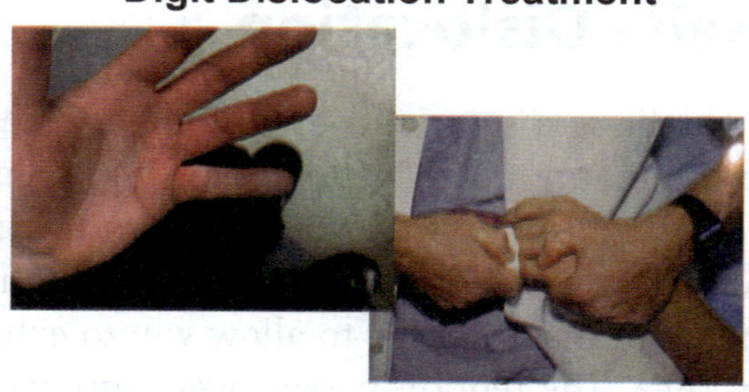

"Slowly but firmly pull the end of the finger in the direction it is pointing and then, while maintaining traction, swing it back into normal position."

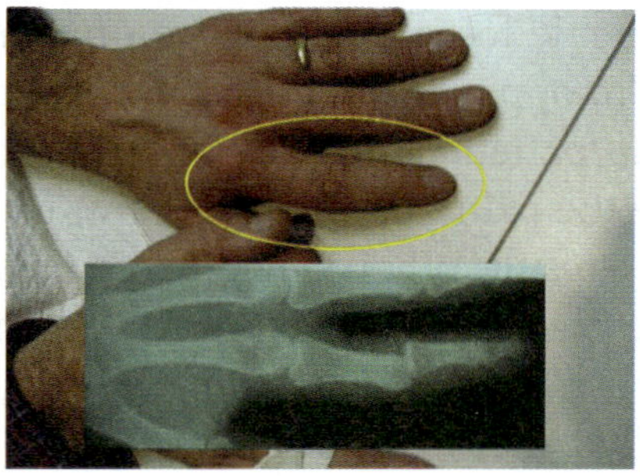

"Sometimes, a dislocation is not so obvious without being able to see an x-ray. However, the complete loss of mobility of the joint is diagnostic."

After manipulation, test passive range of motion to be sure that reduction was successful. The joint will likely be a little swollen and sore with reduced active range of motion. Splint the joint in the mid-range, or by padding and taping the finger to the one adjacent (buddy taping). Remember to check CSM before and after reduction. Pain should improve with your treatment. Medical follow-up should occur within a week, if possible.

Difficult Dislocations

In the backcountry, any dislocation that resists your efforts at reduction can become a serious problem. Pain may be severe, and the potential for tissue damage due to ischemia increases with time. If CSM is significantly impaired and cannot be restored by traction and repositioning, immediate evacuation to medical care is warranted.

Hip dislocations are difficult to distinguish from hip or pelvis fractures in the field. Pulling on a hip or pelvic fracture could lead to increased deformity and bleeding. Even if the diagnosis of dislocation is clear, significant analgesia and sedation are required for a successful reduction.

Elbow dislocations are notoriously painful to reduce and there is a high incidence of long term complications. Like dislocations of the hip, pain medication and sedation are required. Manipulation of either in the field should be performed only to restore distal circulation in an ischemic limb.

Risk Versus Benefit

Dislocation reduction is a medical procedure usually reserved to licensed practitioners. Some emergency physicians even defer the procedure to orthopedic surgeons. That luxury does not often exist in the remote setting. Fortunately, reduction as described here is a low-risk procedure for a high-risk problem.

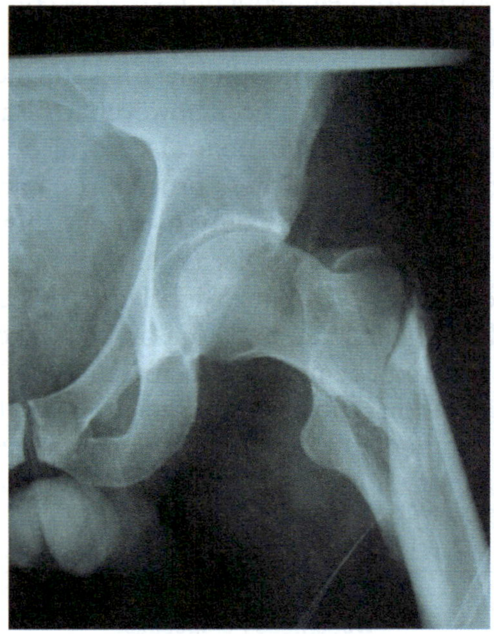

Without the X-ray, it would be difficult to distinguish a hip dislocation from this intertrochanteric fracture of the femur. The leg of this patient was shortened and rotated.

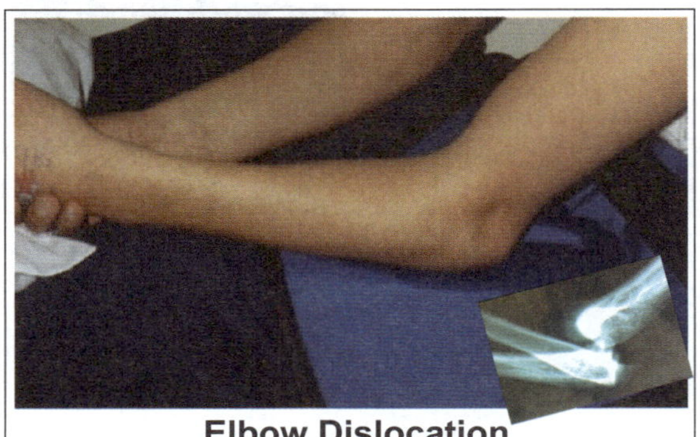

Elbow Dislocation
x-ray inset

Although most medical control physicians are more comfortable with time and distance criteria for field reduction, for example two hours from definitive care for a dislocated shoulder, there is little reason to prolong pain and disability any longer than necessary. There is clear benefit to early reduction of simple dislocations, and the incidence of complication is extremely low. The risks associated with prolonged dislocation include ischemia and infarction of joint structures and the distal extremity. There is also increased risk to the patient and rescuers in the urgent evacuation of a disabled patient in severe pain.

Protocols for field reduction are now common in wilderness medical training and approved by many medical control authorities. It is still incumbent on the medical officer, however, to be aware of local statutes and medical control policies regarding the use of these procedures, particularly when working in a duty-to-act situation like emergency medical service (EMS).

The example techniques detailed in this chapter all use gentle manipulation on an awake and cooperative patient. Some increase in pain with manipulation is normal; severe pain is not. If the patient cannot tolerate the procedure, you need to stop and try something else or evacuate to medical care.

Dislocations

Wilderness Perspective

High-Risk Problem:

- Persistent impaired CSM
- Failed reduction
- Critical System Injury
- Hip or elbow
- Dislocation from direct force
- Compartment syndrome

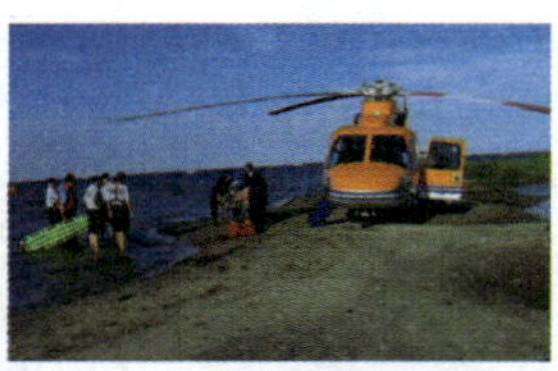

Some techniques used in the hospital employ considerable force, such as two or more people pulling in opposite directions to reduce a shoulder. The patient is usually sedated enough to tolerate the pain, but unable to give useful feedback as a result. When viewing this, bear in mind that the practitioner has seen X-rays and knows exactly what they are dealing with, and there are skilled staff available to minimize the risks associated with sedation. The same technique in the field setting would carry much greater risk. Fortunately, considerable force is rarely necessary in any setting.

Chapter 14 Review:
Dislocations

- Dislocation is complete disruption of joint structure. It involves stretched or torn ligaments and can involve bruised or fractured cartilage and bone.
- A dislocation is diagnosed by a positive mechanism of injury, gross deformity, and complete loss of active range of motion. Pain is usually severe. Obvious impaired distal CSM is common.
- Dislocations from indirect force of the shoulder, patella, and digits are generally simple and easy to reduce in the field. There are many techniques for shoulder reduction. Low-risk techniques for field use are slow and gentle and require patient cooperation and relaxation. Simple external rotation, the baseball position, and scapular manipulation are three examples.
- A patella dislocation is reduced by sitting the patient and gently extending the knee. Manual reduction may be necessary if the dislocation does not reduce by the time the knee is fully extended.
- Digit dislocations are reduced by gentle Traction into Position.
- If reduction is successful and CSM is intact, there is no emergency. Protection from further injury and non-emergent medical follow-up are the treatments.
- A failed reduction is a high-risk problem and requires urgent evacuation.
- Dislocations from direct force and dislocations of the ankle, elbow, and hip are high-risk injuries and are manipulated only to restore circulation or to reduce the risk and complexity of evacuation.

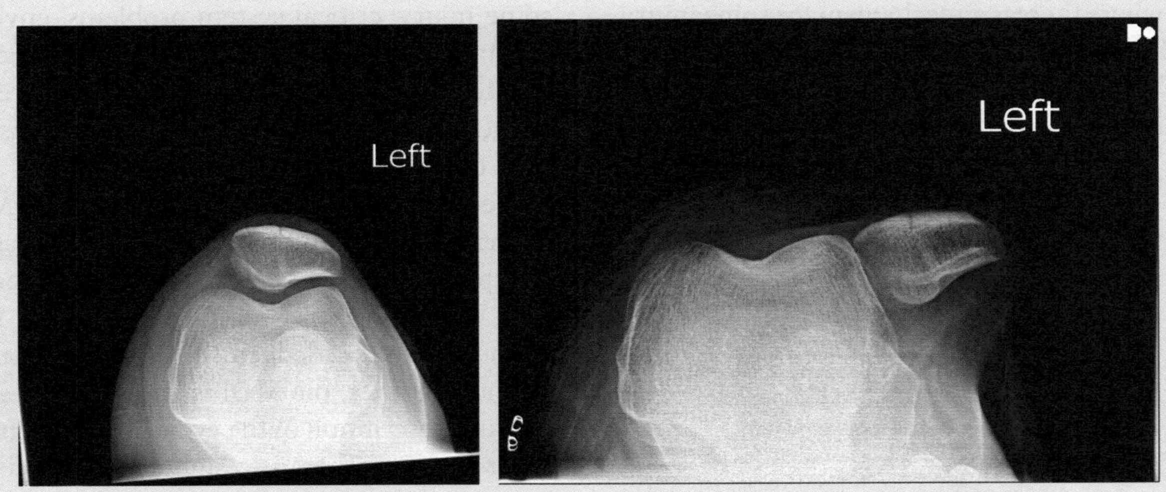

The patella in its normal position (left), and dislocated (right).

Chapter 15: Spine Injury

Stabilizing the spine has been a standard of care in trauma management for emergency medical services (EMS) since the early 1970s. The chief concern was similar to that with other musculoskeletal trauma: an unstable injury to the bones and ligaments of the spinal column could exacerbate injury to the surrounding soft tissue. In the case of the spine, the soft tissue of greatest concern is the spinal cord and its associated blood supply. In the conventional EMS setting, it was protocol to align, stabilize, and package a patient in all situations where there is a mechanism for spine injury (MOI). This was considered a "better safe than sorry" practice that was perpetuated for decades with little acknowledgment of the associated risks.

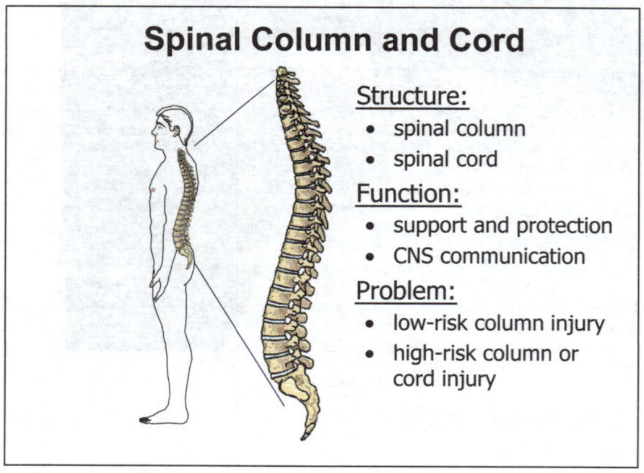

In recent years, however, the practice has been used much more selectively, especially in the wilderness or technical rescue setting where full-body stabilization can substantially increase the complexity of medical care, evacuation, and risk to rescuers and the patient. In most jurisdictions pre-hospital providers have been given the responsibility and freedom to identify those patients for whom this risk is clearly justified, and to avoid increasing risk where there is little or no benefit. This judgment is based on the severity of spine injury, critical system problems, environmental factors, available resources, and the difficulty of evacuation. The goal is to reduce risk to the entire patient and the rescue effort as well as to the spine itself.

The term positive mechanism of injury (MOI) describes any event that could cause damage to the spinal column or cord. A 6-meter fall onto a rock ledge is a positive MOI. A stiff neck from sleeping on a rock ledge is not. For less straightforward injuries, the MOI is based on the scene size-up, description of the event, and presence of other injuries. There is a significant association between traumatic brain injury and spine injury. Severe chest and abdominal trauma should also raise the suspicion of associated spine injury. If you believe that enough force was involved, it is a positive MOI.

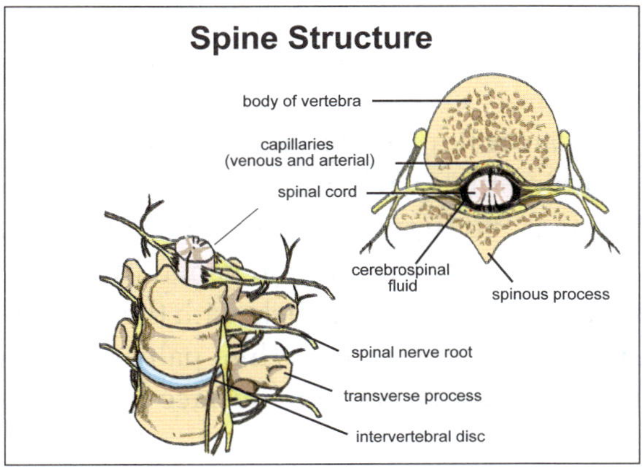

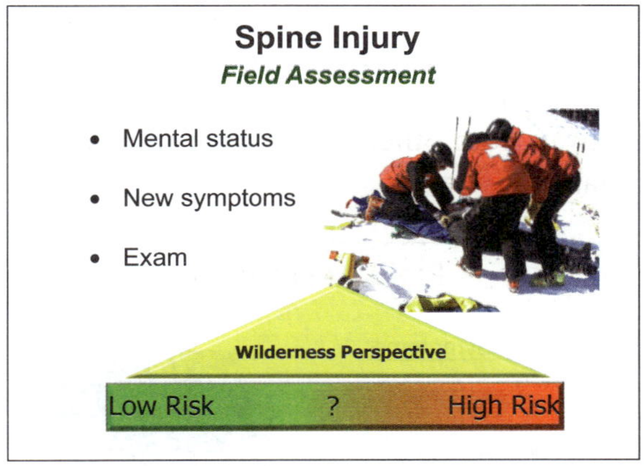

The trauma patient with a positive MOI and altered level of consciousness (V, P, U on AVPU) is considered to have a spine injury until proven otherwise. Treatment should include protecting the spine from further trauma as best you can while managing other medical and logistical problems. However, it should not take priority over airway control and ventilation, bleeding control, or preservation of body core temperature. Stabilization protocols should not interfere with rapid extrication from an unstable scene like avalanche terrain or cold water. The procedure should not substantially increase risk to rescuers. This is one of many areas where blind obedience to conventional protocol can kill people in the unconventional setting!

Field Assessment of Spine Injury

The trauma patient who is A on AVPU offers an opportunity to refine our problem list and risk vs benefit analysis. In any case, spine assessment is not an emergency treatment; it is a specific and meticulous examination performed after the scene is stabilized and critical system problems have been treated or ruled out. Until you are very comfortable with your routine examination you should perform the spine exam separately rather than incorporated into the rest of your secondary assessment. The first step is to determine how reliable the exam will be.

A patient who is awake and cooperative with normal mental status can be considered reliable and will report pain or neurologic symptoms. It is highly unusual for a significant spine injury to go unnoticed if the patient is talking to you, even in the presence of other painful injuries. However, the patient with altered mental status from acute stress reaction or traumatic brain injury may not reliably report signs and symptoms and may not follow your instructions when performing motor and sensory tests. Even then, a spine exam can still be useful if the patient can demonstrate normal motor and sensory function.

If you are an experienced emergency practitioner, you have likely adopted a neurologic exam that is comfortable, familiar, and complete. If not, the WMAI Spine Assessment Criteria can serve that purpose. Conscientiously applied, it will reliably detect all significant spine injury.

Each element of the WMAI Spine Assessment Criteria is important. You are looking for evidence of injury to the spinal column as well as injury to the spinal cord. You are also trying to determine how serious an injury might be to help you judge the risks and benefits of treatment and evacuation.

Your spine assessment really starts with your first impression. The patient who is up and walking around may still have a spine injury, but at least you know that moving and bearing weight is possible. A patient who is splinting (holding the neck and back stiffly) may be involuntarily protecting a spinal column injury. A patient will full mobility, no splinting, and no apparent discomfort is very unlikely to have a spine injury at all.

You should ask specifically about new symptoms. "Does your neck or back hurt? Do you have any numbness or tingling anywhere? Do your legs or arms feel weak?" Be direct and attentive, these are important questions and you want the patient to really think about the answer. You may have to focus the patient's attention on the neck and back and away from other concerns or injuries to get a reliable answer.

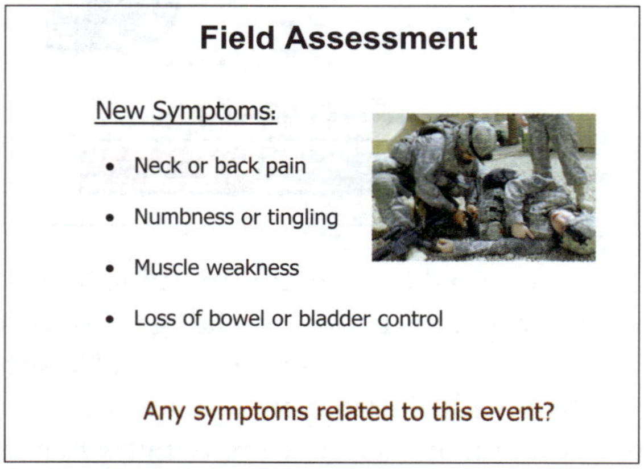

The physical examination of the spinal column involves firm palpation or gentle percussion of the midline spine from the base of the skull to the tailbone. You are looking for tenderness that may indicate column injury. If the patient has already complained of back or neck pain, be gentle but continue with the exam to determine location, severity, and the presence of any deformity. It may be useful and necessary to distinguish midline spine tenderness from paravertebral muscle tenderness.

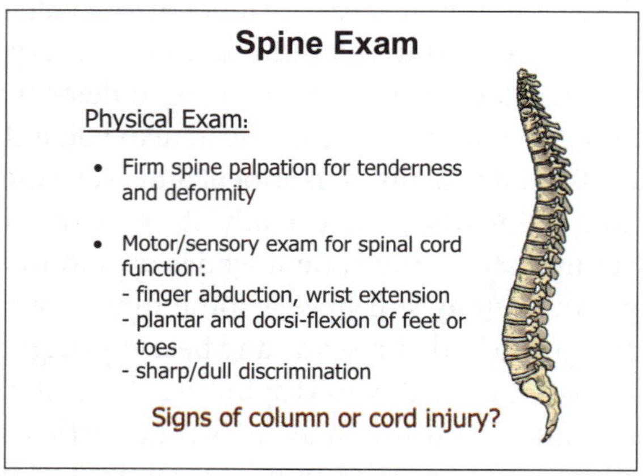

Hands on stabilization of the head and neck before and during the exam is unnecessary unless the patient is having trouble maintaining position on their own. Nodding or shaking of the head while answering your questions is not harmful. A reliable patient will not hurt themself. If you or the patient is uncomfortable with neck movement, ask them to remain still until you have completed your exam.

You can roll a supine patient onto their side to examine their back. Providing head and neck alignment and support to the patient while doing this is more comfortable and generally safe. It is also safe for the patient to help with the roll if they can do so without pain. While palpating, don't forget to examine the skin surface for bruising or abrasions.

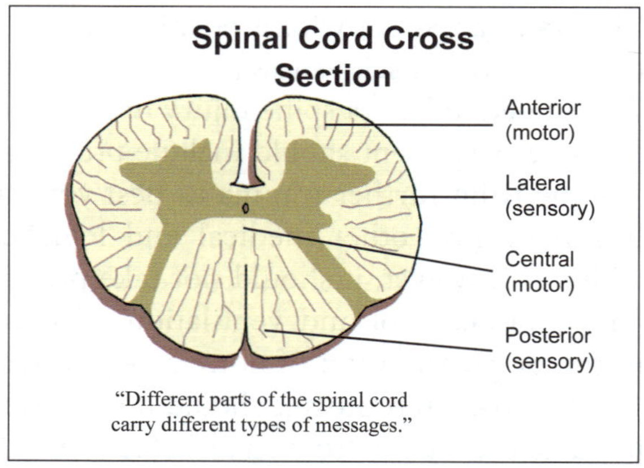

The physical examination of the spinal cord uses motor and sensory function to detect injury or ischemia. The motor examination tests the strength of specific muscle groups. In the upper extremities we test finger abduction (spreading fingers apart) or wrist extension against resistance. In the lower extremities we test plantar flexion and dorsiflexion of the feet or extension of the big toe against resistance. Strong and symmetrical muscle strength is a normal response.

Sensory pathways in the spinal cord are tested by assessing the patient's ability to distinguish between sharp and dull touch on all four extremities. An ideal tool for this exam is a cotton swab where the cotton end is used to apply the dull stimulus and the cut shaft is used as the sharp stimulus.

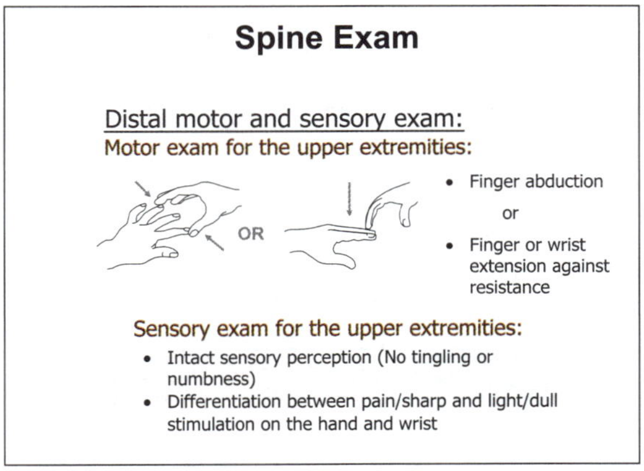

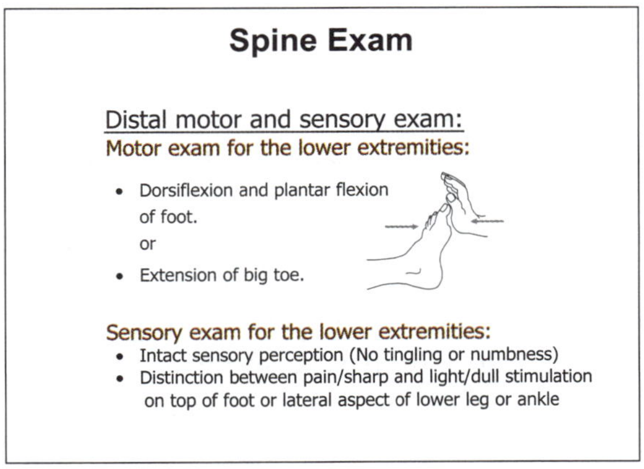

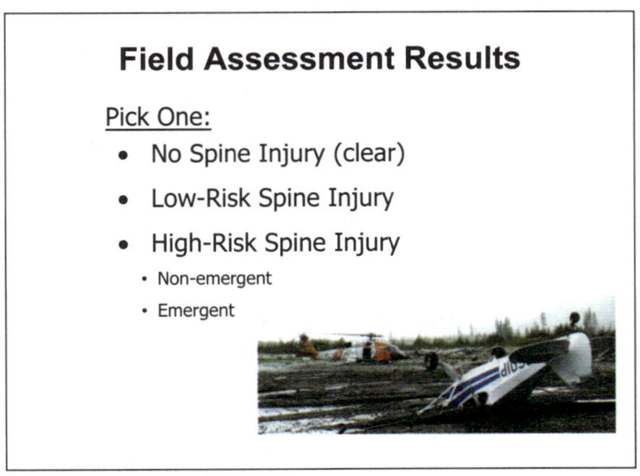

The patient is asked to distinguish, without looking, one end from the other when pressed against the skin. The upper extremities are tested on the ulnar and dorsal aspect of the hand.

The lower extremities are tested on the lateral aspect of the foot or lower leg. An asymmetrical response where one side is very different than the other would be considered abnormal. Calluses or cold extremities may prevent a precise response every time, so you may need to perform repeated tests in different places to confirm your results.

No Spine Injury

If the spine assessment is normal (negative) the spine is clear, and you can remove spine injury from the problem list. Be aware that it is common for trauma patients to develop various minor aches and pains as swelling and inflammation increases over several hours. A stiff neck or back is one of these common late occurring symptoms. If you were able to clear the spine initially, this does not indicate a significant injury.

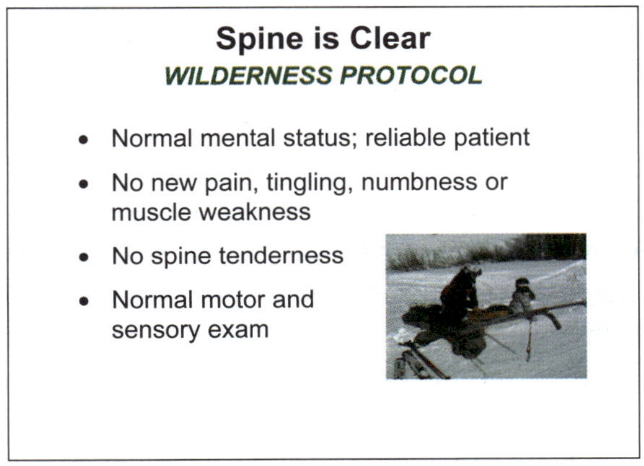

Low-Risk Spine Injury

Any positive findings during the assessment such as persistent pain, tenderness, unequal muscle strength or asymmetrical sharp versus dull discrimination mean that you should presume that the spine is injured. Later examination during evacuation or in the hospital may clear the spine, but for now you should protect the spine from further injury as best you can under the circumstances.

Now the question becomes: Is this presumed spine injury serious or not serious, high risk or low risk? This will determine the urgency of evacuation and how much risk is acceptable in executing it. Fortunately, most spine injuries are at low risk for complications from normal activity and can be evacuated on a non-emergent basis, often by walk-out. The few high-risk injures that do occur in the field should, ideally, be stabilized comfortably and carried out.

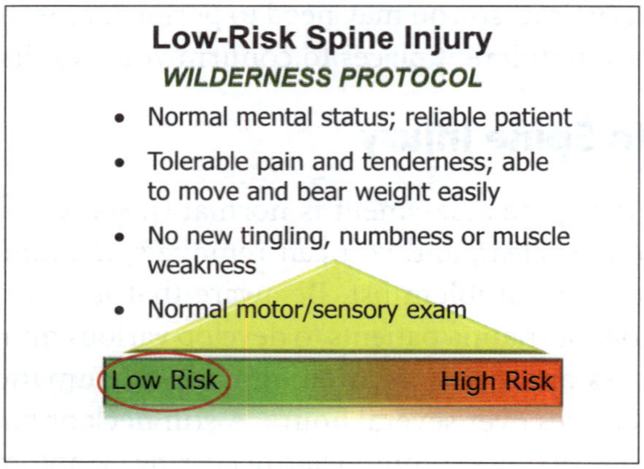

In a low-risk spine injury, pain and tenderness are mild, the patient can move and bear weight easily, and the motor and sensory exam is normal. This is the person who can stand up and sit down without assistance and without screaming in pain. This patient is at low risk for complications if another fall can be prevented.

As always, we try to avoid high-risk evacuations for low-risk problems. Evacuation of the low-risk spine injury is non-emergent and usually does not require a carry. However, to reduce the probability of further trauma, the patient probably should not get back on the horse or mountain bike. A walk out may be the safest plan for all concerned, and be sure to recommend follow-up medical care.

High-Risk Spine Injury

The signs and symptoms of high-risk spine injury are the same as those for other unstable musculoskeletal injury: severe pain and tenderness, deformity, or the inability to move or bear weight. The pain and disability of serious spinal column injury is usually evident immediately in the patient's complaint. High-risk spinal column injury carries the anticipated problem of spinal cord injury in the event of further trauma or rough handling. Fortunately, just like a fractured leg, an unstable spinal column injury may be high risk but is not necessarily an emergency. If the patient is neurologically intact, careful handling and protection is more important than speed.

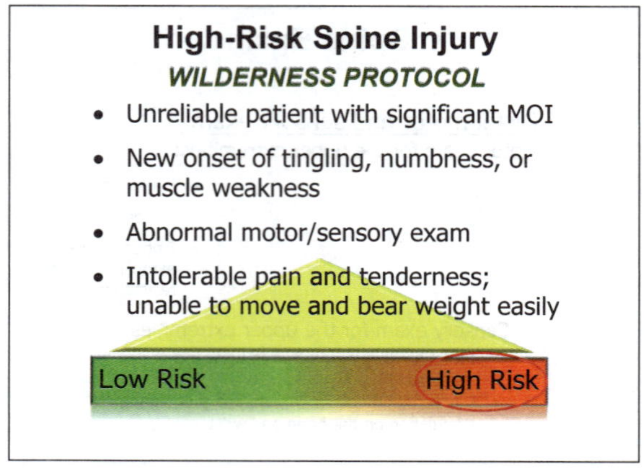

Spinal cord injury, however, *is* an emergency. Persistent neurologic signs or symptoms following significant trauma may indicate ischemia of the spinal cord that will result in infarction if perfusion is not restored. Early surgical intervention may save spinal cord tissue. You will probably choose the helicopter evacuation to the trauma center over the slow carry out to the local hospital, even if the risk in doing so is a bit higher.

Evacuating a high-risk spine injury usually requires a rugged improvised or commercial litter and a large team to carry it. While awaiting the proper equipment, the patient can be stabilized on a foam pad on the ground with packs or other gear positioned to restrict head motion if necessary. The patient must be monitored for symptoms of any developing pressure sores caused by prolonged skin ischemia. Helping the patient to move and shift position periodically may be necessary.

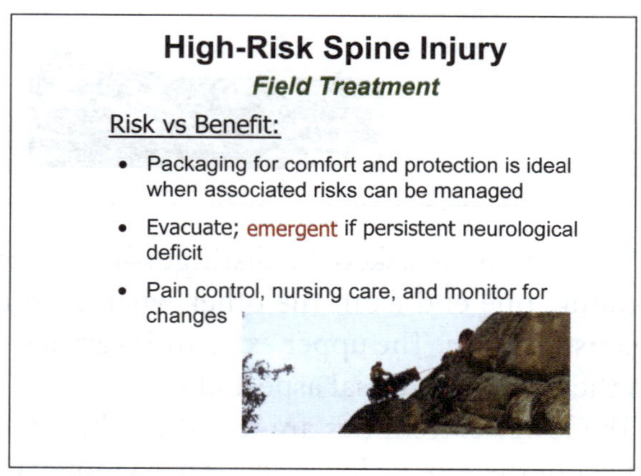

High-Risk Spine Injury
Field Treatment

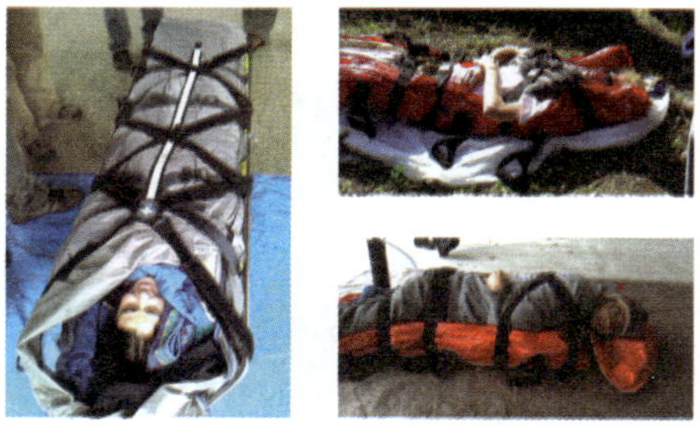

Spine Packaging
Risk vs Benefit

Stabilization can increase other risks:

- Increased time and complexity of evacuation
- Delay in treatment of other problems
- Impair airway control, thermoregulation, and survival efforts
- Cause skin and soft tissue ischemia

During transport, soft stabilization in the lateral or recovery position in a well-padded litter or vacuum mattress is ideal. Rigid cervical collars and unpadded backboards are not recommended for field use. Acceptable cervical spine stability can be accomplished with clothing and other padding. The old ski patrol horse collar technique that uses a blanket, sleeping bag, or jacket is effective, comfortable, and warm.

The use of analgesics and anxiolytics to help an uncomfortable patient tolerate a long carry is appropriate and humane. The dose should be titrated to provide some relief without putting the patient to sleep. If something is going wrong inside the package you will want your patient to tell you. Be aware that opioids and other medications can inhibit shivering or interfere with temperature control.

Risk Versus Benefit

There are many rescue situations in which the risk of full body stabilization exceeds the presumed benefit. Examples include patients or rescuers threatened by wildfire, avalanche, hypothermia, or a difficult technical rescue. In a high-risk environment, the best patient and spine protection may include crawling, walking, running, or swimming. When you have no choice but to move immediately, or to walk rather than carry a patient out, you can take comfort in the knowledge that an unstable spine injury is rare and the probability of further injury is remote.

One of the most common challenges to spine protection is an unsecured airway in a vomiting patient. In a rescue scenario it can be extremely difficult to prevent aspiration of vomit, secretions, or blood into the lungs of a patient stabilized supine on a backboard or litter. It is sobering to realize that aspiration of vomit carries a mortality rate of 20% to 60% depending on which studies are cited. It may be necessary to defer ideal spine protection until you can reduce this high level of risk. Whenever airway problems are anticipated, it is best to package the patient on their side, in the recovery position, or sitting up with their head turned to keep the airway clear.

Another vexing problem for rescuers is the combative patient with TBI where there is a positive mechanism, you must assume spine injury, and the patient will not tolerate spine stabilization. Wrestling a patient like this into a litter is a high-risk treatment. The best spine protection may be to allow the patient to assume whatever position is most comfortable or, if necessary, to apply soft extremity restraints only.

Spine Packaging
Ideal to Real

Consider:

- Assisted walking, crawling, swimming
- Package in sitting or recovery position
- No packaging or splinting if mobility is needed for survival

"There are situations in wilderness and rescue medicine where the risks of spine stabilization exceed the presumed benefit."

The decision to defer spine stabilization in a high-risk injury to reduce some other risk may not be an easy one to make. The thought of a rescuer being responsible for permanent spinal cord damage is appropriately frightening. However, the risk is minimal compared to the often-substantial dangers in wilderness and technical rescue, and to the morbidity and mortality associated with aspiration, hypothermia, and delayed treatment of critical system problems.

If you choose to defer ideal protection, the reasons should appear in your problem list. You might note that problem 1 is a spine that cannot be cleared. Problem 2 might be the fact that the temperature is 20° below zero with 30 knots of wind, and you and your patient are going to freeze to death if you stay where you are.

Spine Injury Summary

WILDERNESS PROTOCOL

Clear:

- Reliable patient
- No spine pain, tenderness, neurological deficit

Low Risk:

- Reliable patient
- Tolerable pain and tenderness; moves easily
- No neurological deficit

High Risk:

- Persistent neurologic deficit (emergent evac)
- Severe pain or tenderness; cannot or will not move
- Unreliable patient with significant MOI

Chapter 15 Review:
Spine Injury

- Any traumatic event capable of damaging the spinal column is a positive mechanism for spine injury.
- Injury to the spinal column without cord or nerve root injury is the most common. Like other musculoskeletal injury, spinal column injury may be stable or unstable.
- Unstable column injury increases risk of injury to the spinal cord and nerve roots. Full body stabilization and evacuation is the ideal treatment.
- The spine assessment criteria are used in cases where a positive or uncertain mechanism of injury exists, but spine injury may or may not have occurred.
- A clear spine means no spine injury. This is a calm, cooperative, sober, and alert patient with no new spine pain or tenderness and an intact motor and sensory exam without new symptoms.
- A low-risk spine injury presents with tolerable pain and tenderness, the ability to move and bear weight easily, and the ability to self-protect. There is no neurological deficit.
- A high-risk spine injury is a positive MOI with altered level of consciousness or severe pain, persistent neurologic deficit, and the inability to move or bear weight.
- The ideal treatment for high-risk spine injury is whole body stabilization and urgent evacuation.
- High-risk spine injury with persistent neurologic deficit is a high-risk problem worthy of an emergency evacuation.
- Full-body spine stabilization may increase other risks. Ideal protection may be deferred or modified until other risks are minimized.
- All patients with an uncleared spine require a follow-up evaluation with an advanced-level practitioner, even those you decide to walk out because of a difficult evacuation and an evaluation consistent with a low-risk injury.

Chapter 16: Wounds and Burns

The skin is the largest of the body's organs. It performs the remarkable function of protecting your sterile and sensitive internal organs from the flora, fauna, heat, and chill of the wild outdoors. It is also a major component of the thermoregulatory system.

The skin is composed of several layers, the outermost being the epidermis. The outer surface of the epidermis is called the stratum corneum, which is a layer of dead skin cells and bacteria. These cells are continuously being generated and shed at an impressive rate—some 50 million per day. This process, like the continuous flow of mucus from the respiratory system, is part of how we protect ourselves from the billions of microbes with which we share our existence.

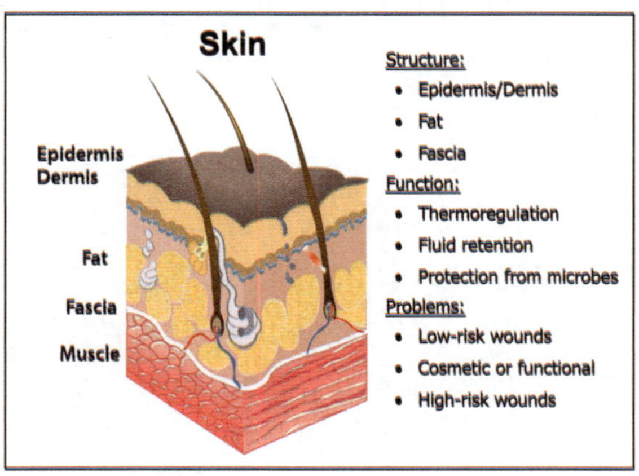

The dermis is the next layer; it contains larger blood vessels, sweat glands, hair follicles, and most of the nerve endings of the skin. Sweat and oil excreted onto the skin surface help with protection by killing some bacteria and reinforcing the skin's barrier effect. The total thickness of the dermal layer varies from a half of a millimeter on the eyelids to three or four millimeters on the palms and soles.

The blood vessels in the dermis are capable of a dramatic change in volume as they constrict or dilate for thermoregulation or the need to maintain core perfusion pressure. When fully vasodilated, the skin can hold up to three liters of blood; when fully vasoconstricted, as in severe shell/core effect, the skin may retain as little as 30 milliliters of blood.

Under the dermis is a layer of fat. In some places, like the buttocks or belly, this layer can be many centimeters thick. In other locations, like the back of the hand, it may be only a few cells thick. Below the fat lies a layer of tough connective tissue called fascia. This is typically dull-white and fibrous in appearance, and covers underlying muscle, bone, organs, and joints.

Wounds

Problems begin when the protective outer layer of skin is damaged and the soft tissue beneath is exposed. This allows microbes to invade unprotected tissue and lets body fluids escape. Deep wounds where the fascia is interrupted are at high-risk for infection. Extensive soft-tissue injury can cause shock and hypothermia.

All wounds damage blood vessels and cause bleeding. The body attempts to control blood loss by automatically constricting blood vessels at the injury site. Chemical components called clotting factors interact with platelets in the blood to form a blood clot. Under most circumstances, bleeding will stop within 15 minutes. Sometimes it needs a little help in the form of direct pressure or other bleeding control techniques including tightly packing a wound.

After the blood loss has been stopped, the slower process of wound repair begins. The initial stages of natural wound cleansing occur over a period of several days. The clot surface dries, forming a natural bandage in the form of a scab. Underlying tissue is further protected by the process of inflammation that provides a protective barrier beneath the injury.

Contaminants like dirt and bacteria are flushed out as the wound drains. By the third or fourth day, the protective barriers are established, and cleansing is well underway. Redness, warmth, swelling, and pain begin to decrease as the normal inflammatory response subsides.

After 6 to 10 days, the wound is very resistant to contamination. Wound edges migrate together as the collagen fibers within the clot contract. Scar formation and complete healing continue over the next 6 to 12 months.

Wound Assessment

There are many terms—such as laceration (slice), avulsion (skin flap or tissue removed), and abrasion (scuff or rubbed off)—used to describe wounds. For field purposes, wounds can be assessed generically as low risk or high risk. Simple low-risk wounds offer no risk of life-threatening bleeding and do not represent a significant risk of infection. They can be managed in the field, with evacuation to medical care as convenient.

Wound Assessment

Wilderness Perspective

- Low Risk (simple)
- Cosmetic or Functional Risk
- High Risk

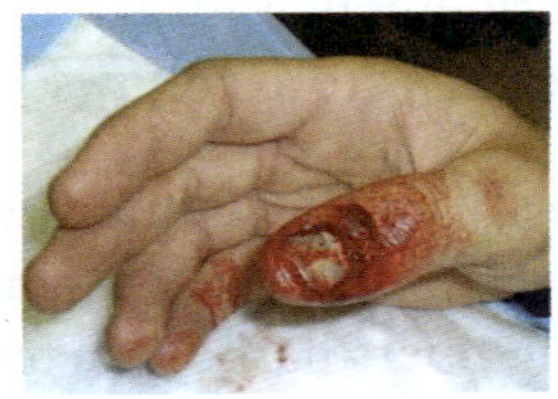

Low-Risk Wounds

Low-risk wounds may involve the dermis and subcutaneous fat, but they do not penetrate the fascia. There is no contamination of muscle, bone, tendon, or joint structure. These wounds are clean and free of devitalized or macerated tissue. A superficial cut from a clean knife is an example.

Wound Assessment

Low Risk (simple):

- Dermis and subcutaneous fat only
- Clean, straight, no devitalized tissue
- Low risk of infection

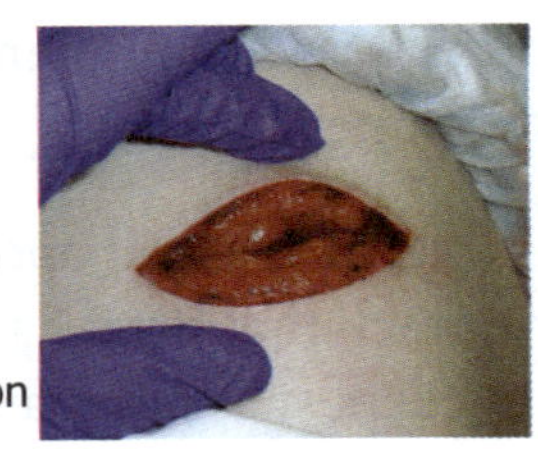

"A superficial cut from a clean knife is an example."

Some wounds have the potential to cause cosmetic or functional defects as they heal. Examples include wounds of the face, hands, and genitalia. You may choose to refer these wounds for immediate care when the risk of evacuation is low. The best results will be obtained when wound repair is accomplished within several hours, but acceptable wound repair can be accomplished days later, if necessary.

High-Risk Wounds

High-risk wounds are those that carry a significant risk of infection or are likely to cause functional problems during early healing. Wounds associated with life-threatening bleeding or critical system injury are also considered high risk. Aggressive field treatment and early evacuation for debridement is ideal. Some examples of high-risk wounds are as follows:

Grossly contaminated. Injuries with imbedded foreign material, such as gravel, sawdust, or clothing fibers harbor bacteria that is difficult to dislodge.

Mangled. Wounds that involve crushed, shredded, or dead tissue provide a growth medium for bacteria.

Deep. Wounds that penetrate the fascia to expose joints, tendons, and bones are difficult to clean adequately, and are prone to serious infection.

Bites (from humans or other animals). Mouths harbor a wide variety of virulent organisms. Human and cat bites are among the worst. Any wound exposed to human or animal saliva constitutes a bite wound.

Punctures. A small opening in the skin with a wound track that extends through several layers of tissue deposits bacteria in areas that are unable to drain properly.

Wound Assessment

High Risk:

- Penetrates fascia, involves deep structures
- Critical system involvement
- Contaminated, crushed, devitalized tissue
- Open fractures
- Deep punctures
- Bite wounds (animal saliva)

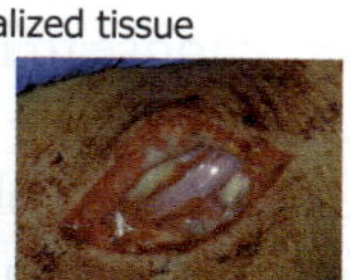

"High-risk wounds are those that carry a significant risk of infection or are likely to cause functional problems during early healing."

Wound assessment is an important skill. Some wounds can appear simple, involving only the dermis and fat layers. On closer inspection, you may find that the fascia is interrupted, and deep structures are contaminated. A good field examination may take some time and involve careful probing with instruments or fingers. You should consider all wounds to be high risk until proven otherwise.

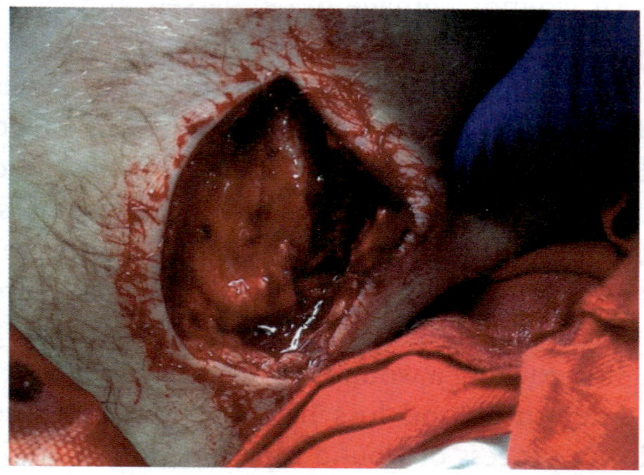

Wounds involving deep structures like this knee laceration into the joint space are considered at high risk for infection.

The fascia is easily identified as a tough, dull-white layer of tissue resembling unfinished fiberglass. Underlying structures like tendon, bone, and joint surface appear shiny and white or yellow. Muscle underlying the fascia appears deep red, like a raw steak.

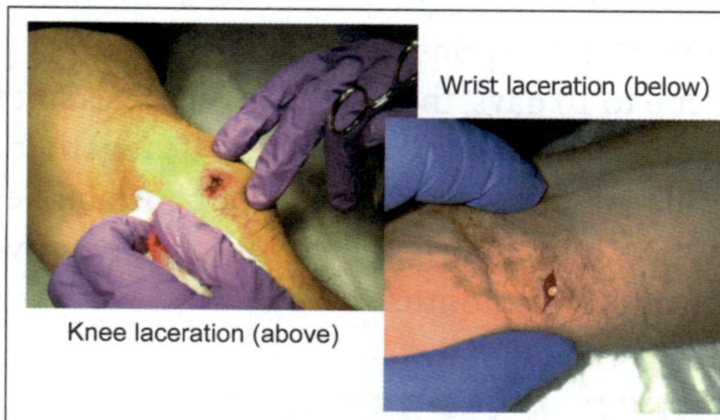

These wounds are small, but penetrate far enough to lacerate tendon sheath and tendon. These are high-risk wounds.

The depth of the wound in millimeters is far less significant than the layers penetrated. An eyelid laceration a few millimeters deep may be high risk, whereas a wound on the buttocks several centimeters deep is considered low risk. Puncture wounds often appear very benign on the surface but carry a substantial risk of infection to deep structures. Avulsion flaps should be lifted, inspected for debris, and probed for deep structure involvement.

Wounds to the chest or abdomen may enter the organ cavities. In such cases, there is sometimes an obvious hollow space, visible or probed. These carry a very high risk of life-threatening infection and often involve critical system injury. Early administration of antibiotics and emergency evacuation to surgical care can be lifesaving.

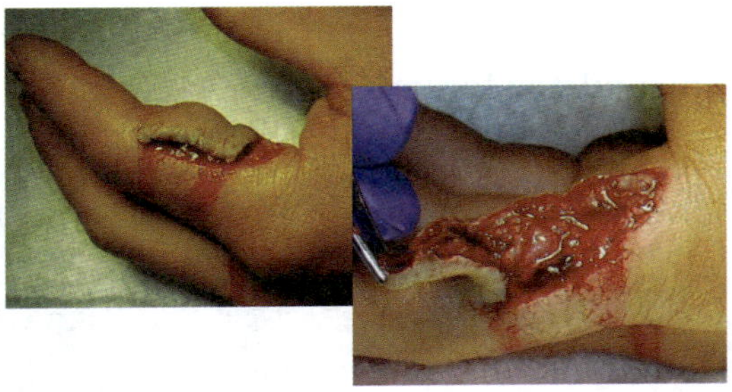

"Avulsion flaps should be lifted, inspected, and probed for deep structure involvement."

Remember that wounds also present risk to the examiner. Don't forget to protect your eyes, skin, and mucous membranes from contact with blood and exudates. Wear gloves and eye protection, and keep your mouth shut or wear a mask.

Field Treatment of Wounds

The initial field treatment of both low- and high-risk wounds is the same: Stop the bleeding, inspect, clean, dress, and monitor for infection. Evacuation should be initiated for high-risk wounds.

Bleeding is best controlled with direct pressure and will usually stop within 15 minutes as the clotting mechanism is activated. If bleeding persists, it is usually because the pressure is not firm enough, is applied in the wrong place, or is not being applied for enough time. A tourniquet may be used temporarily to slow major bleeding while you find and dress the bleeding site, or in cases in which you are too busy managing other critical system problems. A proper tourniquet is composed of a wide (4–5 cm), soft band applied 5–10 cm proximal to the injury. Enough pressure must be applied to stop arterial blood flow, or else venous congestion and edema will develop.

A tourniquet can be left in place for at least an hour without causing significant damage from ischemia. If severe bleeding resumes it will need to be reapplied and left in place during evacuation. Be sure to note the time of application. A tourniquet can also be used for short periods to allow for adequate visualization for wound cleaning. It is a very useful tool and is dangerous only when left in place too long.

Long-term management of any wound requires early wound cleaning to help prevent infection. The use of prophylactic antibiotics is limited in the civilized setting but should be considered for the wilderness context due to the greater difficulties involved in wound care. The initial dose should be administered as soon as possible after the injury has occurred.

Cleansing a wound usually restarts some bleeding by disturbing the clot, so you should not attempt to clean wounds that are associated with life-threatening bleeding. Wash the skin around the wound with soap and water and/or a disinfectant like povidone iodine. Clean a wide area of skin, being careful not to allow soap or disinfectant into the wound itself. Irrigate the wound with copious amounts of clean water. Tap water is fine at home. In the field, water filtered or disinfected for drinking is suitable for wound irrigation. When water supplies are limited, using a 1% solution of povidone iodine may reduce the incidence of infection. There is no significant advantage to using sterile saline or specialty wound irrigation solutions.

Wound Treatment
WILDERNESS PROTOCOL

Low-Risk Wounds:

- Clean surrounding skin surface.
- Irrigate with copious amounts of clean water or 1% PI solution.
- Explore wound and remove foreign bodies.
- Cut away dead tissue.
- Dress and monitor daily.

"Proper wound cleaning can take quite a bit of time. Make yourself and your patient comfortable and do a thorough job."

Wound Treatment
WILDERNESS PROTOCOL

High-Risk Wound:

- Clean per protocol except punctures and wounds at risk for life-threatening bleeding
- Early evacuation
- Consider antibiotics if authorized
- Contact local health department about rabies risk in mammal bites

"Gentle probing…may reveal a previously unnoticed laceration of the fascia exposing muscle or joint space to contamination."

There is an advantage, however, to applying a little pressure to the irrigation stream. Studies demonstrate that the ideal irrigation pressure is generated by a steady stream from a 30–60 cc syringe and an 18-gauge catheter. You are not trying to sterilize the wound, just flush out debris and reduce the bacteria count to levels that can be managed by the body's immune system. Be sure that the irrigation fluid can easily flow out of the wound; otherwise, the pressure will only drive contaminants deeper into the tissues. It is usually impossible to irrigate puncture wounds effectively without this happening.

It is harmful to irrigate a wound with full-strength iodine preparations (typically 10%) or hydrogen peroxide. Iodine and peroxide kill both bacteria and body cells, leaving a partially sterilized wound lined with dead tissue. This can actually increase the risk of infection, as does soaking a wound in a basin of saline or iodine as is still practiced in some clinics and hospitals.

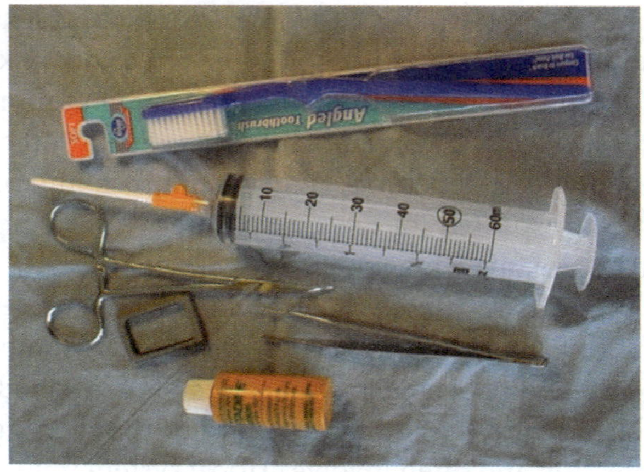

Only a few lightweight and inexpensive instruments are required for wound cleaning in the field.

For irrigation, use only clean water or saline, a 1% povidone iodine solution, or a product specifically formulated for use in open wounds.

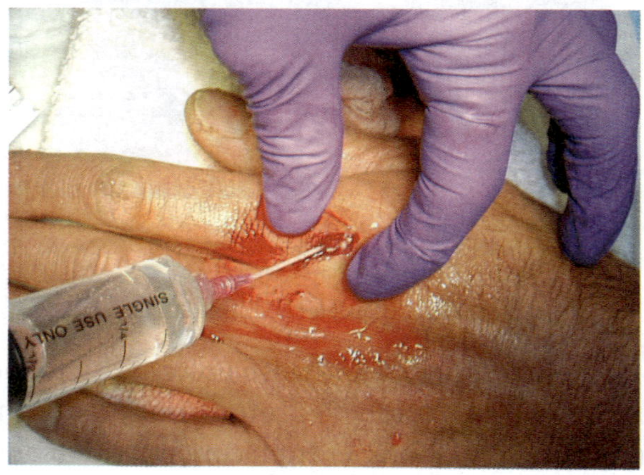

The ideal wound irrigation device is a syringe with an 18-gauge catheter.

Continue cleaning by removing any imbedded debris that was not flushed out by irrigation. A soft toothbrush, forceps, scissors, and a head-lamp are useful tools for this. Cut away any dead tissue or loose fat. These are likely to become a site for bacterial growth.

Proper wound cleaning can take quite a bit of time. Make yourself and your patient comfortable and do a thorough job. It may be inconvenient, but it will save you a lot of time and trouble by preventing an infection.

Once cleaned, the wound should be carefully inspected to determine the extent and depth of the defect. Gentle probing with a sterilized instrument or gloved finger may reveal a previously unnoticed laceration of the fascia that exposes muscle or joint space to contamination. Treatment and evacuation for high-risk wound care would then be a priority.

In most cases, the wound is then covered with a sterile dressing to prevent outside contamination and to absorb wound drainage. Allowing for drainage is important to normal healing. Wound closure with tape, sutures, staples, or glue can create an obstructed hollow space prone to infection. In the backcountry or offshore setting, the risk in wound closure usually outweighs the benefit. Early wound cleaning is essential; early wound closure is not. Wound repair or scar revision can be safely delayed for days or weeks if necessary.

The exception would be simple wounds that do not penetrate the full thickness of the dermis. These may safely be closed after cleaning. This is mostly a matter of convenience. Steri-Strips, butterflies, and wound closure glue are equally effective but will require protection from moisture and contamination. Temporary wound closure with tape might also be indicated for functional reasons, such as taping wounds on the hand to allow paddling or on the feet for hiking. This type of functional taping should be removed at the end of the day.

Wound Treatment

Dressing and Bandaging:

- Prevent contamination
- Allow for drainage
- Avoid causing ischemia
- Allow for wound inspection
- Keep warm and moist
- Preserve and enhance perfusion

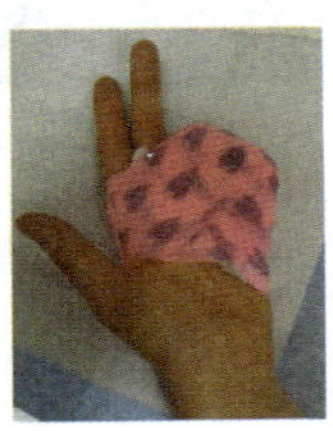

"It should not come as a surprise that products developed for use on livestock, or in nursing homes and home health, are particularly useful in wilderness medicine."

Impaled Objects

Ideally, any significant impaled object is best removed by a surgeon in a hospital but evacuating a patient with an impaled object will often risk more tissue damage than pulling it out will. If the object remains imbedded in the tissue, infection is inevitable. In most cases, impaled objects should be removed in the field and the wounds cleaned like any other.

Having said that, we must acknowledge the other reality; sometimes removing an impaled object is impossible, impractical, or dangerous. If you are going to do significant damage trying to remove the object, or be unable to control the bleeding that results, you must stabilize it in place and evacuate as quickly and carefully as you can. Consider prophylactic antibiotics en route.

Finally, we hope to never have to remove an impaled object from the globe of the eye. The fluid inside the eye cannot be replaced, and any amount lost will doom the patient's vision. Cover both eyes if possible and evacuate urgently to medical care. Pain control and patient care and protection will be challenging.

Wound Treatment

WILDERNESS PROTOCOL

Remove Impaled Objects Unless:

- Impaled in the globe of the eye
- Removal will cause significant problems:
  - tissue destruction
  - severe bleeding
  - unmanageable pain

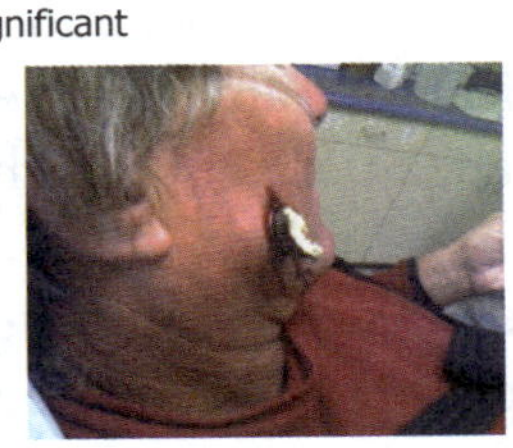

Bandages and Dressings for a Hostile Environment

The combination of bandage and dressing should allow for wound drainage while preventing contamination. The goal of long-term wound care is to preserve and enhance oxygenation and perfusion of the tissue, and to prevent infection. Prolonged shell/core effect or local vasoconstriction of the hands and feet in wet and cold conditions are typical impediments to healing. Altitude is also a problem. Wound healing is significantly delayed at 3000 meters and is almost impossible above 6000 meters.

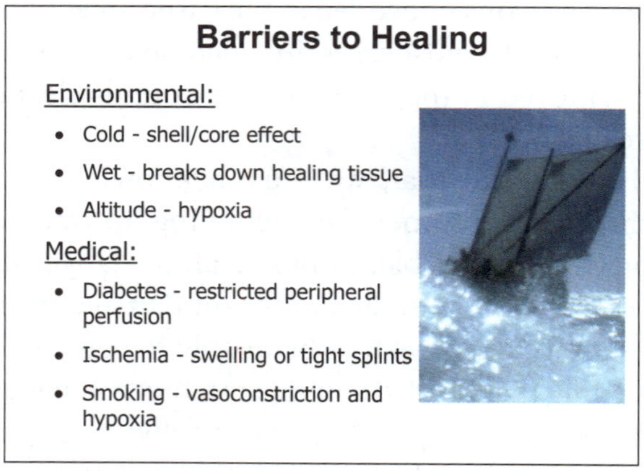

High-risk wounds with exposed soft tissue, bone, or other deep structures are best dressed with a moist, antibacterial surface next to the wound. Drying will further damage tissue. Covered Xeroform or silver-impregnated dressings are ideal, but a dressing soaked with dilute povidone-iodine solution will suffice.

The surface in contact with the open wound should begin sterile and should remain that way for as long as possible. The bandage should not impair circulation or prevent wound examination. Meeting these criteria on a wet and dirty expedition or evacuation can be quite a challenge. Typical first-aid kit adhesive tape and white roller gauze perform poorly in the backcountry or marine environment.

Newer dressings designed for long-term care of open wounds offer medical practitioners some good options for backcountry use. A sterile, transparent, semi-permeable membrane can be left in place for several days. Semi-permeable membranes are also combined with colloidal dressings to absorb exudates, keep the wound moist, and prevent external contamination even in very wet and dirty situations. The dressings are expensive, but far superior to the standard-issue first aid supplies.

An inexpensive roller bandage known as vet wrap, originally developed for veterinary use, can be used for splints or to hold dressings in place far more effectively than tape or an elastic bandage. It is water resistant, self-amalgamating, and reusable. However, it does not store or perform well in extremely hot conditions.

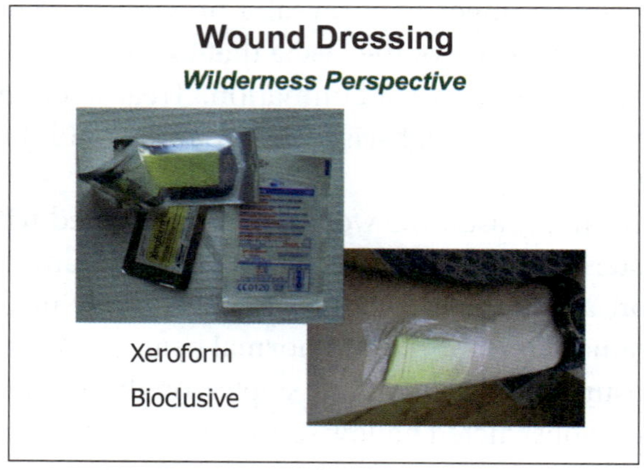

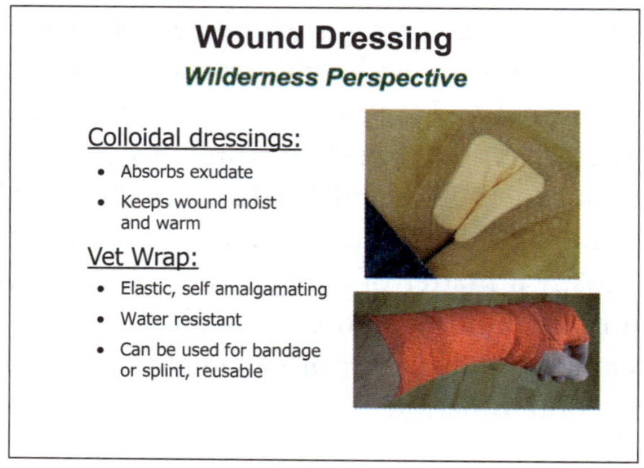

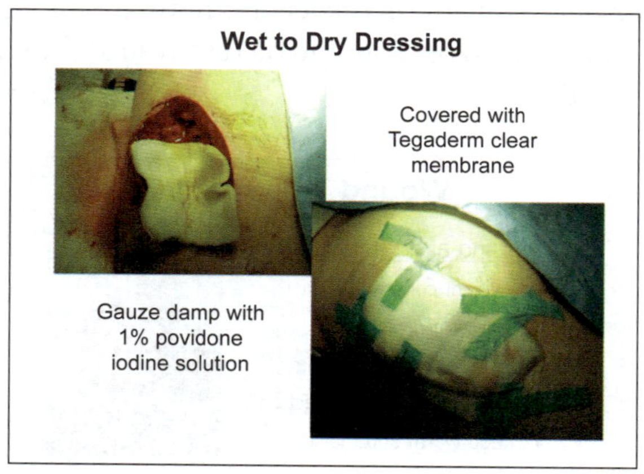

Abrasions and shallow wounds in which only the superficial layers of skin are affected can be dressed with antibiotic ointment alone or with an easily removed sterile dressing. Since the most common anticipated problem with abrasions is infection, frequent cleaning and inspection is a priority. Antibiotic ointment can also be used alone in difficult-to-bandage places like eyelids and ears. Wounds over or involving joints should be splinted if conditions and travel allow.

A tetanus vaccine booster should be given to anyone with an open wound who has not had a vaccination within ten years, or within five years in cases of high-risk wounds. This is ideally done within 24 hours of injury but does not warrant an evacuation if the person has already been immunized at some point. You can keep this from becoming a problem by keeping your routine tetanus vaccinations up to date and ensuring that everyone else in your group does the same.

Monitor the wound for signs of infection whether you choose to evacuate or not. You should also monitor the circulation, sensation, and movement (CSM) distal to the injury as you would with a musculoskeletal problem. Bandages, splints, and swelling can create ischemia there as well.

Evisceration

Internal organs protruding from an abdominal or chest wound is a gruesome scenario, but possible with penetrating trauma to the abdomen or thorax. Eviscerated organs should be covered with wet gauze or occlusive dressings like plastic wrap, and the patient evacuated to surgical care as rapidly as possible. Allowing a bent-knee position in the litter will reduce the tension of the abdominal wall and help prevent ischemia of the extruded organs.

Abdominal Evisceration

- Do not push the organs back inside.
- Apply moist or occlusive dressings.
- Position with knees bent.
- Emergency evacuation, anticipate:
  - Shock
  - Hypothermia
  - Systemic infection
  - Organ ischemia

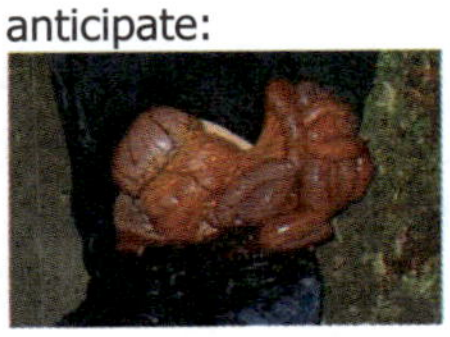

Positioning the patient for transport may result in spontaneous reduction of the evisceration, or you may attempt gentle manipulation that allows the organs to slide back inside. No attempt should be made in the field to *push* the organs back into the body cavity. Systemic infection, shock, and death are inevitable without surgical care. Hypothermia is an anticipated problem during evacuation.

Traumatic Amputation

Full or incomplete amputations should be treated with the expectation that replantation is possible, or at least that tissue and skin from the amputated part can be useful in repair of the stump. Successful replantation has been accomplished after as much as 24 hours. The surgeon should decide which injuries are candidates for replantation; your job is to get your patient and the amputated part to the appropriate facility as soon as possible.

The ideal field treatment is to wrap the amputated part in a gauze sponge soaked with saline, place it in a plastic bag, and float the bag in ice water. Bleeding from the patient's amputation site should be controlled only with direct pressure, and the wound maintained with moist dressings. Tourniquets and clamps should be used only if bleeding cannot be controlled otherwise.

In the absence of ice and sterile saline to preserve the amputated part, a dressing moistened in clean water or 1% PI solution will suffice. Keep the part as cool as possible without freezing and continue with the evacuation. Partially amputated extremities are treated the same way while still attached to the patient. Do not cut the part free.

Treatment of Traumatic Amputation

If managed correctly, an amputated extremity is not a life-threatening injury. Despite the drama and urgency of the situation, do not risk the lives of the patient and rescuers to preserve the possibility of replantation. A live patient with an artificial limb confirms a successful rescue. A fatality during the evacuation does not.

Traumatic Amputation

- Wrap the part in sterile, moist, dressing.
- Keep the part cool, transport with patient.
- Control bleeding with direct pressure or tourniquet.
- Do not complete partial amputations.
- Splint the extremity.
- Emergency evacuation.

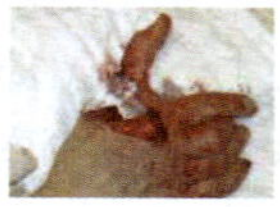

If the scene is more remote, replantation is not in the plan. Manage the stump as a high-risk wound; antibiotics, daily dressing changes, medical care when possible. Bury the dismembered tissue. In such cases, completing a partial amputation may be reasonable.

Rabies

Rabies is a viral infection nearly always fatal in humans. It is transmitted via the saliva of an infected animal, usually from biting or licking. It is most common in bats, dogs, and cats, and in mesopredators like raccoons, foxes, and skunks. Most of the time, an exposure is obvious. With bats, a bite or other exposure to saliva may go unnoticed. The mere presence of a bat inside a house may be reason enough to give rabies post-exposure prophylaxis (PEP) to the human inhabitants. Consult the Centers for Disease Control and Prevention (CDC) or an experienced practitioner for advice. Because rabies vaccine may not be available in low resource areas, vaccination may be indicated before long voyages and travel in developing countries.

Post-exposure prophylaxis consists of immediate and vigorous wound cleaning with warm water and soap, followed by irrigation with povidone-iodine solution. In animal bite wounds, the benefit of killing a potentially fatal virus justifies the risk of tissue damage caused by the soap or solution. The patient should then be urgently transferred to a medical facility equipped to provide rabies immune globulin and vaccine.

Wound Infection

In normal wound healing, the pain, swelling, redness, and inflammation decrease quickly within the first 2 or 3 days. If the wound becomes infected, these signs and symptoms begin to increase instead. Pus develops as the cellular debris and edema fluid accumulate in the wound. Infection is a possibility in any wound at any time during the healing process but is most likely to develop within 2 to 4 days after injury.

If a local infection spreads, it will ultimately enter the general circulation and cause a systemic infection. This is referred to as blood poisoning, lymphangitis, or sepsis. The symptoms of this whole-body inflammation include fever, skin redness, body aches, general malaise, and ultimately septic shock (a form of vascular shock). Even simple wounds like blisters that become infected present some risk of progressing to life-threatening sepsis.

Wound Infection

Local Infection:

- Increasing redness, pain, warmth, swelling
- Most likely to develop days 2–4
- Drainage or accumulation of pus (abscess)

Systemic Infection:

- Fever, malaise, regional swelling
- Lymphangitis (red streaks)
- Vascular and volume shock

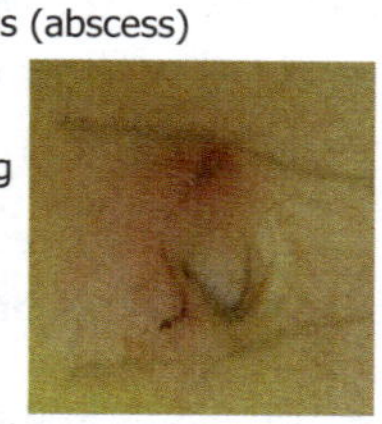

Treatment of Wound Infection

If the infected wound has been closed with tape, sutures, or staples, it should be opened, irrigated, and allowed to drain. Avoid forcefully squeezing the purulent material from the wound or else you may drive bacteria through the protective barrier into healthy tissues. At some point in your past, you've probably seen a minor pimple become a large abscess because of this practice.

If an abscess has formed in the dermis close to the surface, it can be safely opened with a sharp blade, and then irrigated and allowed to drain.

Clean the skin surface with antiseptic or soap and nick the pus pocket. In the field this procedure is reserved for those cases where the pus pocket is obvious and superficial. Do not attempt to incise anything in the deeper layers of the skin or soft tissue.

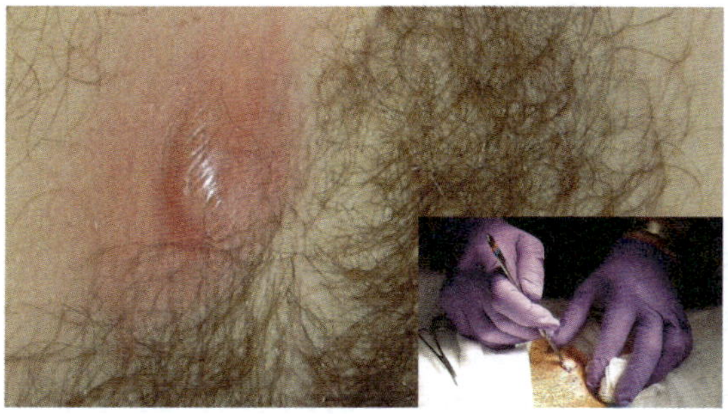

A superficial abscess like this 2 cm lesion in the axilla could be safely incised with a scalpel or sharp knife.

Applying heat to the infected area will increase circulation and help the body fight the infection locally. Use as much heat as your patient can comfortably tolerate against normal skin for 30 minutes at a time, as often as five to six times a day. Heat can be applied in the form of hot soaks or through contact with a warm rock or hot water bottle.

Local Infection

Treatment:

- Incise and drain superficial abscess
- Irrigate and dress
- Allow for drainage
- Hot soaks 4x a day
- Antibiotics
- Evacuation

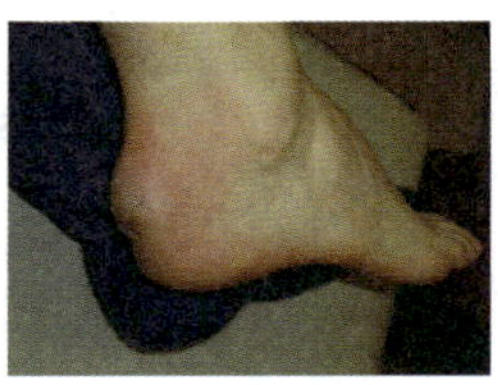

"Field treatment may improve S/Sx, but continue to monitor for systemic infection."

Drainage and heat applications often cure a wound infection, but antibiotics are considered to be part of the ideal treatment whenever surgical care is unavailable. Although not usually within the scope of practice for emergency medical responders (EMRs) and EMTs in the urban context, these drugs may be a worthy addition to your wilderness treatment protocols. If your duties take you days away from medical help, consider obtaining formal authorization and instructions from a medical practitioner.

Although the routine use of prophylactic antibiotics is controversial, and often of limited benefit, it should be considered for high-risk wounds in settings where surgical follow-up may be delayed for days or weeks. Deep punctures, open fractures, and multiple bites (especially to the hand) are good examples. To be most effective, antibiotics should be administered within 2 hours of injury.

Any evidence of systemic infection should be considered a medical emergency. Broad-spectrum antibiotics should be started immediately. Some oral medications can be just as effective as those given by injection and are easily used by wilderness EMRs and EMTs with the proper authorization. Urgent evacuation is required. Septic shock is an anticipated problem.

Burns

For field management, we need to know the depth and extent of burns, as well as their location. The extent is described in terms of body surface area (BSA), and critical locations include hands, feet, genitalia, and the respiratory system. The circulatory system can also be affected because burns can cause rapid fluid loss, resulting in shock. Hypothermia is an anticipated problem in large burns.

Burns

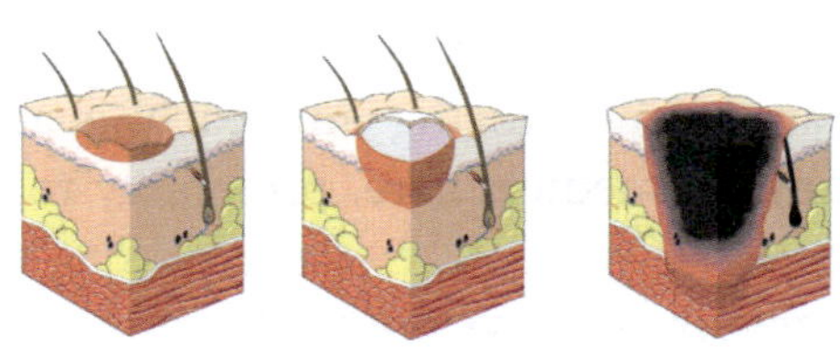

Superficial
- Intact sensation
- Red - inflamed
- No blisters

Partial Thickness
- Intact sensation
- Red and inflamed
- Blisters

Full Thickness
- Reduced sensation
- No blisters
- Black or leathery

Estimates of irregular burns can be made using the entire palmar surface of the patient's hand, which is about 1% of the body surface area. The depth of burn refers to how deep the damage goes. This can be difficult to estimate, particularly where different areas are burned to different depths.

In superficial (first degree) burns, skin integrity is not disrupted. Capillaries and nerves are intact. Inflammation occurs with redness, pain, and warmth. An example of a superficial burn is typical sunburn.

In partial-thickness (second degree) burns, the skin surface is damaged, but the injury is limited to outer layers. These are characterized by intact blisters and reddened or pink skin. Surface capillaries are damaged, but deeper skin, blood vessels, and nerves are intact. There is fluid loss, redness, warmth, and pain.

Full-thickness (third degree) burns penetrate the dermis to involve the subcutaneous soft tissues. Skin blood vessels and nerves are destroyed. The burned area may appear charred black or gray. The area may not be painful due to loss of nerve endings. Normal inflammation cannot occur, and as a result, blisters do not develop. Small full-thickness burns may appear to be less serious because of this.

As with other injuries, look first for potentially life-threatening problems. These will usually come in the form of volume shock, respiratory distress, or toxic exposure to carbon monoxide. High-risk burns are those that include anticipated major problems with critical body systems, severe pain, infection, or scar formation.

High-Risk Burns

The following signs and symptoms should motivate careful monitoring and early evacuation to definitive medical care, preferably to a burn center:

Any respiratory system involvement. Burned respiratory passages develop the same inflammation, blisters, and fluid loss that are seen on the skin. Signs and symptoms include singed facial hair, burned lips, sooty sputum, and persistent cough. Respiratory distress may develop from pulmonary edema or from swelling and obstruction in the airways. It can develop quickly or slowly over a period of hours. Respiratory burns carry a mortality rate of about 20%.

Partial-thickness burns of the face, genitalia, hands, and feet. Any significant burns in these areas can cause problems with swelling and ischemia in the short term, and mobility and scarring in the long term.

Circumferential burns. Burns that completely circle an extremity can cause distal ischemia as swelling develops.

Burns > 10% BSA. Large burns carry the anticipated problem of volume shock and hypothermia.

Any full-thickness burn. Any full-thickness burn is at high risk for infection.

Chemical burns. It can be difficult to fully arrest the burning process because some chemicals react with the skin. Damage can continue for hours afterward.

Electrical burns. Skin damage may be minor, but human-made electrical current can cause extensive injury to internal organs and tissues. Lightning tends to cause only superficial burns and internal electrical injuries are rare.

Burns of very young or very old patients. Infants and the elderly have a more difficult time compensating for injury.

High-Risk Burns

- Grossly contaminated
- Cosmetic or functional risk
- Circumferential Burns
- Full thickness
- Respiratory burns
- Chemical burns
- > 10% BSA partial or full thickness

Treatment of Burns

The initial treatment for burns is to remove the heat energy. The fastest way to do this is to immerse the patient, or injured part, in cool water but not ice; 20 minutes will suffice. Fortunately, this is almost instinctive as it serves to relieve pain as well. If the burn is greater than about 10% BSA, limit your cooling to prevent hypothermia. For most chemical burns, continued irrigation with water will not only cool the area but help remove the chemical itself. Irrigation of chemical burns should continue in cool water for at least 20 minutes.

If the burn is not a life-threatening emergency, clean and dress it with antibiotic dressings like you would for a minor abrasion or use a long-term wound care product. This can be done along with the application of cool soaks for pain relief. Monitor for infection as you would with any open wound.

Dressing a burn is generally similar to any other open wound. For burns specifically, the Xeroform type of gauze or other occlusive dressing will reduce pain by excluding air. For a temporary dressing, simply covering it with plastic wrap will work.

Burn Treatment

- Immediate cooling
- Continue cooling for several minutes
- Irrigate with water or 1% PI solution
- Remove dead skin
- Decompress blisters only if necessary
- Dress to prevent contamination
- Monitor for infection
- Hydration

If the burn falls under the category of high-risk, plan to have the patient to medical care within 48 hours if possible. If the burn involves significant damage to the respiratory or circulatory system, emergency evacuation should be initiated with early access to advanced life support (ALS). Ideally, transport the patient directly to a burn center.

In a wilderness setting, even sunburn can be a significant problem if it occupies a large area of skin surface. Ultraviolet radiation causes inflammation of the dermis and epidermis, inhibiting skin function and causing pain and redness. You should anticipate all the same problems inherent in any large surface area burn: volume shock, thermoregulatory problems, pain, and infection.

Dressing a large surface area burn can be difficult. The goal is to minimize contamination and to reduce evaporative cooling. An improvised dressing can consist of a clean cotton t-shirt, covered with a waterproof clothing layer or plastic kitchen wrap. Immediate attention should be given to maintaining hydration and body core temperature. The patient will need food, fluids, and protection during evacuation. Prophylactic antibiotics may be indicated for large or contaminated burns. Aloe vera gel is useful to relieve pain, and to provide some topical antibiotic and anti-inflammatory effect.

Blisters

Blisters, like the kind you get on your heel while hiking, are caused by the heat generated as your boots and socks rub against your skin. The damage results in swelling and inflammation. Although a blister is only a superficial wound, it can become a major transportation problem.

Blisters progress through three stages, beginning with a hot spot, progressing to a partial-thickness burn, and then bursting to become a contaminated superficial wound. The stage at which you confront blisters, and your logistical situation, will determine your treatment. Generally, blisters are treated the same as other partial-thickness burns.

Treatment of Blisters

If you can stop the friction, you can prevent a blister from forming. Advise your patient to change their socks, adjust shoelaces, and cover the sore area with a liner sock, smooth surface tape, gel dressings, or mole skin. You can also apply antibiotic ointment to lubricate the area and reduce friction.

If a blister does form, it is important to remember that a blister is a sterile wound until it breaks. The best treatment is to leave the overlying skin intact until healing can start. Small blisters can be covered with gel dressing. Larger ones usually cause some degree of disability unless you can take the pressure off.

Blisters

Prevent Friction and Heat:

- Moleskin, donut dressing
- Smooth tape
- Gel dressings

Treatment:

- Unroof blister if it appears infected
- Drain blister if it prevents travel
- Dress as partial thickness burn

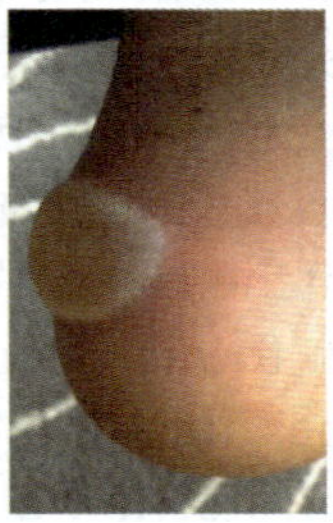

If the blister has formed in a challenging spot, like the back of the heel, you may have to drain it to allow the patient to keep moving. As in draining an abscess, clean the skin around and over the blister with soap and water or antiseptic. Sterilize a sharp knife blade using flame or iodine. Make a small incision in the blister at the lower margin and allow the fluid to drain out. Leave the skin over the blister intact to act as its own sterile dressing. Cover the area with antibiotic ointment and dress it as you might a hot spot. Like any open wound, it must be cleaned and dressed daily, and monitored for signs of infection. Avoid draining blood-filled blisters.

Open blisters occur when a blister has broken into a non-sterile environment. An open blister should be treated like an abrasion. Cut away the dead skin and irrigate to remove debris. Cover the wound with antibiotic ointment and sterile dressings. Clean daily and monitor for infection. Fix the source of friction with padding or tape.

Blisters

Specialized Dressings:

- Maintain moisture and sterility
- Protect from abrasion
- Relieve pain

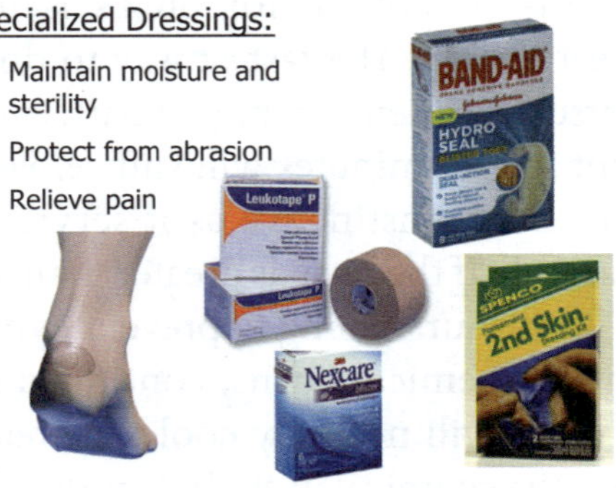

Risk Versus Benefit in Wound Care

Early wound cleaning is a low-risk procedure for a high-risk problem. Conscientious inspection, debridement, and irrigation has been shown to substantially reduce infection rates, especially when accomplished immediately after injury. Early wound closure with staples or sutures does not carry the same benefit and does not justify a high-risk evacuation to a hospital or clinic. Prophylactic antibiotics may reduce the risk of infection in some wounds and should be seriously considered in any high-risk wound. Like wound cleaning, early treatment will yield the best protection.

Wounds and Burns

Wilderness Perspective

High-Risk Problem:

- Large surface area burns
- Systemic infection (lymphangitis, fever)
- Pain out of proportion to apparent injury
- Uncontrolled bleeding or fluid loss
- Respiratory involvement in burn
- Rapidly progressing local infection
- Distal ischemia

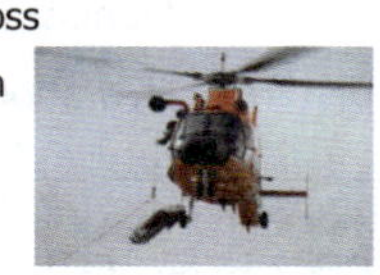

Chapter 16 Review:
Wounds and Burns

- Life-threatening wounds are those that can cause shock, respiratory failure, or brain failure. This includes severe bleeding, penetrating abdominal or chest wounds, respiratory burns, and large surface area skin burns.
- Wounds are described with a variety of terms. For field assessment, the important distinction is low risk or high risk?
- High-risk wounds have the potential to become serious, primarily due to the anticipated problem of infection. These include deep, grossly contaminated puncture and bite wounds and any full-thickness burn.
- Early wound cleaning and dressing can reduce the risk of infection, preserve the wound for later repair, and promote wound healing. Prophylactic antibiotics are sometimes useful to reduce the risk of infection.
- Impaled objects are removed in the field unless the procedure will cause more tissue damage, severe bleeding, or unmanageable pain. Do not remove an object impaled into the globe of the eye.
- The initial treatment for burns is immediate cooling. Burns are then treated like other wounds.
- Hot spots are best treated before becoming blisters. Blisters are treated and protected like other wounds. Blisters are unroofed when contaminated or when necessary for function.
- Bandages and dressings should protect from outside contamination, allow for drainage, avoid causing ischemia, and keep the wound warm and moist.

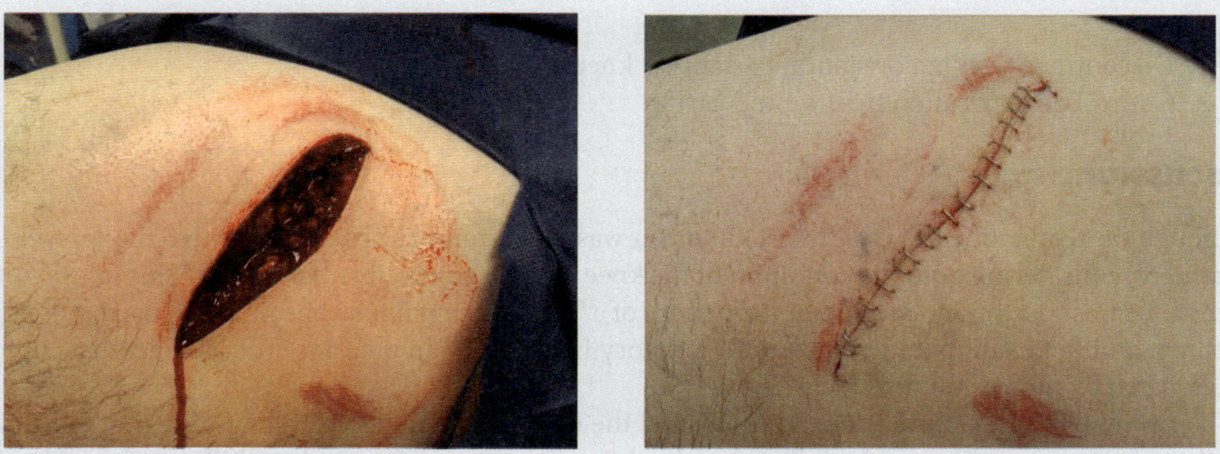

A large but simple thigh wound; clean, straight, and a good candidate for closure with staples in a clinical setting.

Case Study 7: Summer Ski Trip

SCENE
A guided ski trip to a popular summer snowfield in the Canadian Rockies. The guide suffers a knee injury in a fall while leading his group out of the high country in the face of rapidly developing afternoon thunderstorms. The scene is exposed alpine tundra 1 kilometer from the trailhead. At 1605 hours the weather is cloudy with light rain and approaching lightning. Winds are west at 10 m/s and the temperature is 10°C and rapidly falling.

S: A 43-year-old man complains of pain and instability of the left knee after he caught an edge, causing a tumbling fall. He felt a pop and a brief burning pain. On attempting to stand, the knee "gave out." He did not hit his head and has no neck pain. He has full memory of the event. He has an allergy to Vicodin, takes ibuprofen for headaches, has never injured the knee before, and has no significant past medical history. His last meal was 40 minutes ago. The descent was at the end of the day, with only a kilometer to go. He attempted to ski further, but the left knee "gave out" when he tried to stand and became more painful and began to swell. Weight bearing became very uncomfortable.

O: The guide was found sitting upright in stable position with the left knee flexed. He was fully alert, warm, and reasonably dry. He had no spine tenderness. The left knee was tender and moderately swollen. He was able to flex and extend the knee somewhat with moderate discomfort. Distal CSM was intact. There was no other obvious injury. Vital signs at 1610 were normal.

A:

1. Unstable injury left knee
   A': Distal ischemia due to swelling
   A': Pain and further injury from continued use
2. Decaying weather
   A': Lightning strike
   A': Hypothermia

P:

1. Discontinue walking or standing; stabilize knee at the vehicle.
2. Controlled extrication by slide and carry.

Discussion:

Although the temptation to limp the last kilometer was very strong, the patient agreed to the appropriate treatment, considering both the condition of the knee and the environmental threats. This injury fit the criteria for unstable injury because of the history of a "pop" during injury, the sense of instability, rapid swelling, and the inability to bear weight. This story is typical of an anterior cruciate ligament rupture exacerbated by further injury.

The risk of lightning strike and cold motivated the deferral of further examination and stabilization until a safe zone could be reached. Fortunately, the evacuation route was downhill on snow, allowing the clients to remove the guide quickly by sliding him on a tarp almost all the way to their vehicles. The guide's knee will require surgery and months of rehabilitation but will recover. The guide's pride may not.

Case Study 8: Mountaineering

SCENE
A group mountaineering course in the Torres del Paine National Park. A student suffers a hand injury during the descent of a talus slope 8 kilometers from the trailhead. The group is on an independent route-finding exercise, trailed at a distance by their instructor. Alarmed by the response of the patient to the injury, the group has activated their emergency beacon. At 0910 hours the weather is partly cloudy with light winds and a temperature of 12°C.

S: A 17-year-old girl caught her right index finger between loose rocks. She was able to dislodge herself but complained of immediate pain. Shortly afterward, she became dizzy and nauseated, then unresponsive for at least a minute. When the instructor arrived on scene at 0920 hours he was told that the patient did not fall and was not struck by anything. She has no allergies, is not on medication, and has no significant past medical history. She had breakfast 1 hour ago. She had been walking without difficulty prior to the accident and was well rested and hydrated. The rock was stable, but the weather was cool and windy.

O: The patient was found lying against a large rock. She was pale and sweaty, but oriented and responsive. The right index finger was very tender with obvious deformity at the proximal interphalangeal joint. The patient was unable to demonstrate any range of motion. There was no other injury. Vital signs at 0930: BP: unknown, P: 64, R: 24, Skin: pale, cool, moist, T: feels cool, C: A on AVPU with confusion and disorientation, improving.

A:

1. No critical system injury. Unnecessary beacon activation.
2. Dislocation right index finger
   A': Ischemia to infarction
   A': Pain and disability
3. Acute stress reaction now resolved

P:

1. Deactivate beacon
2. Reduce finger dislocation, buddy splint. Monitor CSM.
3. Reassurance

Discussion:

The finger was immersed in a cold stream to relieve pain. The joint was reduced with minimal traction. She was encouraged to lie in a sleeping bag and calm down. Her vital signs rechecked at 1000 were normal. The finger was splinted by taping it to the third finger with a gauze pad between the fingers. The girl was instructed to keep the finger elevated as much as possible and to use cool soaks for swelling and pain relief during rest stops. She was cautioned to check circulation and sensation at the fingertip frequently. She would be referred to medical care when the group reached town in three days.

Although this patient was displaying very frightening signs and symptoms immediately after the injury, there was no mechanism to explain it except acute stress reaction (ASR). The changes in mental status rapidly resolved with rest, reassurance, treatment, and pain relief, leaving only an unhappy girl with a sore finger. Activation of the beacon was inappropriate and could have caused an unnecessary, expensive, and risky rescue response.

Case Study 9: Sail Training Offshore

SCENE

Sail training and research vessel in the Gulf Stream approximately 300 m SE of Cape Cod. The weather was mild but was expected to deteriorate over the next 24 hours.

S: A 23-year-old student was struck on the head by a swinging davit when a cable lowering oceanographic instruments parted. He was found sitting on deck with a large and freely bleeding laceration across the top of his head. He remembered everything about the event. He denied neck pain, and he had no other complaints. He denied allergies, was taking no medications, was well-fed and warm, had no significant medical history, and was up to date on his tetanus vaccination.

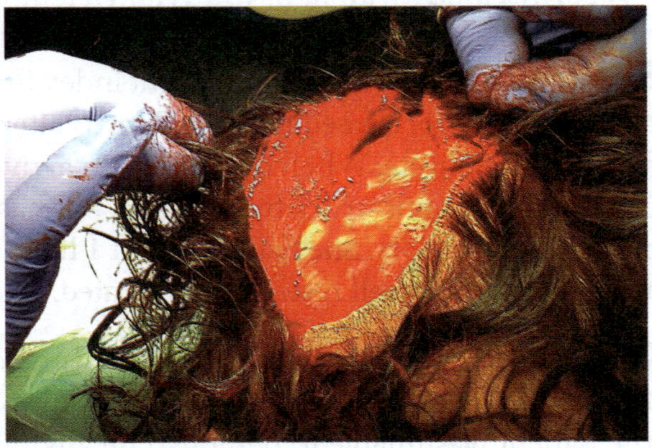

O: Awake, oriented, and cooperative man holding a blood-soaked kerchief on his head. Blood covered his left shoulder and chest, and there was a large pool of it on the deck. He had no neck deformity or tenderness, had full range of motion, and had normal sensation of extremities with no numbness or tingling. The scalp had a 4 cm laceration, clean and straight, through the skin and subcutaneous tissue to the skull. No depression or bone fragments could be seen or felt. Vital signs at 1805: BP: 112/78, P: 88, R: 16, C: awake and oriented, T: normal, Skin: normal color and temperature.

A:

1. Scalp wound
   A': Wound infection (unlikely)

P:

1. Direct pressure to stop bleeding
2. Wound irrigation and dressing
3. Monitor for infection, change dressings daily
4. Follow-up in Bermuda on planned port call in three days

Discussion:

The scalp did just what it was designed to do by absorbing enough of the force of the impact to protect the skull and brain. There was no traumatic brain injury, just a scalp wound. As is common with the scalp, bleeding was profuse but easily controlled with direct pressure. Although it looked like a lot of blood, vital signs showed that not enough was lost to produce shock. Because of the rich blood supply in the scalp, even deep scalp wounds usually heal well with a very low incidence of infection. There was no serious medical problem here.

Section V: Environmental Medicine

Chapter 17: Thermoregulation

The core of the human body operates most efficiently at or very near a temperature of 37°C. The brain automatically adjusts heat production and retention based on information from temperature sensors in the skin and body core. This thermoregulatory system uses muscles to generate heat, the skin to dissipate heat, and the endocrine system to control metabolism. Blood vessels in the skin dilate to dissipate or release heat or constrict to preserve heat. Sweat glands release fluid to enhance cooling by evaporation. Shivering produces heat with involuntary exercise. You can watch this compensation mechanism work, but it is not under your direct control.

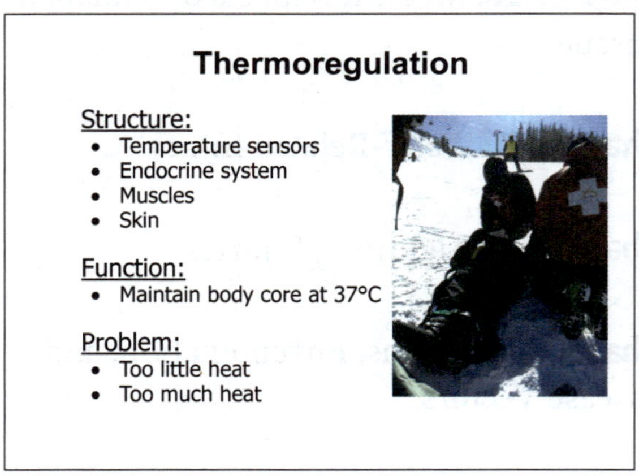

Because your body core is always at a temperature of about 37°C, your conscious perception of hot or cold comes from sensors in your skin. When heat energy is released into your skin by contact with a warm object, you *feel* warmth. When heat energy is removed from your skin, you *feel* cold. In the healthy individual the perception of being warm or cold, and the need to produce or dissipate heat, is based primarily on conditions affecting the body shell.

A number of things can influence this perception. Alcohol in a beverage, for example, is a vasodilator that allows more warm blood to perfuse the skin surface, reversing the shell/core compensation. It impairs normal shivering and inhibits effective thermoregulatory sensation and response. Additionally, too much alcohol will impair a person's ability and desire to care for themselves in cold weather.

This example reminds us that our conscious efforts are important to thermoregulation, too. Even the best body morphology will not keep you healthy if you do not pay attention to hydration, calories, and shelter. Problems with heat and cold often have their origins in poor judgment.

Problems with thermoregulation can also develop when the function of the system is impaired by illness, injury, toxins, or medication. The system can also be overwhelmed by environmental extremes. Maintaining the function of the thermoregulatory system is a key element of patient care in the wilderness setting.

Hypothermia

Cold response is a normal reaction to feeling cold and starts long before the body core temperature begins to fall with the onset of hypothermia. Shell/core compensation reduces heat loss to the environment, while shivering increases heat production from muscle activity. The discomfort you feel by being cold motivates your conscious effort to add layers of clothing and get out of the weather. If the system works normally and is not overwhelmed by an extreme challenge, normal core temperature and mental status is preserved.

Nobody can mount an effective cold response when short on food and fluids. Shivering is a very efficient form of heat production but requires a tremendous amount of energy. Living outside in a cold environment can require more than 6,000 calories a day. Adequate glycogen stores and easily digested food must be available to maintain the effort. Normal body fluid volume is also required to generate and distribute heat effectively.

Normal Body Compensation

Heat Response:

- Vasodilation
- Sweat

Cold Response:

- Shivering
- Vasoconstriction
- Cold diuresis

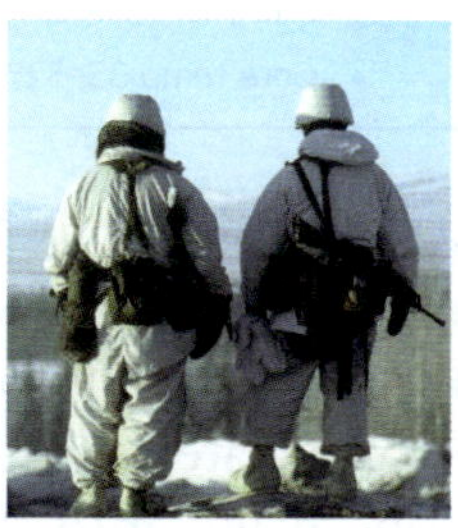

"You can watch these mechanisms work, but they are not under your direct control."

An anticipated problem associated with the cold response is cold diuresis. This is the tendency of the body to produce more urine when shell/core compensation occurs. As blood is shunted from the shell into the core, the kidneys sense an increase in fluid volume in the central circulation and act to get rid of some of it. Cold diuresis and the logistics involved in obtaining fresh water in an extreme environment can lead to dehydration.

Although cold response is normal and healthy, it carries the anticipated problem of hypothermia. Several factors can accelerate the process. A patient who is immobilized by injury will not be able to exercise or consciously act to retain heat. Drugs that cause vasodilatation of the skin result in greater heat loss. Chronic endocrine system problems like hypothyroidism or diabetes can impair the body's ability to sense or respond to temperature changes. Elderly people have less muscle mass and a reduced ability to perceive and respond to heat loss. Children tend to have less body fat and a greater surface area to mass ratio, which also increases the rate of heat loss.

Impaired Compensation

- Immobilized by injury, unable to generate heat
- Multiple trauma, volume shock
- Illness that impairs circulation, metabolism, sweat production, or temperature sense
- Drugs that inhibit temperature regulation: cocaine, methamphetamine, diuretics, behavioral medications, pseudoephedrine.
- Extremes of age
- Sunburn

Reversing cold response requires insulation, protection, calories, and fluids. To reverse a cold response most effectively, you need to understand the physics of heat production, retention, and dissipation. Heat energy flows from warmer objects (like your patient) to colder objects (like the ground or litter). The mechanisms are conduction, convection, evaporation, and radiation. In protecting and packaging your patient, you must consider the combined effect of all these forms of heat loss.

Conduction is heat transfer between objects in contact. The denser the object, the faster heat energy is transferred. Your patient will lose heat more quickly to the cold hard ground they are lying on than to the low-density foam pad that you should have placed under them.

Convection is heat transfer via moving fluids, including air and water. Although air is the least dense substance, there is an infinite supply of it. Heat lost to wind or even to the air billowing in and out of loose clothing can be considerable. Water works the same way, just 25 times faster.

Evaporation refers to the heat energy absorbed by water as it turns into water vapor. The body uses this very efficient mechanism for cooling in the form of sweat. Water evaporating from the skin will cool your patient very efficiently whether they need it or not.

Radiant heat energy is emitted and absorbed by all objects, including your patient. This is long-wave electromagnetic radiation well below the frequency of visible light. This energy is the warmth you feel from sunlight or a campfire. Radiant heat from your body can be absorbed by dense or thick clothing or reflected to you by a foil covering.

Transfer of Heat Energy

Conduction: by direct contact

Convection: by wind or moving water

Radiation: by long-wave energy

Evaporation: by water absorbing energy as it evaporates from skin

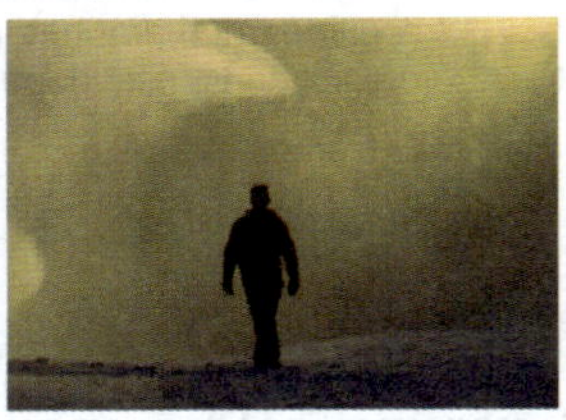

Noncompressible insulation such as a closed-cell foam pad should be used to protect the patient from conductive heat loss to the ground or other cold objects. High-loft, low-density insulation such as a synthetic or down sleeping bag forms a dead air space around the patient, reducing convective heat loss and trapping the radiant heat being emitted by the patient.

A waterproof vapor barrier around the insulation prevents wetting of the package from rain or snow and reduces the evaporative cooling from moisture already on the patient.

Support for heat production is equally critical. Your patient needs calories and fluids to fuel shivering. Simple sugars are best at first. They are absorbed and converted into energy quickly. Complex carbohydrates, fats, and protein can be added later to maintain heat production.

Adding heat in the form of warm liquids or heat packs is comforting, but not as useful as the calories, hydration, and exercise. The heat energy in a cup of hot tea is minimal compared to the heat that is produced when the patient burns the four tablespoons of honey you put into the tea. Do not delay food and fluids while waiting for your stove to heat up.

Most of the time, your rewarming efforts will be successful. Sometimes, the system fails or is overwhelmed by environmental conditions, resulting in a drop in body core temperature. Shell/core compensation persists, shivering continues, and your patient's mental status begins to decay. Your anticipated problem has become the existing problem.

Mild Hypothermia

Mild Hypothermia

Mechanism:

- Heat loss exceeds heat production
- Onset can be acute or sub-acute

Signs and Symptoms:

- Early brain failure with mild to moderate mental status changes
- Shivering
- Shell/core effect
- Core temp 35–32°C

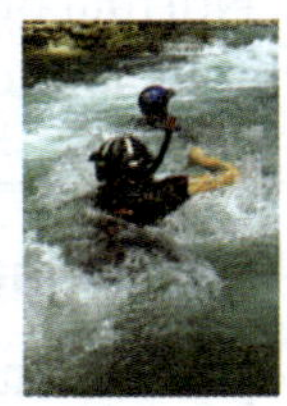

Rescuers will certainly think of hypothermia in cases of obvious and extreme exposure such as cold-water immersion. Even dressed for cold weather, ice water can kill you within an hour or two. Nobody will miss the diagnosis in situations like this.

In most backcountry situations, however, the onset of hypothermia is more often insidious than dramatic. It progresses slowly and quietly in a patient who is just a little cold for a long time. In this case, the problem is easy to overlook.

Hypothermia may be the primary problem you are treating or a side effect of environmental conditions. It is a common complication in trauma cases in which a patient has remained immobile for hours while waiting for evacuation. It also develops in rescue team members waiting hours for instructions.

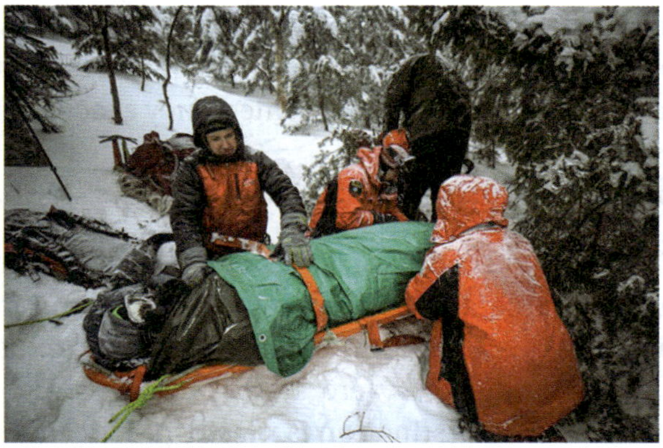

Hypothermia is a dangerous complication in trauma cases where patients may lay immobile for hours awaiting evacuation.

In rapid onset cases such as cold water immersion, there is often a marked difference in temperature between the cold body shell and the still relatively warm body core. People often become incapacitated by cooling of extremity muscles before they become severely hypothermic. Generally, the patient has not had time to become significantly dehydrated or glycogen depleted. This is called acute hypothermia, and spontaneous rewarming is usually possible once the patient has been removed from the water, dried, and insulated.

In slow onset cases, called subacute hypothermia, glycogen stores and blood sugar have been depleted. The patient is usually dehydrated. The temperature difference between shell and core is not as dramatic. These patients are not able to rewarm without help. In fact, rewarming efforts can be lethal without hydration and food.

Mild Hypothermia: Acute

- Rapid onset, minutes to hours (cold water)
- Usually not dehydrated or calorie depleted
- Spontaneous rewarming is usually possible

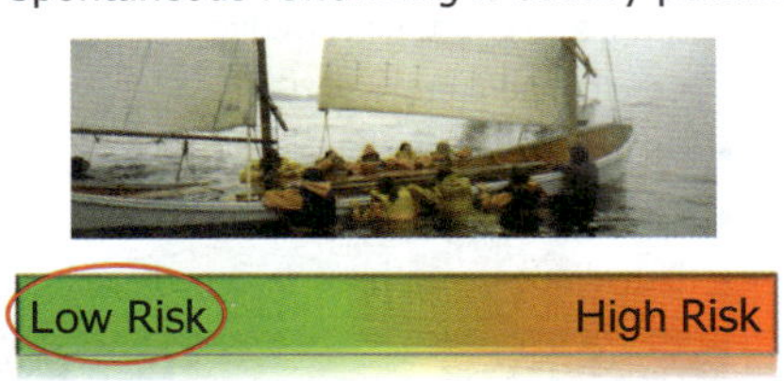

Mild Hypothermia: Sub Acute

- Slow onset, hours to days
- Dehydrated and calorie depleted
- Will not rewarm spontaneously

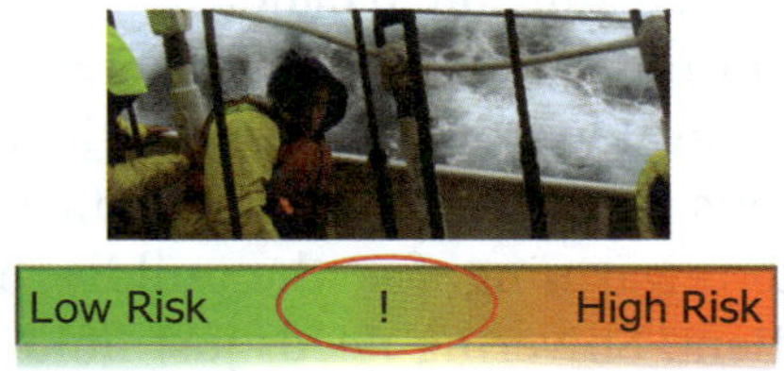

The most obvious signs of mild hypothermia are mental status changes and shivering. The patient may be lethargic, withdrawn, confused, or exhibit other personality changes. The skin is pale and cool, and there may be some loss of dexterity in the extremities as the shell/core compensation reduces blood flow. Body core temperature measures below 35°C. Shivering can be mild to severe. If the patient is not already dehydrated, cold diuresis may continue with the patient producing relatively dilute urine.

Vital Signs in Mild Hypothermia:

- **Pulse:** Normal to slightly elevated
- **Blood pressure:** Normal
- **Respirations:** Normal
- **Temperature:** Between 32° and 35°C
- **Consciousness:** A to V on AVPU; mild to moderate mental status changes
- **Skin:** Shell/core compensation

The most accurate body core temperature measurements are made by esophageal probe, which is not usually available for field rescue. Rectal measurements would be the next most useful. A special low-reading clinical thermometer is required for measuring core temperature below 34°C. Oral, ear, and skin surface measurements are frequently inaccurate in hypothermia.

Treatment of Mild Hypothermia

Mild hypothermia is a serious problem requiring immediate and aggressive treatment in the field. The anticipated problem, severe hypothermia, will be much more difficult to handle. The treatment is essentially the same as that for cold response: protect from heat loss and restore calories and fluid.

Vigorous shivering is the most efficient form of field rewarming for the mildly hypothermic patient. Shivering needs just fluid and fuel. Adding external heat with hot water bottles or body heaters is generally safe and certainly more comfortable, but no attempt to mobilize and exercise the patient should be made until obvious improvement in mental status is noted, especially in cases of subacute hypothermia.

Mild Hypothermia

Treatment:

- Immediate field rewarming
- Food and fluids
- Trap heat generated by shivering
- Insulate from convection, conduction, radiation
- Dry skin and clothing to reduce evaporation
- Exercise only when improvement is noted
- Package and evacuate if not improving

All hypothermic patients experience some degree of afterdrop, where the body core temperature continues to decrease even after rewarming has begun. This is due to the physics of heat transfer through any medium, but it is exacerbated by vasodilatation of the body shell and circulation of blood through the cooler extremities as the patient rewarms. As a result your patient may get a little worse before getting better, especially if you exercise them too soon, which seems to cause a greater degree of afterdrop. It may require over 40 minutes of shivering, sugar, fluids, and aggressive external rewarming before an improvement in symptoms indicates that it is safe to allow the patient to exercise.

In many cases field treatment for mild hypothermia will be definitive and evacuation will not be necessary. Remember, however, that mild hypothermia that cannot be fixed will eventually become severe hypothermia. Inadequate response to field treatment warrants emergency evacuation.

Severe Hypothermia

For hospital treatment, several distinct stages of hypothermia are defined to guide the resuscitation effort. Most commonly these are referred to as mild, moderate, severe, and profound. For field treatment the distinction is mostly practical: can the patient cooperate with your treatment or not? A very cold patient who is not awake and/or is not shivering and cannot cooperate with treatment is treated as severely hypothermic. An accurate measurement of core temperature is not required.

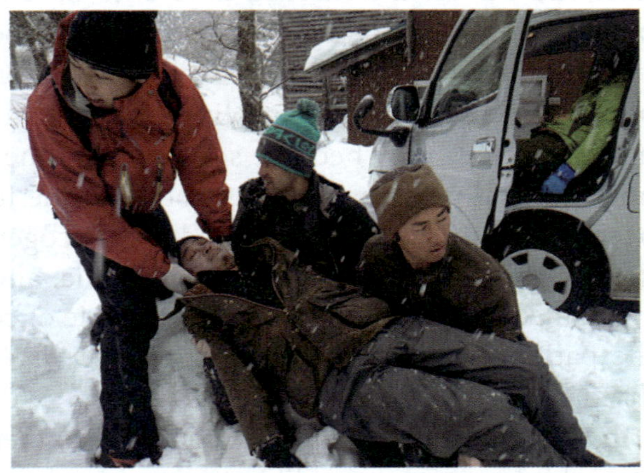

As the core temperature falls below 32°C mental status changes are followed by a drop to V, P, or U on the AVPU scale. This is quite different from the subdued but awake mild hypothermic. Shivering stops as muscles are deactivated by shell cooling and lack of calories to burn.

Severe Hypothermia

Signs and Symptoms:

- Brain failure (V, P, or U on AVPU)
- Shell/core effect, no shivering
- Core temperature < 32°C
- VS may be undetectable
- Cardiac irritability
- Dehydration, metabolic derangement

Low Risk High Risk

Treatment of Severe Hypothermia

The ideal treatment for severe hypothermia is controlled rewarming in a hospital, preferably a Level 1 trauma center. Take the time to package the patient properly before initiating a gentle but urgent evacuation. This should include heat sources such as warm water bottles or a charcoal heat pack applied to the thorax. This minimizes heat loss and may begin rewarming, improving the stability of the cardiovascular system. Rough handling can cause the cold heart to go into ventricular fibrillation. Keep the patient horizontal.

Positive pressure ventilation with heated air will help reduce heat lost to respiration. Because the patient's oxygen demand and production of CO_2 is decreased, the rate can be reduced to about six breaths per minute. The best source of heated and humidified air in the backcountry is probably going to be your own breath supplied through a pocket mask. If available, intravenous normal saline warmed to 40°C can restore fluid volume without contributing to heat loss.

In extremely cold patients, pulse and respiration may not be detectable. It is quite possible to mistake severe hypothermia for death. Anecdotal experience and animal studies suggest that even patients in apparent cardiopulmonary arrest may be salvageable if the body core temperature is above 10°C and definitive medical care can be accessed within a reasonable time. However, any significant risk to rescuers will not be justified by the low probability of success.

Severe Hypothermia

Evacuation:

- Package with added heat source to begin rewarming
- Urgent but gentle evacuation to hospital maintained in horizontal position
- PPV with heated and humidified O2, 6/min
- Warmed IV if available
- No chest compressions if it will delay transport or put rescuers at risk.

Most authorities recommend that CPR be performed on all patients without a palpable pulse. However, we believe that performing CPR on a hypothermic patient during a backcountry evacuation is counterproductive and may be harmful, especially if it delays access to definitive care. In addition, chest compressions may cause a very slow but functional cardiac rhythm to decay into ventricular fibrillation. For these reasons, we recommend attempting only rewarming and PPV during a litter or toboggan transport.

If you are waiting at a helicopter landing zone or trailhead, continuous CPR may be beneficial. As the science of hypothermia resuscitation continues to evolve, several cases have documented success with high quality CPR and timely access to advanced medical care. How long CPR can continue pending helicopter or ambulance transport will likely be determined by resources and rescuer endurance.

If evacuation from the field is impossible, rewarming a severely hypothermic patient in place can be attempted. Find shelter and apply heat to the patient any way that you can, but try to avoid aggressive external rewarming like immersion in a hot spring or exposure to a hot engine room. This may produce vasodilatation and shock. Add sugar orally if the patient rewarms enough to protect the airway. Dextrose can also be added to an IV. If you succeed in improving level of consciousness and mental status, recognize that metabolic derangement may be significant and evacuation to medical care is still the ideal plan when it can be accomplished.

If the patient is in apparent cardiac arrest, try to warm them enough to produce detectable vital signs. Perform CPR if you have the resources to do so. If no pulse or other life signs (including organized electrical activity on a monitor) are observed after 30 minutes of external heat and warmed PPV, the effort can be discontinued.

> **Severe Hypothermia**
> ***Wilderness Perspective***
>
> Do Not Resuscitate:
> - Obvious lethal injury
> - The chest is frozen
> - The core temperature is below 10°C
> - Submerged underwater more than one hour
> - Airway packed with snow in avalanche burial > 35 minutes

If an AED is available, we recommend one shock if prompted and one round of medications per protocol if the body core temperature is above 25°C. Rewarming efforts and CPR should be resumed, and a measurable increase in temperature observed, before trying defibrillation and medications again. How long advanced level field resuscitation should continue is the subject of some debate. Real field experience is very limited, but one hour is probably a generous maximum. In any case, do not put yourself and your group at risk by continuing a resuscitation effort to the point of exhaustion.

Heat-Related Illness

Because vital organs work best at a temperature around 37°C, the body conserves only as much heat as it needs to keep it at that temperature and gets rid of the rest. Your primary mechanism for heat dissipation is skin vasodilatation and sweat. When sweat evaporates, it absorbs a tremendous amount of heat energy from the skin surface. This is a very effective cooling system if there is enough blood and sweat to keep it going. The body constantly sacrifices fluid to maintain normal temperature in hot environments.

Like cold response, heat response is a normal process. If heat dissipation is not overwhelmed by heat production and retention, the body core temperature will remain within an acceptable range. Eventually, continued heat stress will result in diminished performance and less heat production, especially in people not acclimated to the conditions. It can take two weeks or more to fully acclimatize to a hot environment.

Heat response carries the anticipated problems of heat exhaustion and heat stroke. It can be reversed by reducing heat exposure and production, and by fluid replacement as needed. Although urine output and color are often mentioned as the best field indicators of fluid status, thirst is probably more reliable. Thirst almost always precedes significant volume depletion and is a good reminder to drink before you have a fluid problem.

Heat Exhaustion

Heat exhaustion is the term used for a heat related condition characterized by elevation of core body temp above 38°C and non-specific symptoms that can include fatigue, weakness, nausea, headache, often making continued exertion nearly impossible. For field purposes, heat exhaustion is diminished performance due to heat stress. Heat exhaustion may also signal impending heat stroke.

The heat exhausted patient is awake with normal mental status, but complains of nausea, headache, and weakness. The history may reveal inadequate time to acclimatize to a new environment or increased work load. The patient may report low food and fluid intake and reduced urine output. Body core temperature is normal to slightly elevated.

Fatigue is the primary problem and there may be some degree of dehydration. If addressed early this is not a serious problem, but it requires immediate treatment in the field. The progression of heat illness must be halted and reversed.

Treatment of Heat Exhaustion

The treatment of heat exhaustion is the same as it is for heat response, just more urgent. Move the patient into a cooler area and stop physical exertion to reduce heat production. Begin active cooling if not improving.

If fluid replacement is needed, oral fluids are usually effective, but IV is faster. If the patient is vomiting, oral replacement is still possible by giving fluid frequently in small amounts. Without IV fluids, it may take more than 12 hours to bring the dehydrated patient back to normal. Look for less thirst, increased urine production, and an improved sense of well-being as an indication of success. In most cases, field treatment for heat exhaustion will be definitive and evacuation will not be necessary.

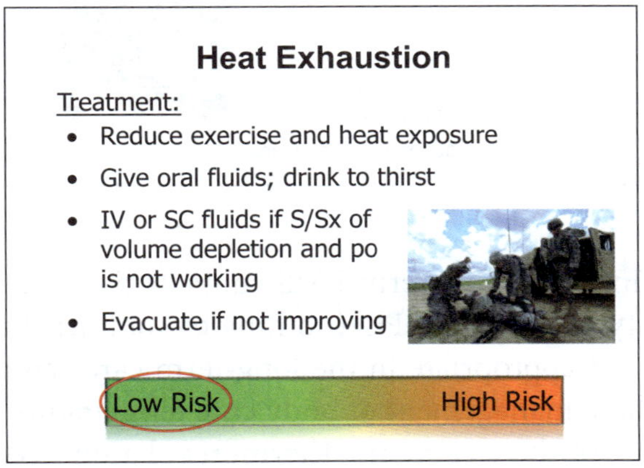

Heat Stroke

Heat stroke is a serious critical system problem requiring immediate field treatment. The primary problem is dangerously elevated body core temperature, which is capable of significant damage to the central nervous system and other vital organs. Aggressive cooling is required. The patient may also be in volume shock from dehydration, but this is not the focus of immediate field treatment.

The mechanism of injury may be extreme heat production from vigorous exercise or exposure to high ambient temperatures and confining clothing. Generally, it is some combination of the two, like wildland firefighting or a forced march in hot weather. The patient may have become heat exhausted first or progressed directly to heat stroke. Medications can also play an important role. People taking diuretics and psychotropic medications are at greater risk of developing heat stroke and other heat-related problems.

A person can maintain normal mental status for a brief period with a body core temperature as high as 40.5°C. But eventually, mental status changes will develop followed rapidly by a drop on the AVPU scale. The skin may have the classic hot, red, and dry appearance, but this is not always the case. With extreme heat exposure, a critical rise in core temperature can occur before the patient has time to become dehydrated. The skin may be still wet with sweat. The patient will feel hot.

Treatment of Heat Stroke

In the field, a hot patient with altered mental status has heat stroke and immediate and aggressive cooling is required. Immersion in cold water is ideal. As an alternative, you can maximize heat loss from the entire body surface by evaporation, conduction, and radiation if available. Just applying ice to the neck, armpits, and groin is insufficient. Look for an improvement in level of consciousness and mental status to indicate the return to a more normal temperature.

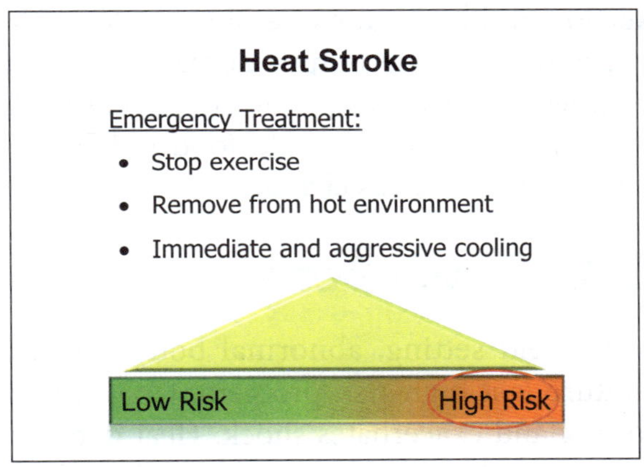

Fluid replacement is part of the treatment but only after core temperature is effectively managed. IV fluid replacement is ideal but oral fluids may work if the patient can cooperate and protect their airway. The high temperature may have caused brain injury with the anticipated problem of elevated intracranial pressure (ICP). A condition called rhabdomyolysis may develop, leading to kidney failure. Advanced life support (ALS) intervention is a priority and emergency evacuation is justified. These patients are best served by treatment and observation in the hospital.

Heat Stroke

Continued care after cooling:

- IV or PO hydration for normal urine output
- Food as tolerated
- Protect from heat challenge
- Evacuate to hospital, urgent if abnormal mental status or abnormal urine output

Where immediate evacuation would be high risk, transport may be deferred if mental status and other vital signs promptly return to normal. Field care should include rest and enough oral hydration to maintain normal urine output. Avoid exertion and heat exposure. Reconsider urgent evacuation if urine output decreases or urine becomes red or brown, or if the patient begins to feel worse, is unable to take food and fluids, or exhibits mental status changes.

Risk Versus Benefit

In the field setting, abnormal body core temperature is a high-risk problem. Cold inhibits clotting and exacerbates shock. Heat denatures protein, leading to tissue damage, kidney failure, and elevated ICP, contributing to vascular and volume shock. Maintaining normal body core temperature is part of routine treatment that will vastly improve outcome, even in critically ill or injured patients. Hypothermia as therapy, even with post-cardiac arrest patients, remains controversial. In any case, therapeutic hypothermia is reserved for carefully controlled EMS or hospital environments.

Heat-Related Illness
Wilderness Perspective

High-Risk Problem:

- VS do not return to normal
- Persistent altered mental status
- Decreased urine output
- Urine color becomes red or brown
- You cannot prevent exposure to heat
- The patient is getting worse

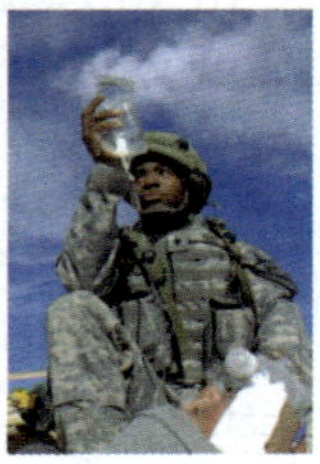

In most short-term EMS contacts the patient is typically kept NPO (nothing by mouth). This is not appropriate in the long-term care setting where management of body core temperature is part of the treatment. Thermoregulation needs fluid and calories. Oral intake is acceptable if airway protection is not a problem.

The need to control fever in systemic illness (as opposed to heat stroke) is debatable. Generally, if a fever is making the patient uncomfortable you should act to lower body core temperature with acetaminophen, ibuprofen, or cool water. Fever associated with altered mental status indicates a critical system problem and the need for emergency evacuation.

Chapter 17 Review: Thermoregulation

- Heat energy is transferred by conduction, convection, radiation, and evaporation. All are important to consider when assisting a patient with thermoregulation.
- The key signs and symptoms of mild hypothermia include cold and pale skin, uncontrollable shivering, and altered mental status.
- Acute hypothermia is rapid onset with less dehydration and calorie depletion. Spontaneous rewarming is possible. Subacute hypothermia develops over hours or days and is accompanied by dehydration and calorie depletion. Insulation, rehydration, and restoration of energy stores are necessary for rewarming.
- The key signs and symptoms of severe hypothermia are a cold person who is V, P, or U on the AVPU scale or shivering has stopped. The pulse may be slow or undetectable. Body core temperature is below 32°C.
- Severe hypothermia should be considered an emergency. The ideal treatment is controlled rewarming in a hospital. Evacuation should be gentle but expeditious with rewarming around the thorax en route.
- If evacuation is impossible, severe hypothermia can be rewarmed in the field by applying heat around the thorax. Sugar can be given under the tongue as a paste or gel when the patient is positioned to protect the airway. Warmed IVs and dextrose may be given. Urgent but gentle evacuation should be accomplished when it becomes possible.
- CPR may cause cardiac arrest in a severely hypothermic patient. CPR should be initiated only when a palpable pulse or monitored rhythm is lost and/or it will not interfere with efficient evacuation to definitive care.
- Because vital organs work best at a temperature of around 37°C, the body conserves only as much heat as it needs to keep it at that temperature and gets rid of the rest, primarily through skin vasodilatation and sweat.
- Heat exhaustion is extreme fatigue from heat stress. It may be associated with dehydration.
- The field treatment for heat exhaustion is shade, rest, and adequate hydration.
- Heat stroke is a major critical system problem requiring immediate and aggressive cooling. The primary problem is dangerously elevated body core temperature, which is capable of significant damage to the central nervous system and other vital organs.
- It is ideal to evacuate any heat stroke patient to hospital care once temperature is controlled. Patients who recover quickly in the field to normal mental status and have normal urine output may be considered less urgent for evacuation.

Chapter 18: Cold Injuries

Frostbite injures tissue through a complex process involving ischemia to infarction, metabolic derangement, cellular dehydration, ice crystal formation, blood clots, and inflammation. Trench foot is tissue damage from prolonged cold-induced vasoconstriction, resulting in ischemia and associated pain, inflammation, swelling, and secondary infection.

Because nerves are the first to be affected by ischemia, the earliest symptom of cold injury is often numbness, explaining why it is easy to ignore at first. Not only can the tissue damage be a serious medical problem, but the loss of use of hands or feet can be a challenge to survival in a difficult situation.

Frostbite

Contact with subfreezing air, rock, or ice is required to produce frostbite. It is unlikely to occur above a temperature of -15°C unless heat loss is accelerated by the evaporation of a volatile liquid like gasoline. Tissue will not freeze if the ambient temperature is at or above 0°C, even with wind chill.

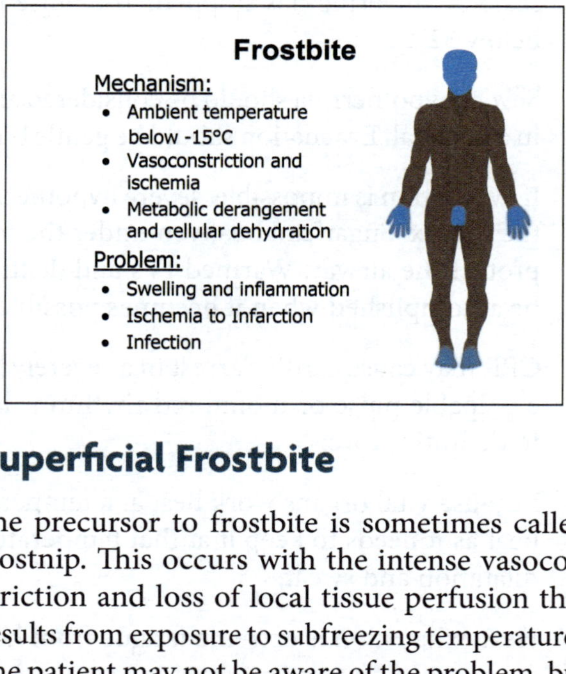

Superficial Frostbite

The precursor to frostbite is sometimes called frostnip. This occurs with the intense vasoconstriction and loss of local tissue perfusion that results from exposure to subfreezing temperatures. The patient may not be aware of the problem, but sensation to touch is usually intact and occasionally painful. The area appears pink or white, but still feels soft to the touch. Ice crystals may form on the surface, but not within the tissue.

In frostnip, only the outer layers of skin are affected. Damage is minimal and prompt rewarming at this stage does not result in disability or tissue loss. Simply covering the area and warming the patient to reverse shell/core compensation is usually enough. The patient may experience mild inflammation and pain. There is no blister formation, but the area may be more susceptible to cold injury for a while.

Frostbite Field Assessment

Frostnip and Superficial Frostbite:

- Soft, pale, cold, numb
- Involves dermis only
- Moves freely over subcutaneous tissue

Deep Frostbite:

- Hard, pale or blue, no sensation
- Frozen into subcutaneous tissue
- Involved joints do not move

Superficial frostbite occurs when the water in skin cells begins to freeze. Sensation is dulled, and the area appears white or blue but still feels soft or doughy to the touch. Because subcutaneous tissue is not yet involved, the skin still moves easily over joints and soft tissue. At this point, however, the damage has begun. Because water expands in volume as it solidifies, cells and blood vessels suffer mechanical trauma during the freezing process.

Like frostnip, the treatment for superficial frostbite is immediate field rewarming. Cover the area and feed, hydrate, and warm the patient. The rewarmed area will likely be red and sore and may develop superficial blisters. Continued care includes wound management and protection from trauma and refreezing. Blisters should be left intact unless drainage is required for mobility and survival. Long-term disability is unlikely, but scar formation in the injured tissue can cause an increased lifelong susceptibility to frostbite.

Frostbite Field Treatment

Frostnip and Superficial Frostbite:

- Immediate field rewarming
- Reverse shell/core effect
- Protect from refreezing
- Leave blisters intact
- Protect from trauma

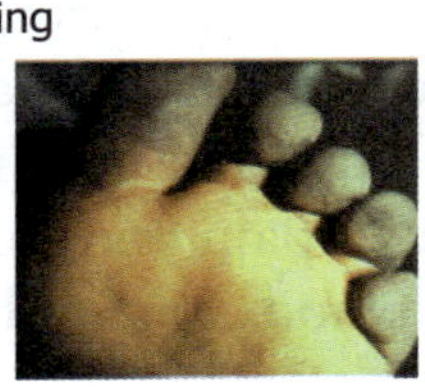

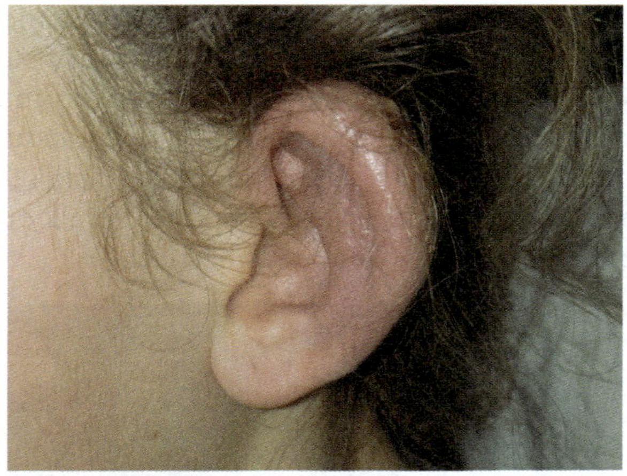

Rewarmed superficial frostbite.

Deep Frostbite

Deep frostbite is a serious injury worthy of emergency evacuation. The skin and underlying tissues are frozen solid. The area is white or bluish and hard to the touch. The skin does not move over joints or underlying tissues. Ice crystals are usually visible on the skin surface, and there is a complete loss of sensation. The digit or extremity feels like a club.

Frostbite: Field Treatment

Deep Frostbite:

- The *ideal* treatment is evacuation to controlled rewarming in a medical facility
- No field rewarming if evacuation can be accomplished within 24 hours
- Protect patient and injured extremity to prevent further freezing

"A patient can walk or ski on frozen feet. Once rewarmed, a carry-out or air evacuation will be necessary."

Deep frostbite is ideally rewarmed under controlled conditions in a medical facility. Much of the tissue damage from prolonged or very deep freezing occurs during and after rewarming. There is demonstrated benefit to early treatment in the hospital with thrombolytics and vasodilators to improve perfusion and oxygenation of rewarmed tissue. Consultation with a burn center familiar with the treatment of deep frostbite is ideal.

Inflammation, pain, and infection are anticipated problems. Rewarmed tissue is very susceptible to further injury, even from normal use. Refreezing is devastating. Allowing tissue to remain frozen for several hours during a self-evacuation is better than attempting to walk out on painful and swollen rewarmed feet.

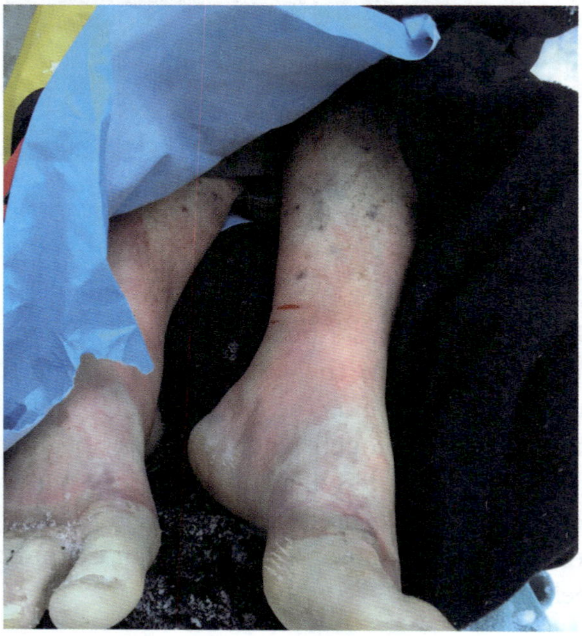

In deep frostbite the skin and underlying tissues are frozen solid. The area is white or bluish and hard to the touch.

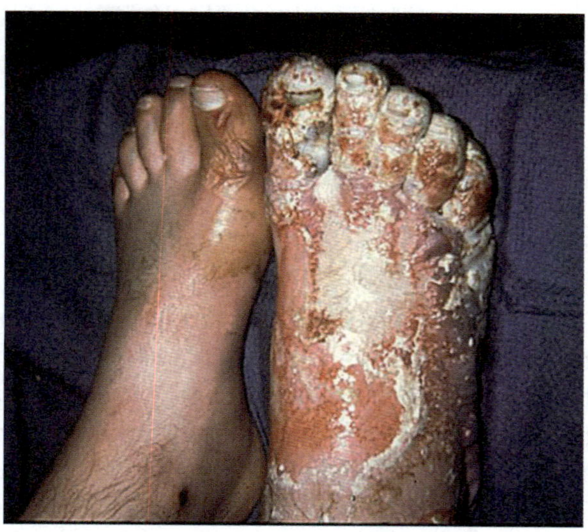

The foot on the right was frozen, rewarmed, and frozen again before hospital admission. The left foot remained frozen until controlled rewarming was performed.

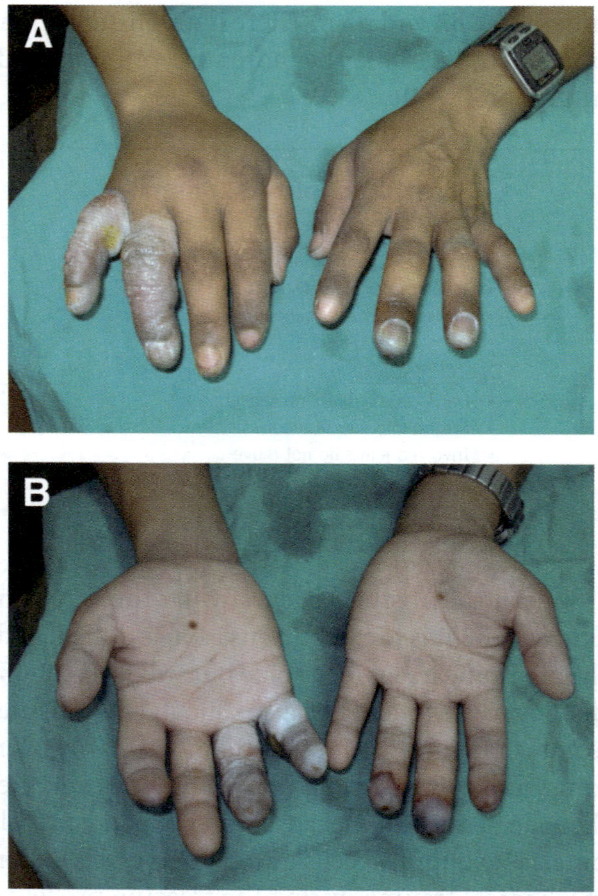

Figure A: Ecchymotic frostbitten lesions on ventral aspect of fingers on both hands. Figure B: Swollen right 4th and 5th fingers showing ruptured blistering at the base of 5th finger.

Subedi BH, Pokharel J, Thapa R, Banskota N, Basnyat B. Frostbite in a sherpa. Wilderness Environ Med. 2010;21(2):127-9. Reprinted with permission from the Wilderness Medical Society. ©2010 Wilderness Medical Society.

Field rewarming of deep frostbite is less than ideal but should be considered if evacuation will be dangerous or prolonged. You must have the necessary shelter and equipment and be able to prevent refreezing. *Do not rewarm in the field if use of the extremity will be necessary for survival and evacuation.* Set up a secure shelter, and be sure your patient is warm, dry, well fed, and hydrated.

Premedicate with an anti-inflammatory drug like ibuprofen (800 mg) taken by mouth. This reduces pain and inflammation and helps prevent blood clots in the rewarmed tissue. Giving stronger pain medication may be necessary during the process.

Rewarming is performed by immersing the frozen extremity in water warmed to between 37° and 39°C. The water should feel warm to normal skin, but not uncomfortable. Keep adding warm water to the pot to maintain the temperature as the thawing process continues. Avoid direct exposure to dry heat like a camp fire. Rewarmed tissue will appear red and blue and feel soft to the touch. Blisters may form early and be clear, red, or blue depending on the fluid inside.

Once the part is rewarmed, it is vital to protect it from trauma. This means no use of the digit or extremity. Sterile dressings should be placed over and between digits, and the extremity should be bandaged and splinted to restrict movement. Absolutely never allow the part to refreeze. If the feet are affected, a carry-out or air evacuation is necessary.

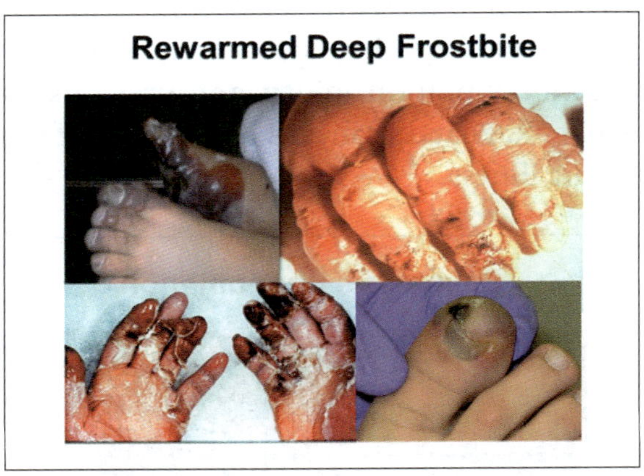

Monitor frequently to ensure that splints or bandages do not constrict circulation as swelling develops. If possible, keep the part elevated. Continue regular doses of ibuprofen at a minimum of 12 mg/kg divided twice daily. This may be increased to a maximum of 2,400 mg divided four times daily if the patient is experiencing pain. If you have it, cover the area with aloe vera gel or ointment, which has been shown to have both anti-inflammatory and antibacterial properties.

Rewarmed frostbite is a high-risk wound. Early surgical referral is indicated. Blister formation will occur over hours to days, and the sloughing of dead tissue will continue for weeks. With competent treatment, most of the damaged tissue can be salvaged.

The spontaneous rewarming of deep frostbite without the benefit of warm water immersion has been shown to produce a worse outcome but may be the side effect of rewarming and protecting a cold patient. As a treatment, it is a last resort. However, most experts agree that it is better than intentionally keeping a foot or hand frozen while the rest of the patient is rewarmed.

Prevention of Frostbite

Anything that restricts the circulation of warm blood to tissues allows freezing to occur more readily. In people who are already a little chilled, shell/core compensation reduces perfusion to the extremities to maintain core temperature. Constricting clothing such as ski boots or a splint tied too tightly can reduce blood flow as well. Cigarette smoking is an additional core temperature factor, infusing the body tissues with nicotine, which is a powerful vasoconstrictor.

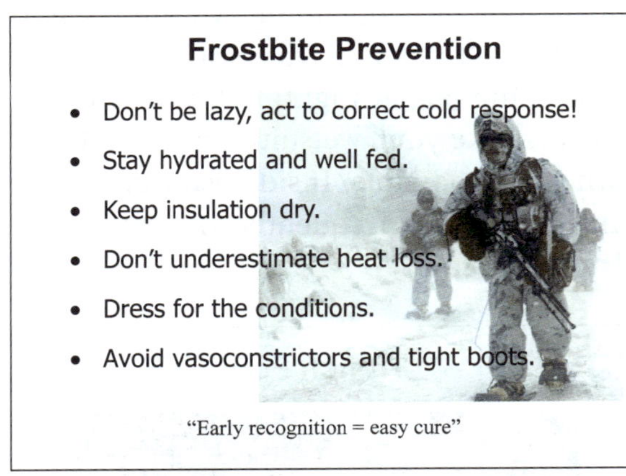

Certainly, well-insulated and fitted boots, gloves, and a face mask can go a long way toward preventing frostbite in extreme conditions. But equally important is maintaining an active and warm body core. This ensures a good supply of warm blood to the extremities. That is why proper nutrition and warm clothing are so important.

Trench Foot

Trench foot is an example of one of the several conditions that develop with prolonged exposure to cold and wet conditions above freezing. It is not limited to feet and often involves the hands of paddlers, fishermen, and others working or playing on the water. Inflammation results from prolonged vasoconstriction and tissue breakdown, an example of ischemia to infarction. Blisters can develop, with the possibility of secondary infection where the dermis has been exposed.

Treatment of Trench Foot (or Hand)

Because the mechanism for trench foot is ischemia from being wet and cold, the ideal treatment is to improve perfusion by keeping the feet warm and dry. Treat any open wounds to prevent infection and allow for healing. Ibuprofen may help with inflammation and pain. Like rewarmed frostbite, tissue damage can be exacerbated by further use. Walking may be difficult or impossible.

Prevention is well worth the trouble. In "trench" conditions, try to give your hands and feet several dry and warm hours each day. Reverse shell/core compensation by maintaining hydration, calories, and activity. It's okay to dry your wet socks in your sleeping bag at night, but not while wearing them. Take your wetsuit booties and gloves off whenever possible. Inside waterproof boots, change your socks frequently to keep your feet as dry as you can.

Trench Foot

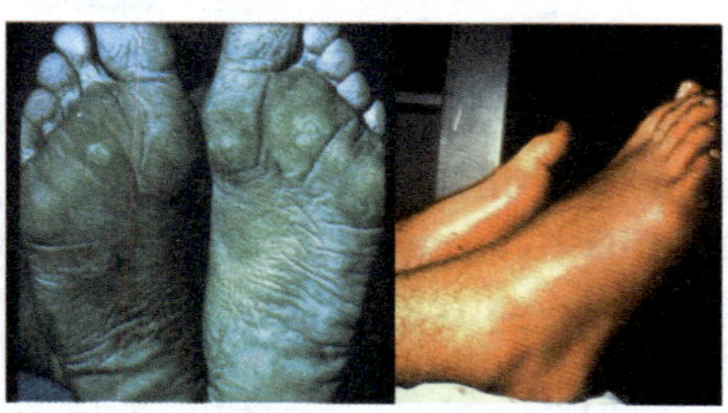

Inflammation results from prolonged vasoconstriction and tissue breakdown, an example of ischemia to infarction.

Trench Hands

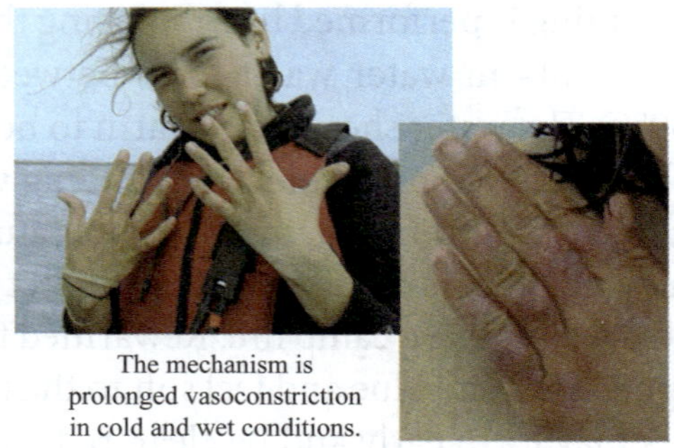

The mechanism is prolonged vasoconstriction in cold and wet conditions.

Raynaud's Phenomenon

Raynaud's is a disorder of the blood vessels near the skin, most often affecting the hands and fingers and aggravated by cold exposure. Profound vasoconstriction causes temporary ischemia, with the typical white or blue appearance and numbness and tingling. Raynaud's is usually self-limiting if the extremity is protected from further cold exposure. Predisposing factors include repetitive use injury, vibration injury, and previous cold frostbite. Raynaud's can also be a feature of other systemic illness.

Raynaud's Phenomenon

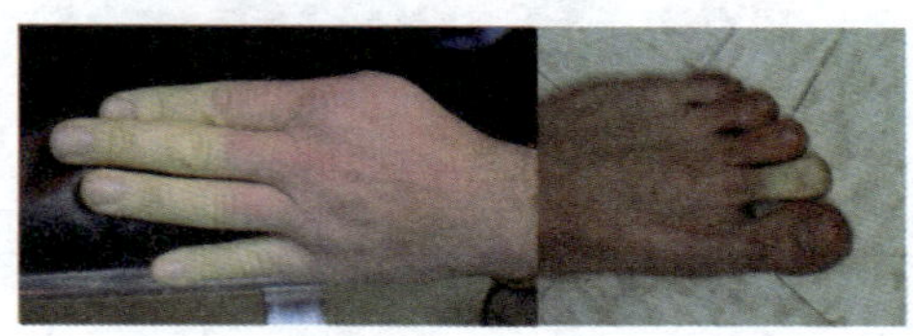

"With Raynaud's, profound vasoconstriction causes temporary ischemia, with the typical white or blue appearance and numbness and tingling."

Of primary concern in backcountry medicine is that Raynaud's patients are at high risk for frostbite in freezing weather and for prolonged ischemia in cool weather, with accompanying tissue breakdown and inflammation. These people need to be especially conscientious about wearing gloves and staying warm and well hydrated. Definitive treatment is prolonged and may involve the use of medication and desensitizing exposure to cold and hot stimulus.

Risk Versus Benefit

Rewarming deep frostbite is a high-risk field treatment primarily because you will have rendered your patient incapable of using their hands or feet. This can be a real survival problem in some situations. Even so, it can be difficult to convince a person not to rewarm when the opportunity presents itself. It may be counterintuitive, but the discovery of fully frozen feet is not an invitation to warm up by the campfire. It is a mandate to return to the trailhead and find a hospital immediately.

The formation of blisters and swelling in rewarmed frostbite is an indication of moderate tissue damage that would become devastating with additional mechanical trauma or refreezing. Continuing use of an extremity in this condition risks permanent damage and infection, yet people routinely overlook this to finish a race series or bag one more peak. This is unwise under any circumstance and can be lethal if critical mobility becomes impaired. The prevention of frostbite is not just a convenience; it is an essential survival skill.

Chapter 18 Review:
Cold Injuries

- The precursor to frostbite is sometimes called frostnip. This occurs with the intense vasoconstriction and loss of local tissue perfusion that results from exposure to subfreezing temperatures.
- Superficial frostbite occurs when the water in skin cells begins to freeze. Sensation is dulled, and the area appears white or blue and feels soft to the touch.
- Deep frostbite is a serious ischemia to infarction problem. The skin and underlying tissues are frozen solid. The area is white or bluish and hard to the touch. Deep frostbite should be evacuated emergently to a medical facility for controlled rewarming.
- Field rewarming of deep frostbite is a high-risk treatment and is carried out only when evacuation is impractical and the equipment and shelter is available.
- Rewarmed frostbite should be treated as a high-risk wound and should never be allowed to refreeze.
- The prevention of frostbite is an essential survival skill and requires insulation, protection, and a warm body core.
- Trench foot is an injury that develops with prolonged exposure to cold and wet conditions above freezing. It is not limited to feet and often involves the hands of paddlers, fishermen, and others working or playing on the water.
- Raynaud's is a disorder of the blood vessels near the skin, most often affecting the hands and fingers and aggravated by cold exposure. Profound vasoconstriction causes temporary ischemia, a white or blue appearance, and numbness and tingling. There is no field treatment, but it is a predisposing factor of frostbite.

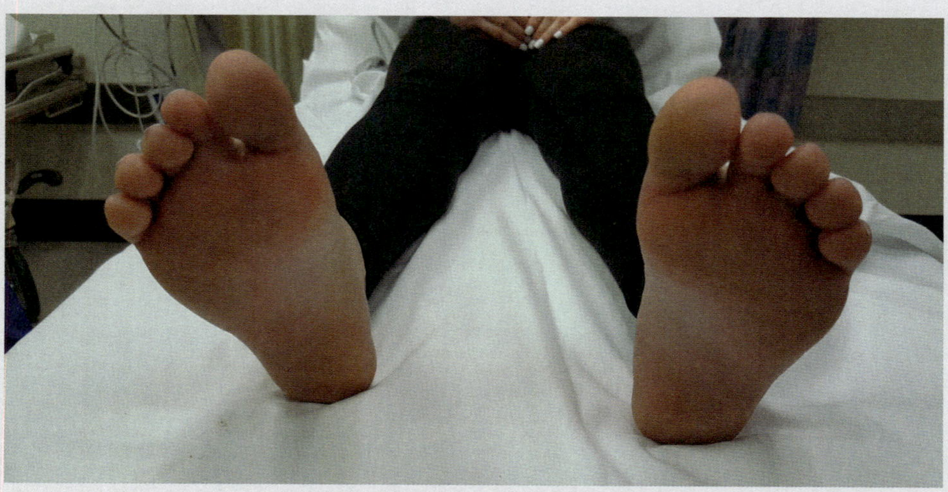

Rewarmed superficial frostbite.

Chapter 19: Altitude Illness

As you climb in elevation the atmosphere becomes less dense which decreases available oxygen, reduces water vapor, and allows greater ultraviolet penetration. It is the decrease in available oxygen that causes the most serious altitude-related symptoms.

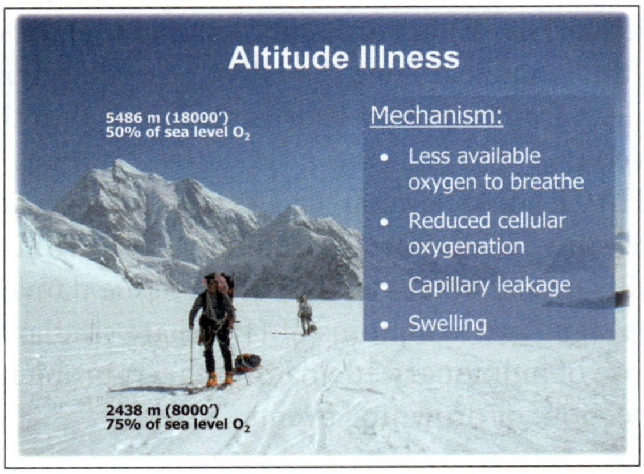

As altitude increases normal oxygen saturation decreases. At sea level, a healthy respiratory system will fill the hemoglobin in the red blood cells with oxygen, yielding an oxygen saturation measurement of 98–100%. At an altitude of 3,000 meters, oxygen saturation in a healthy individual typically measures 90–96%. For most people from sea level, this represents mild hypoxia that can result in a noticeable decrease in performance and at least minimal symptoms of altitude illness.

Initially, the body compensates with mild hyperventilation and increased cardiac output. This is observed as an increased respiratory rate, increased pulse rate, and elevated blood pressure. This allows for a person to ascend, within limits, without a significant reduction in cellular oxygenation.

One side effect of the body's compensatory effort is respiratory alkalosis; a rise in blood pH due to blowing off too much carbon dioxide. Respiratory alkalosis produces some of the commonly felt altitude symptoms as well as a periodic depression in respiratory drive that results in episodes of hypoxia and sleep apnea. Carbon dioxide is a waste product of cellular metabolism and is transported as a dissolved gas in the blood plasma. Getting rid of more of it might seem beneficial, but carbon dioxide has an important role in maintaining the acid/base balance in the blood, normally kept at a pH of 7.43.

Under normal conditions, your brain monitors changes in pH as the primary method of controlling respiratory effort. The brain responds to a rise in pH by reducing the rate and depth of respiration to retain more carbon dioxide. But at altitude, this response conflicts with the need to extract more oxygen from thinner air. The result is often a disturbance in the breathing pattern, particularly during sleep when breathing normally slows. It also inhibits the adjustment process.

Compensation at Altitude

Short Term:

- Hyperventilation
- Tachycardia and increased blood pressure
- Kidneys trying to maintain normal pH

Long Term:

- Body produces more red blood cells and hemoglobin
- Capillary beds increase in density

As part of the short-term adjustment the kidneys excrete bicarbonate (a base) to maintain the pH balance despite the increased respiratory rate. This usually takes 2 or 3 days and may or may not be completely successful. Patients can help the process by avoiding climbing higher until adjusted to the new altitude and by maintaining adequate hydration for kidney function. A medication called acetazolamide can help with this process.

Side Effects of Compensation

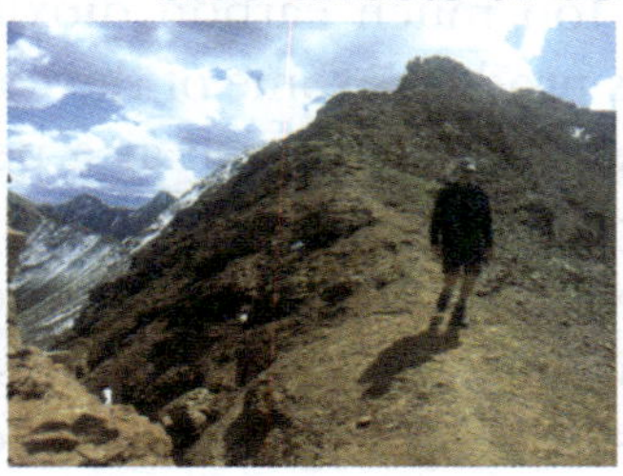

Hyperventilation

Respiratory Alkalosis

Irregular Respiratory Control

Sleep Hypoxia and Delayed Adjustment

Long-term compensation for an individual staying at altitude includes producing more red blood cells to carry oxygen and the development of more dense capillary beds in body tissues. This process can take months to years. The acclimatized individual's oxygen saturation will still read low, but because the carrying capacity of the blood has increased, there is actually more oxygen being transported.

Alpinists can continue to ascend if they allow enough time for short- and long-term adjustment. How quickly this occurs and how high a person can ultimately go, depend on health, fitness, and genetics. Eventually, the ability to compensate is maximized and inadequate cellular oxygenation prevents further ascent.

Cerebral and Pulmonary Edema

Reduced oxygen in the blood and body tissues results in edema due to capillary dilation and leakage. This generally occurs as oxygen saturation falls below about 90%, but can occur with saturation measuring in the normal range. The mechanism is not completely understood and is different in the brain than in the lungs. But, the signs and symptoms we worry about most are the same as those seen in cerebral or pulmonary edema from other causes.

High-altitude cerebral edema (HACE) is caused by vascular changes that result in capillary leakage of fluid into the brain. High-altitude pulmonary edema (HAPE) is the result of vascular changes in the lungs that have the effect of forcing fluid to leak from capillary beds in the lungs into the alveoli.

HACE looks similar to elevated intracranial pressure (ICP) from a traumatic brain injury (TBI) or any other cause of brain tissue damage. The signs and symptoms of HAPE are similar to those of pulmonary edema from heart problems, infection, or drowning events.

High-Altitude Cerebral Edema

The symptoms of mild HACE are often called acute mountain sickness. A small amount of cerebral edema produces the characteristic headache, loss of appetite, and nausea associated with the slight increase in ICP. These are the same symptoms one might expect following a mild TBI. Acute mountain sickness generally develops within a few hours of arrival at moderate altitudes and resolves within 48 hours for most people.

High-Altitude Cerebral Edema

Mechanism:
- Capillary dilation and leakage leading to increased ICP

Signs and Symptoms:
- Mild HACE (AMS) – mild headache, fatigue, nausea
- Moderate HACE – severe headache, vomiting
- Severe HACE – brain failure (mental status changes, ataxia)

Treatment is largely symptomatic. Aspirin, ibuprofen, or other aspirin-like drugs reduce pain and may reduce cerebral edema. Hydration is important to kidney function, and the patient should avoid alcohol and narcotic medication that would depress respiratory drive. The prescription drug acetazolamide can be used to reduce symptoms by maintaining a more normal blood pH.

HACE Medications

Acetazolamide (Diamox):
- Prophylaxis 125mg q12h (5 mg/kg/day in 2 divided doses for kids)
- Treatment 250mg bid or tid

Dexamethasone (Decadron):
- 8 mg loading dose, then 4 mg q12h for emergency treatment of moderate and severe sx (IM, SC or PO)
- Prophylaxis for high altitude rescue teams

Oxygen:
- Titrate to patient response
- 1–2 liters per minute may suffice

Ideally, a climber should not continue to ascend until symptoms have resolved. However, schedules often interfere with ideal prevention and treatment. Pushing through symptoms to a higher altitude or level of activity can make the situation much worse.

Moderate HACE is increased ICP due to brain swelling. The patient shows early mental status changes and begins to vomit. The headache may not respond to NSAIDs. The ideal treatment is supplemental oxygen and an immediate descent of at least 300 meters.

If the patient is trapped at altitude by weather or terrain, treatment in place includes rest, pain medication, supplemental oxygen, and fluid to maintain hydration. For a short time under emergency circumstances a corticosteroid medication can be used to reduce the symptoms of cerebral edema. An example is the drug dexamethasone given by mouth or intramuscular injection.

Altitude Illness Prevention

- Above 3,000 meters, ascend 300–1,000 meters per day
- Rest days every 1,000–1,500 meters in ascent
- Carry high, sleep low
- Avoid CNS depressants
- Stay hydrated and well fed
- Be alert to early symptoms
- Prophylactic medications

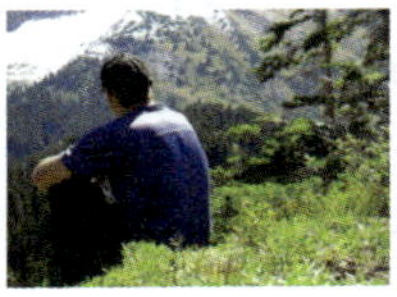

A portable hyperbaric chamber (e.g., Gamow bag) is another emergency treatment occasionally available through rescue teams or cached at popular climbing areas. This device can be used to increase the air pressure around the patient temporarily by about two pounds per square inch, simulating a descent of 1,000–2,000 meters. This may temporarily improve the patient's condition, allowing a walk-out evacuation before debilitating symptoms return.

The symptoms of moderate HACE may improve with treatment and time. However, climbing partners or rescuers must be prepared for an emergency descent if the patient's condition worsens. The practitioner must also be alert to other anticipated problems such as hypothermia and volume shock from dehydration.

Severe HACE is a serious critical system problem. Fortunately, it rarely occurs below 4,000 meters in elevation. One of the common signs is ataxia (loss of muscle control, often seen as an inability to walk straight). The patient also exhibits changes in level of consciousness and mental status that may range from mild to profound. Persistent vomiting and complete loss of appetite are common.

The symptoms of severe HACE can be confused or mixed with those of other problems such as hypoglycemia, dehydration, hypothermia, hyperthermia, and simple exhaustion. All of these problems can cause a decrease in muscular performance and efficiency, and all can cause changes in mental status. Even though your primary concern may be altitude, it is important to include all five problems as possible causes until proven otherwise.

Severe HACE is treated using all the techniques and medications useful for the mild and moderate forms, plus an immediate descent of at least 1,000 meters. Exertion should be minimized, but there should be no delay in descent. A patient in severe HACE is not likely to survive without aggressive intervention.

High-Altitude Pulmonary Edema

Unlike HACE, which develops within 24 hours, HAPE tends to develop several days after arrival at altitude. It can exist without any symptoms of HACE or present long after symptoms of HACE have cleared. At moderate altitudes (2,700–4,000 meters), HAPE tends to occur as an isolated illness.

High-Altitude Pulmonary Edema

Mechanism:

- Capillary dilation and leakage leading to pulmonary edema

Signs and Symptoms:

- Mild – decreased performance, dry cough, mild SOB on exertion
- Moderate – persistent cough, inspiratory crackles, SOB at rest, low grade fever
- Severe – respiratory failure, copious sputum, marked crackles

The early symptoms of HAPE are shortness of breath on exertion, general fatigue, and sometimes a dry cough. It can also produce a low-grade fever. People with an existing or recent respiratory illness seem to be more predisposed to develop HAPE. In fact, many patients will mistake mild HAPE for a worsening pneumonia or bronchitis. In the early stages, fluid in the alveoli may not be audible with a stethoscope.

The ideal treatment for HAPE is supplemental oxygen and immediate descent. Significant improvement or resolution of symptoms can be noted with as little as 300 meters drop in altitude. Mild HAPE can also be safely managed on site if low-flow supplemental oxygen can be given over 24 hours, and if descent will be easy and quick to accomplish if conditions worsen. Acetazolamide at 125 mg twice a day may also help.

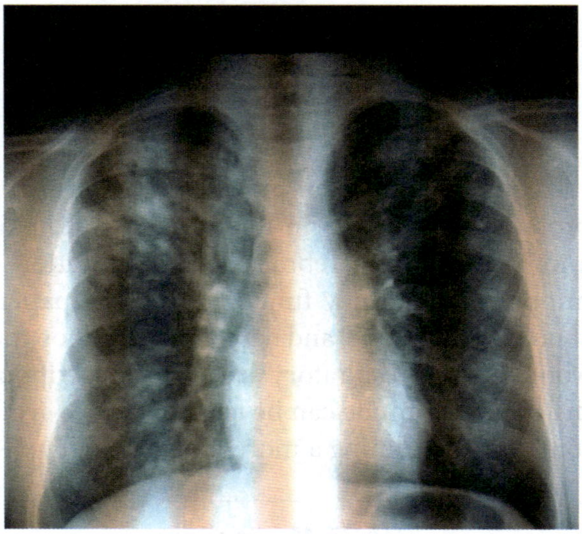

This chest x-ray shows the patchy accumulation of fluid in the alveoli of the right lung that can be heard as crackles with a stethoscope.

If pulmonary edema worsens, the patient experiences shortness of breath, even at rest, and a persistent cough. Crackles on inspiration are audible with a stethoscope or an ear to the chest. Moderate HAPE is a bad sign. The condition tends to progress from bad to worse.

Unfortunately, exertion makes pulmonary edema worse due to an increase in pulmonary hypertension. There may be situations where it would be better to remain where you are rather than perform a strenuous evacuation over a mountain pass. If descent will be delayed, supplemental oxygen and positive pressure ventilations can be lifesaving. HAPE also responds to treatment in a portable hyperbaric chamber.

High-Altitude Pulmonary Edema

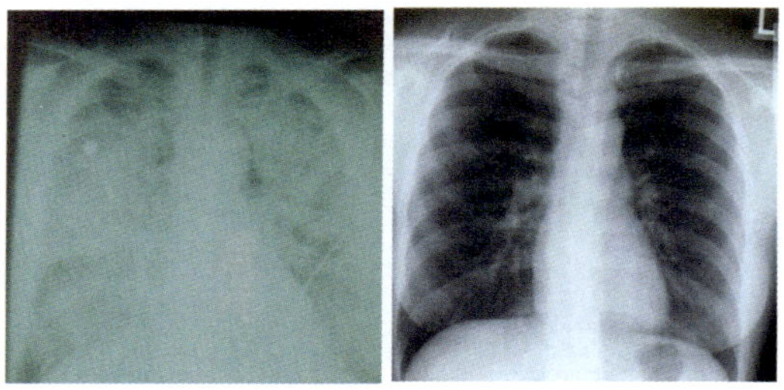

Severe HAPE — Normal Chest X-ray

HAPE Medications

Nifedipine (Procardia, Adalat):

- 30 mg XR po for emergency treatment of moderate and severe sx
- 30 mg q12h for prophylaxis

Oxygen:

- Titrate to patient response, 1–4 L/m may suffice
- High flow may be necessary in severe cases
- CPAP is ideal for emergency treatment

Acetazolamide:

- Prophylaxis, not treatment
- 125mg q12h (5mg/kg/day in 2 divided doses for kids)

Emergency medications for HAPE include oral nifedipine, a smooth muscle relaxer that is normally used to treat high blood pressure. It seems to ease the pulmonary hypertension that is forcing fluid to leak into the alveolar space. Nifedipine is a prescription medication in the United States. Other prescription medications like acetazolamide, tadalafil, sildenafil, and dexamethasone may prevent HAPE in people with a past history of it, although the place for these drugs in emergency treatment is not clear.

High-Altitude Pulmonary Edema

Treatment:

- Mild HAPE – oxygen, rest day, hydration and food
- Moderate HAPE – immediate descent of 500 meters, consider nifedipine or CPAP
- Severe HAPE – CPAP, immediate descent of 500+ meters, nifedipine or PDE 5 inhibitor

Severe HAPE will ultimately result in respiratory failure and death. Emergency treatment includes positive pressure ventilation (PPV), oxygen, nifedipine, and an immediate descent of at least 1,000 meters. Pulmonary edema may persist for several days after descent and require hospital observation and treatment. Unlike HACE, severe HAPE can and does kill people at moderate altitudes.

Other Altitude Illnesses

Although HACE and HAPE are the most dangerous forms of altitude illness, they are not the only manifestation. Capillary dilation and leakage can produce edema anywhere in the body. People traveling at altitude can end up with edematous hands and feet. Swelling in the gut can produce diarrhea. Edema in the mucous membranes of the nose and sinuses can mimic the congestion of a cold or sinus infection. Altitude makes the symptoms of an existing illness worse. The reduction in available oxygen as well as the reduced protective effects of the atmosphere predispose people to other problems as well.

Sunburn at altitude can be quick and extreme due to the lower atmospheric density and less water vapor. The minimum erythematous dose (MED) for unprotected skin can be as little as 15 minutes at 3,000 meters. Many ski and climbing trips have been ruined by the first morning of sun. Apply sunblock early and often.

Snow blindness (solar keratitis) can develop within just a few hours. This condition is not only painful, but results in a debilitating and dangerous loss of vision in a high-risk environment. Treatment with complete shielding, lubricating eye drops, and pain medication usually results in a complete resolution within 2 or 3 days, but prevention of the problem with high-quality goggles or sunglasses is a lot easier.

Risk Versus Benefit

High-altitude mountaineers and trekkers are usually aware of altitude illness and quick to recognize the patterns and trends. Some will push upward anyway and risk turning an anticipated problem into an existing problem. At least they are usually making the decision knowingly and can reduce the consequence with a quick turnaround. It would be very unwise, however, to take such a risk without the benefit of a quick and easy escape to lower elevation.

More troublesome is altitude illness at moderate elevations where there are lots of people skiing, hunting, biking, and hiking who have little or no awareness of the risk. The Chambers of Commerce of mountain resort towns typically don't post headache, nausea, and gasping for breath alongside their lists of amenities. People can spend a long time suffering before discovering that a course of acetazolamide or a night on low-flow oxygen can change everything.

Although HACE is unlikely to become a serious problem at most ski resorts and mountain towns, this is not the case with HAPE. People die in hotel rooms surrounded by cold and flu medications, completely unaware of the real problem. HAPE can kill at elevations as low as 2,500 meters. It is the responsibility of guides, outdoor educators, and resort staff working at altitude to give their clients the risk awareness not provided by the Chambers. This might include a recommendation to acquire prophylactic medication from their health care provider and to spend a night or two acclimatizing before beginning a backcountry trek.

Mountain rescue teams and combat units that travel quickly to altitude have little choice but to use medication preventively to blunt the symptoms of altitude illness long enough to complete the mission. The risk associated with the use of dexamethasone, a medication commonly used for this purpose, are acceptable for the benefit of being functional on scene. This risk versus benefit ratio may not make sense when applied by a climber just trying to meet a schedule.

Chapter 19 Review:
Altitude Illness

- The basic mechanism for altitude illness is swelling caused by hypoxia.
- Mild symptoms are caused by short-term compensation efforts and mild swelling. Serious problems are caused by severe swelling.
- High-altitude cerebral edema (HACE) is caused by capillary leakage of fluid into the brain, resulting in increased intracranial pressure.
- High-altitude pulmonary edema (HAPE) is the result of capillary leakage of fluid into the alveoli, causing respiratory distress.
- The early symptoms of HACE are the characteristic headache, loss of appetite, and nausea associated with the slight increase in ICP.
- The ideal treatment of HACE is immediate descent. If that is not possible, treatment on scene includes rest, pain medication, supplemental oxygen, and fluid to maintain hydration.
- The symptoms of severe HACE include headache, vomiting, and altered mental status. It can be confused with those of other problems such as hypoglycemia, dehydration, hypothermia, hyperthermia, and simple exhaustion.
- The early symptoms of HAPE are shortness of breath on exertion, fatigue, and sometimes a dry cough. It can also produce a low-grade fever.
- As pulmonary edema worsens, a HAPE patient experiences shortness of breath, even at rest, and a persistent cough. Crackles are audible with a stethoscope or an ear to the chest.
- The ideal treatment for HAPE is supplemental oxygen and immediate descent. If that is not possible, treatment on scene includes medications, PPV, and supplemental oxygen.
- Expeditions traveling above 3,000 meters should consider carrying prophylactic and emergency medications and the use of a portable hyperbaric chamber.
- Altitude makes the symptoms of an existing illness worse. The reduction in available oxygen as well as the reduced protective effects of the atmosphere predispose people to other problems as well.

Chapter 20: Medical Aspects of Avalanche Rescue

Most avalanche fatalities are caused by asphyxia. Since snow is mostly air and is very porous the victim may be able to breathe for a period of time. Eventually, the victim's exhaled breath condenses and freezes into a nonporous ice mask around the airway. Although it seems like the cold would play a major role in death by burial in snow, very few victims actually survive long enough to die from hypothermia.

The most important factor in survival of avalanche burial is the speed of recovery. In the first 15 minutes, between 80% and 90% of victims are found alive. This drops to about 30% at 35 minutes and around 3% at 130 minutes. It makes sense that most of the victims that survive are dug out by the people traveling with them, not by rescue teams arriving hours later.

If the victim is wearing an avalanche beacon, other members of the group may be able to find and recover them within minutes. The Recco system, used in many ski areas, is a device that broadcasts a directional radio wave that excites a small metallic tag or sticker sewn into the skier's clothing. The return signal is picked up by the unit's receiver and can be followed directly back to the victim. The device has been known to detect a reflected signal off cellphones, radios, and other metallic objects. In the absence of either technology, the most efficient tool for locating a buried victim is a well-trained avalanche search dog team.

If neither the technology nor dog is available, a quick find is unlikely unless some part of the victim is projecting above the surface of the snow. The backup plan consists of a probe line of rescuers working slowly through the debris field. A live find is far less likely.

Nevertheless, survival of prolonged burial is possible especially in cases where the victim has come to rest in an air space around a tree or boulder or has been partially protected by building debris. User deployed airbag devices, designed to keep a victim afloat during an avalanche, can also create an airspace around a victim who is completely buried. Another device called the Avalung can allow victims to continue breathing under the snow for an hour or more if the user has managed to retain the mouthpiece in place during the slide.

The possibility of a prolonged survival makes avalanche search and recovery a high-priority time-sensitive mission. If a live patient is recovered, the primary problem addressed by the medical practitioner is likely to be respiratory arrest due to asphyxiation. This can occur because of snow packed into the nose and mouth, the formation of an ice mask, or restricted respiratory excursion due to the pressure of the snow pack on the victim's chest. Hypothermia and trauma are secondary considerations.

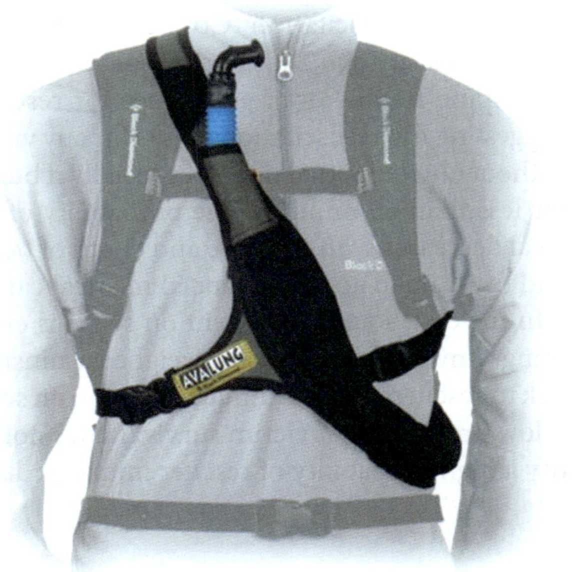

Equipment like the Avalung can allow avalanche victims to continue breathing under the snow for an hour or more.

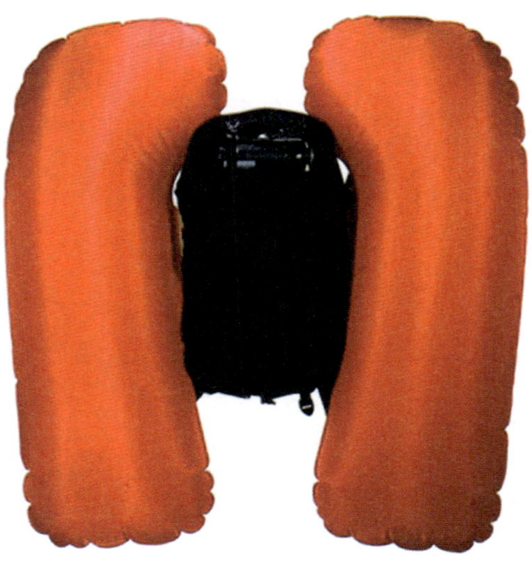

An airspace can be created by an inflatable floatation device installed in a backpack. The increasing use of avalanche survival devices like these increases the probability of a live find in a prolonged burial.

Data indicate that survival is highly unlikely when burial is deeper than 2 meters. That's why most avalanche probes carried by backcountry skiers are less than three meters long. The longer and heavier probes are carried only by rescue teams performing body recovery.

Treatment

The treatment for avalanche survivors includes immediate airway control, positive pressure ventilation (PPV), supplemental oxygen, and evacuation. Once the patient is freed from the insulating snow pack, hypothermia becomes an anticipated problem. Airway control is critical if the patient is less than A on AVPU (Alert, responsive to Verbal stimuli, responsive to Pain, Unresponsive). Increased intracranial pressure (ICP) due to brain hypoxia can also develop but this is likely to occur well after an evacuation has been accomplished.

Live Find

Treat what you see:

- Respiratory failure is likely to be the primary problem.
- Increased ICP is an anticipated problem from trauma and/or hypoxia.
- Hypothermia is not an issue if burial < 35 minutes.
- Once recovered, hypothermia is an anticipated problem.

Do not attempt to resuscitate an avalanche victim in full cardiopulmonary arrest if there is obvious lethal injury or if the effort puts rescuers at risk. Experience shows that the chances of success are minimal after 35 minutes of complete burial with an airway packed with snow. In this case you can assume that breathing stopped at the time the avalanche occurred.

In the absence of obvious lethal injury it can be difficult to decide where to draw the line between treating a patient and performing a body recovery. Equipment like a cardiac monitor and reliable thermometer can help make that decision. If you choose to begin CPR, the effort may be discontinued after 30 minutes of pulselessness unless severe hypothermia is a factor. A cardiac monitor showing asystole in a patient whose core temperature is above 30°C would also confirm that the patient has died.

Cardiorespiratory Arrest

Do Not Resuscitate:

- Effort puts rescuers at risk
- Obvious lethal trauma
- >35 min burial and airway is packed with snow
- Body core temp <10°C

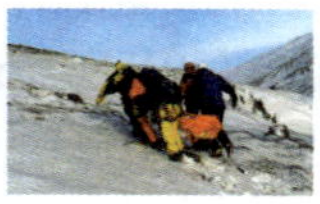

"Drawing the line between treating a patient and performing a body recovery can be a difficult decision to make."

Long Burial

- Survival of prolonged burial is possible.
- Severe hypothermia may be responsible for depressed or undetectable vital signs.
- Treat as severe hypothermia if:
  - clear airway
  - minimal ice mask
  - obvious air pocket or Avalung
  - acceptable risk to rescuers

Hypothermia is rarely an immediate problem or benefit to the completely buried victim. Respiratory failure is likely to kill the victim long before any protective effect of severe hypothermia is realized. There is no demonstrated reason to extend resuscitation beyond the 30-minute CPR protocol. The only exception might be the recovery after a prolonged burial of a severely hypothermic victim wearing an Avalung, or from a buried building, vehicle, or tree well with a preserved air space.

Risk Versus Benefit

Avalanche awareness and search and recovery are major topics in their own right. Practitioners working with search and rescue (SAR) teams in avalanche terrain must be trained and equipped for safe travel and operation. Avalanche recovery represents a considerable risk to rescuers, often in cases where the chance for finding a live victim is minimal.

Various groups and agencies such as the European Resuscitation Council, Wilderness Medical Society, and The International Committee on Alpine Rescue offer guidelines for rescuers suggesting full resuscitation efforts for any victim without obvious lethal injury, especially if buried for less than 60 minutes. The probability of survival decreases with the time and depth of burial, and the time to access advanced medical care.

In the end, sound judgment on scene is everything. Any guideline must be weighed against the risk to rescuers and the unique situation on scene. A low probability of victim survival does not justify a high probability of rescuer injury or death.

Chapter 20 Review:
Medical Aspects of Avalanche Rescue

- Most avalanche fatalities are caused by asphyxia, with trauma being the second most common cause of death. Few die of hypothermia. The most important factor in survival of avalanche burial is the speed of recovery.
- If a live victim is recovered, the primary problem addressed by the medical practitioner will be respiratory arrest due to asphyxiation. This can occur because of snow packed into the nose and mouth, the formation of an ice mask, or restricted respiratory excursion due to the pressure of the snow pack.
- The treatment for avalanche survivors includes immediate positive pressure ventilation (PPV), supplemental oxygen, and evacuation. Once the patient is freed from the snow pack, hypothermia becomes an anticipated problem.
- The decision to perform any treatment on scene should consider the risk of a second avalanche.
- Avalanche rescue is a high-risk activity and requires specialized training and expertise.

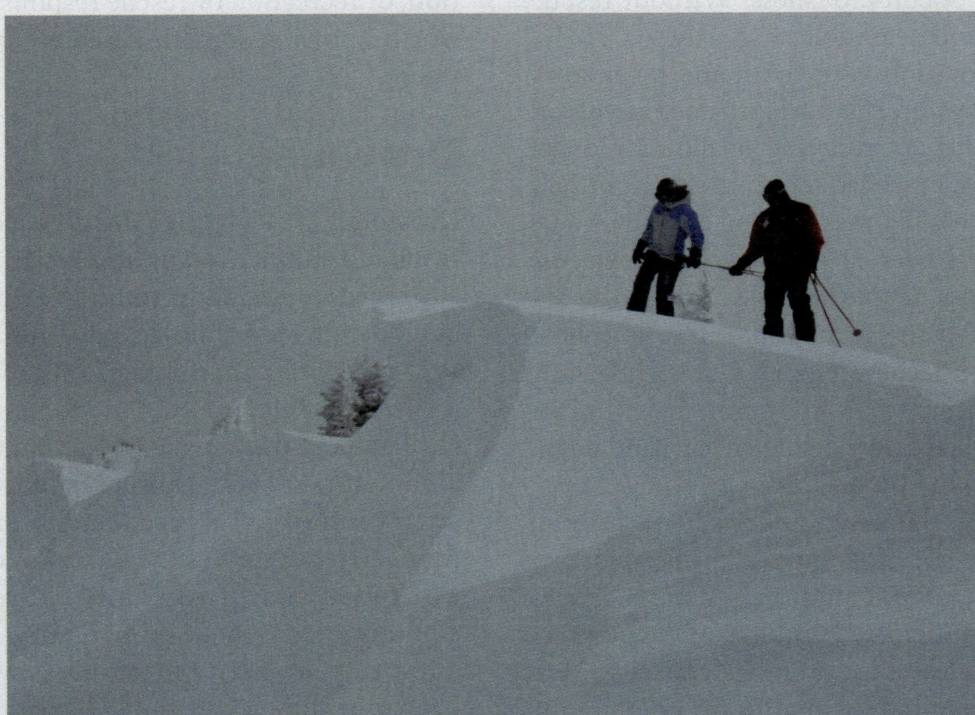

Unfortunately, training in avalanche awareness alone is not enough to prevent an accident. Many people who end up buried are well aware of the avalanche risk.

Chapter 21: Water-Related Injury

Trapped under water, most untrained people will inhale within a minute or two. Laryngeal spasm may protect the lungs for a short period, but ultimately water will infiltrate the alveoli, causing hypoxia and unconsciousness. Without rescue, brain injury and death follow shortly.

You can condition your brain and respiratory system, or temporarily manipulate your blood chemistry by hyperventilating, to allow for longer breath holding. Practiced free divers can routinely achieve breath hold times of 5 and 6 minutes. The world record is over 11 minutes. With extreme discipline, these people are able to resist the diaphragmatic spasms and intense urge to inhale long enough to become hypoxic with significantly altered mental status. At this point, the swimmer usually recognizes the need to surface and begin breathing and the timer stops.

SCUBA (self-contained underwater breathing apparatus) has largely eliminated the need for prolonged breath holding underwater, but it carries its own set of anticipated problems. Compressing air allows for breathing against water pressure but creates the potential for significant pressure differentials across body structures as water pressure increases and decreases with changes in depth. A ruptured ear drum is a minor example; a ruptured lung is a more serious consequence of the same problem.

For humans, water is a high-risk environment, but many of us seem to love being near, on, or under it for work and play. Water also plays a role in many natural disasters. Regardless of your location, or recreation or rescue responsibilities, it is worth knowing something about water-related injury.

Drowning

Drowning is respiratory distress occurring as a result of a submersion or immersion event (from sustained coughing to respiratory arrest). Your ability to swim has little to do with your ability to drown. One common cause of drowning is the loss of muscular coordination due to the rapid shell cooling that occurs in cold water.

Sometimes, sudden immersion in very cold water causes a reflex gasp that fills the lungs and immediately deprives the victim of oxygen. Self-extrication efforts may be hampered by bulky clothing and boots or by being pinned down by a fast current. Even the strongest swimmer can drown in these conditions. Unless interrupted by rescue, the final act is the loss of consciousness and the inhalation of a substantial amount of water. Cardiac arrest and death follows within a few minutes.

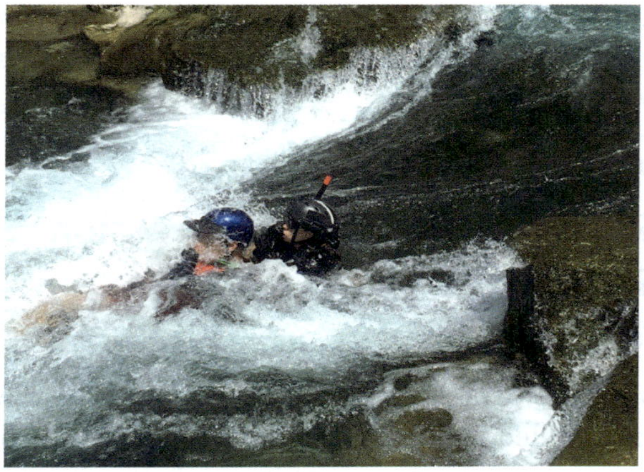

A person's ability to swim has little to do with their ability to drown. Survival efforts are often hampered by bulky clothing and equipment, cold water, and current.

Cases where a patient is rescued and resuscitated are considered to be drowning with injury. The respiratory system and brain are at risk for significant complications, especially if crackles are detected on auscultation of the lungs. Respiratory distress and increased ICP are on the anticipated problem list.

By contrast, the swimmer who did not lose consciousness or experience respiratory distress during the event will not develop drowning injury regardless of how dramatic and scary the event was. These patients may be uncomfortable and scared, but they are not in trouble from water inhalation or hypoxia. You should be most concerned about the patient who lost consciousness and had to be rescued and resuscitated. Nevertheless, don't forget to look for other injuries that may have occurred during the event and rescue.

Treatment of Drowning Injury

If the primary assessment problem is respiratory arrest, then the immediate treatment is positive pressure ventilation (PPV). The treatment does not differ between salt and fresh water submersions. There is no need to drain water from the lungs and foamy sputum does not need to be continually suctioned or cleared unless it interferes with PPV. If the effort is initiated within a few minutes of submersion, the patient may recover spontaneous respiration quickly. After starting PPV, begin chest compressions and if available, apply an AED and shock if indicated.

Once the patient is breathing, consider an urgent evacuation with the anticipated problem of respiratory failure from pulmonary edema, and elevated ICP from hypoxia. Water inhalation causes irritation of the alveoli in the lungs. Hypoxia causes brain injury. In all but the warmest water, hypothermia can also become an issue.

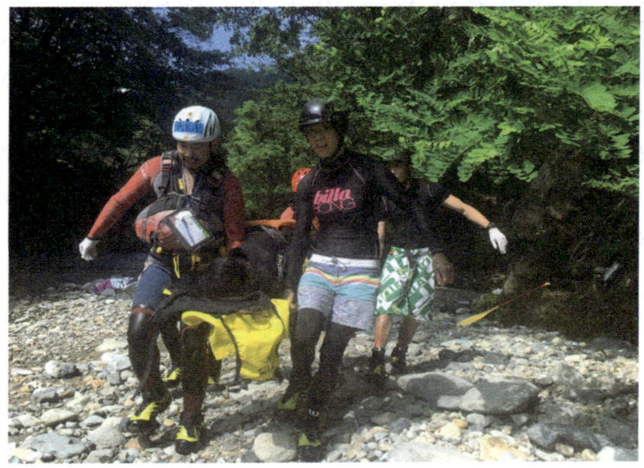

If evacuation is not an option, careful monitoring of respiratory status should be part of the plan, with PPV and oxygen being the anticipated treatment if respiratory failure develops. Patients who remain clear of symptoms for at least 8 hours can be considered at very low risk for further complications.

Drowning with Injury

Problems:

- Respiratory arrest
  A': cardiac arrest
- Water inhalation lung injury
  A': pulmonary edema
- Hypoxic brain injury
  A': Increased ICP

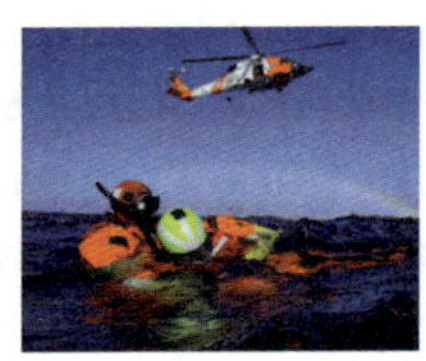

"The initial assessment problem is respiratory arrest and the immediate treatment is positive pressure ventilation."

A successful resuscitation is far less likely if the patient was submerged long enough to go into cardiac arrest. Nevertheless, there are some prolonged submersion survival stories and aggressive resuscitation is warranted if it will not put rescuers at risk. Some research has suggested that there is benefit from the effects of very cold water where rapid cooling of the brain may delay the damage caused by hypoxia. Other studies show that the temperature of the water makes little or no difference. In any case, the best chance for survival rests with early rescue, aggressive resuscitation, and early access to sophisticated medical care.

In a setting remote from advanced medical care, an attempt at resuscitation following prolonged submersion of up to an hour should be made only if it does not place rescuers at risk. Patients who do not respond quickly to basic life support (BLS) will not survive. Resuscitation efforts beyond the 30-minute cardiopulmonary resuscitation (CPR) or automated external defibrillator (AED) protocols are not justified.

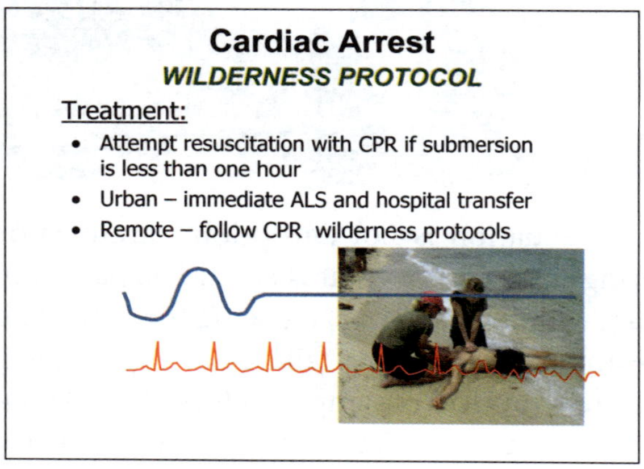

SCUBA Diving Injuries

Hyperbaric injury (associated with an increase or decrease in air pressure) was seen before the invention of SCUBA from the use of diving bells and in workers from pressurized bridge construction caissons. It became more common with the emergence of military and sport diving in the 1940s. It took many years and casualties before the problems associated with breathing gas under pressure were properly identified and understood.

Certified sport and commercial divers are now well trained in the prevention and recognition of hyperbaric injury. However, because SCUBA has become popular as a tool for both recreation and rescue, it is important for all medical personnel working in water rescue and marine environments to be able to recognize and treat diving injuries. This section will serve as a basic overview for practitioners who have not had the benefit of SCUBA training.

Pulmonary Overpressure Syndromes and Decompression Sickness

Dive-related injuries are caused by the behavior of air under pressure. As described by Boyle's Law, an air-filled balloon forced underwater would be compressed to one half of its original volume at 10 meters below the surface, where the ambient pressure is double the surface air pressure. At 20 meters underwater, the balloon will be reduced to a third of its original volume. The same number of air molecules will be present, but they will occupy less space. If the balloon is allowed to return to the surface, it will expand back to its normal size without damage. This is exactly what happens to the lungs of a free-diver not using pressurized air.

To breathe underwater, a diver must be able to expand their lungs against the massive force of water pressure. Doing this more than a half of a meter below the surface requires the assistance of pressurized air. The pressure regulator in the SCUBA system provides just enough air pressure on inhalation to overcome water pressure and allow the diver to expand their lungs to full volume. The result is that at 10 meters below the surface, the diver's lungs contain twice as many air molecules as they would on the surface. (The diver could also use a SCUBA tank to pressurize our example balloon to its original volume, even though it is also 10 meters underwater.)

As the diver swims back toward the surface, our balloon begins to expand as the water pressure decreases. The diver's lungs also begin to expand, but because the diver continues to exhale while ascending, the excess volume of air is vented through the regulator. Since the balloon has no ability to vent, it continues to expand until it ruptures in a cloud of bubbles. This is also what would happen to the lungs of the SCUBA diver if they were to ascend too fast for the expanding air to escape.

Pulmonary Overpressure Syndromes

Mechanism:

- Uncontrolled rapid ascent from depth
- Underwater blast
- Hyperexpansion and rupture of lungs
- Arterial gas embolus

Signs and Symptoms:

- Altered mental status
- Pneumothorax
- Respiratory distress
- Bloody sputum
- Shock

Pulmonary overpressure is the most dramatic and serious hyperbaric injury. The usual cause is a panicked rush for the surface while forgetting to breathe. Expanding air ruptures the lungs, airways, and blood vessels, allowing air to enter the chest cavity, subcutaneous tissue, and circulatory system. Large bubbles of air can cause an arterial gas embolus, producing ischemia in the heart and brain. Air in the chest cavity produces a tension pneumothorax. These are serious critical system injuries and death can be immediate. If the diver survives, emergent medical care is required.

The other major diving injury is decompression sickness, otherwise known as the bends. This is caused by the tendency of air under pressure to dissolve into the blood and body tissues it is in contact with. As stated by Henry's Law, the greater the pressure, the more air will be dissolved.

As a diver descends, the air they are breathing is forced to dissolve into their blood and tissues in direct proportion to water depth. The deeper the diver goes and the longer they stay, the more air is forced into solution. This is why deeper dives are usually kept shorter in duration.

If the diver returns to the surface too quickly, the gas (primarily nitrogen) will come out of solution to form bubbles in the blood. The best illustration of this is a carbonated beverage; when the bottle or can is opened, the pressure is released and the gas bubbles out. In a carbonated beverage, this is good; in the blood, this is bad.

If the diver ascends slowly enough, the emerging gas molecules are expired through their lungs without causing injury. Dive computers and decompression tables are used to determine a safe rate of ascent. This reduces the risk of decompression sickness but does not eliminate it completely. Off-gassing actually continues for many hours after a dive.

If a diver fails to decompress adequately for the depth and duration of the dive, small bubbles accumulate in the smaller vessels, causing microvascular ischemia and inflammation. The early symptoms of decompression sickness, such as skin itching, are caused by injury at the capillary level. These bubbles can cause more significant complications depending on their size and location. Larger bubbles tend to lodge at joints, causing joint pain. Bubbles causing ischemia in the brain can elicit the symptoms of stroke. Bubbles in the spinal cord can cause paralysis. The onset of these various symptoms can be delayed by many hours and are exacerbated by travel to high altitude or by the low cabin pressure in an aircraft.

Treatment of Pulmonary Overpressure and Decompression Sickness

BLS and advanced life support (ALS), including the administration of high-flow oxygen during rapid evacuation to a hyperbaric chamber, is the ideal treatment for both pulmonary overpressure and decompression sickness. If possible, include the patient's dive computer (or the information on it) with your evacuation and communication. The Diver's Alert Network (DAN) can help you find a hyperbaric chamber and is available by phone 24 hours a day by calling 1+919-684-9111. The chamber is the safest place to pressurize the patient to shrink the bubbles that are causing the problems.

Decompression Sickness

Mechanism:

- Prolonged exposure to pressure (e.g. >20m, >60 minutes) or multiple dives
- Insufficient time to decompress
- Bubbles form in blood and tissue from slow dissolution of gas

Signs and Symptoms:

- Itching, tingling, joint pain
- CNS: focal signs, AVPU changes, ataxia
- Respiratory distress and shock in severe cases

Ear Pain and Mask Squeeze

Middle ear barotraumas can affect SCUBA and free divers alike. The tympanic membrane (ear drum) in the ear is particularly susceptible to injury from changes in water or air pressure. As the diver descends, they must force air into the middle ear behind the ear drum to counter the water pressure pushing in from the outside. If the air pressure inside matches the water pressure outside, the ear drum will remain uninjured. If either becomes excessive, the membrane will rupture and allow water to enter the middle ear.

Middle ear barotrauma is usually not an emergency, but it carries the anticipated problem of middle ear infection. The patient should not be permitted to swim or dive until the ear drum has healed. This usually takes several weeks to months. Serious problems can develop when the injury involves the inner ear or facial nerves. Early evacuation to medical care is indicated since there is no real field treatment.

Middle Ear Barotrauma

Signs and Symptoms:

- Pain
- Impaired hearing
- Congestion

Serious:

- Facial paralysis
- Hearing loss
- Tinnitis
- Vertigo
- Fever

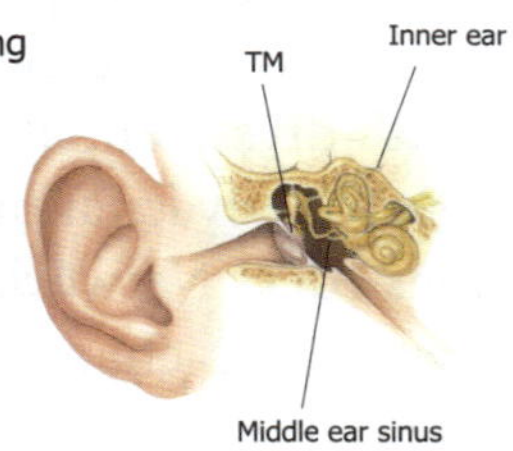

Mask squeeze develops from a failure to pressurize the air space in the face mask during descent. The relative increase in pressure in the vascular system and soft tissue under the mask can cause the rupture of small blood vessels in the conjunctiva of the eye and skin of the face and nose. Although scary looking, it is usually not serious. Treatment is directed at relieving symptoms.

Risk Versus Benefit

Water is a high-risk environment for the injured and the rescuers, especially if it is moving and cold. Water rescue offers an almost unlimited opportunity to create more patients and increase the scale of disaster. Mitigating the risks is the first step in rescue and resuscitation. Considerable training and practice are required. Unskilled rescuers should remain ashore.

A patient in the water is an unstable scene. In all but the most desperate situations, removal of the patient from the water comes before assessment and treatment. In-the-water spine stabilization, for example, is appropriate only in a heated pool with enough rescuers and scene control to ensure the safety of all involved, including the patient.

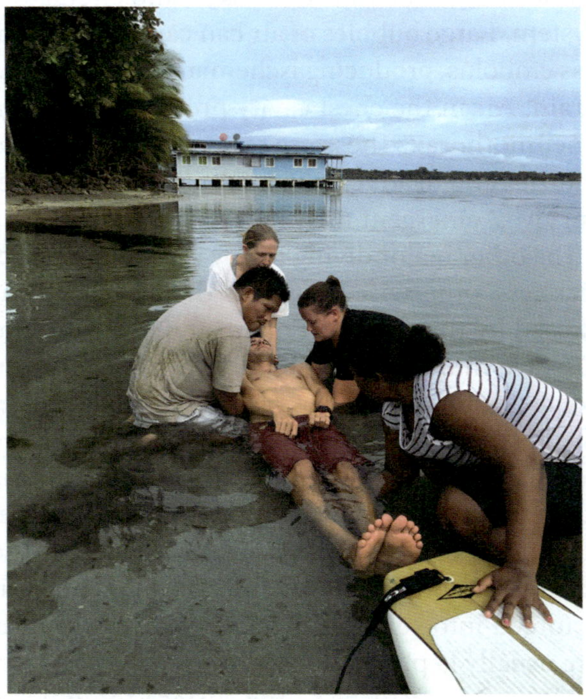

Beware that your treatment does not inhibit your patient's ability to survive in and around water. A patient immobilized on a backboard or litter is completely helpless. Allowing your patient freedom of movement may risk exacerbating an injury but will be of substantial benefit if the raft or small boat capsizes.

Chapter 21 Review:
Water-Related Injury

- A submersion event with self-rescue, no loss of consciousness, and no persistent respiratory symptoms is not likely to result in critical system problems.
- The primary assessment problem with submersion injury is respiratory failure or arrest, and the immediate treatment is positive pressure ventilation (PPV).
- People who are submerged for more than a few minutes will go into cardiac arrest. At that point, successful field resuscitation is highly unlikely.
- Because SCUBA has become popular as a tool for both recreation and rescue, it is important for all medical personnel working in water rescue and marine environments to be able to recognize and treat diving injuries.
- Pulmonary overpressure is the most dramatic and most serious hyperbaric injury. The usual cause is a panicked rush for the surface while forgetting to breathe, preventing rapidly expanding air in the lungs from escaping without causing injury.
- Decompression sickness (the bends) is caused by the release of air previously dissolved under pressure in the blood and body tissues while using SCUBA or other compressed air systems. The accumulation of small bubbles in the circulatory system causes widespread problems with ischemia.
- Basic and advanced life support, including the administration of high-flow oxygen during rapid evacuation to a hyperbaric chamber, is the ideal treatment for both pulmonary overpressure and decompression sickness.
- Middle ear barotrauma is usually not an emergency, but it carries the anticipated problem of middle ear infection.

Chapter 22: Lightning Injuries

Lightning is nature's way of equalizing the difference in electrostatic charge that develops between regions of the atmosphere and between the atmosphere and the earth's surface during violent weather. Convection caused by ground heating, the advance of a cold front, or air passing over hills and mountains tends to cause an accumulation of positive ions in the cloud tops, negatively charged electrons in the mid-level cloud, and a weak layer of positive charges in the cloud base. The more violent the convection is, the more rapidly the charges will develop and the more frequent the lightning.

Cumulus clouds showing progressive vertical development indicate the potential for lightning. As the lower regions of a thunderstorm become more negatively charged, the earth's surface below becomes more positively charged. The tendency of similarly charged objects to repel each other explains why your hair stands on end when you are about to be struck by lightning. Other signs of accumulating electrostatic charge include small rocks jumping about and the buzzing and glowing of the air around metal objects.

A lightning strike occurs when these charges build up enough potential difference to overcome atmospheric resistance. A conductive column of ionized air is created by stepwise progressions of upward streamers, usually from a negatively charged region, that ultimately meet shorter streamers from the opposite side. The connection allows an electrical discharge generating millions of volts and tens of thousands of amperes. Fortunately, about 95% of lightning passes from cloud to cloud, which means that only about 5% of lightning activity involves ground strikes.

Lightning Injuries

Despite its immense power, lightning is extremely brief in duration. The average discharge lasts for only about 0.001 seconds. This is not enough time for much of the electrical energy to overcome skin resistance and enter the body. Fewer than 20% of lightning victims die of their injuries. Most of the current passes over the skin surface on its way to the ground. As a result, the types of internal injuries typical of human-made electrical current are rarely seen with lightning.

The energy in lightning dissipates in the form of heat and light. The instantaneous heating and expansion of the column of air through which the current passes generate the shock wave we hear as thunder. Like any explosion, if you are close enough, the shock wave can rupture ear drums, fracture bones, and damage internal organs. You can also be injured by flying rock, splinters, and other debris.

Lightning Exposure

- Direct strike
- Ground current
- Side flash
- Streamer effect
- Touch Voltage

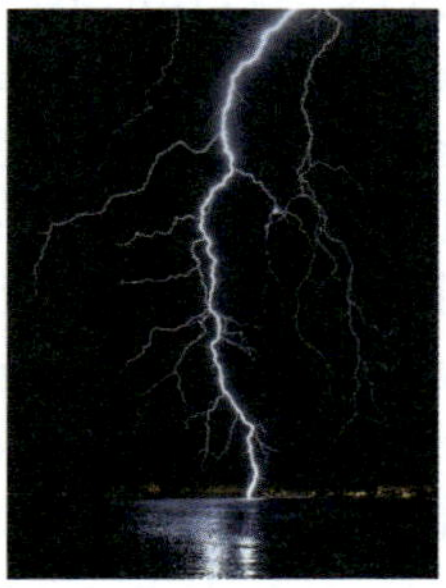

The direct current flow in a lightning strike can disrupt the electrochemical function of the nervous system, causing respiratory and cardiac arrest. The current flowing over the skin heats the moisture on the surface, causing superficial burns and, in some cases, enough explosive force to blow clothing apart.

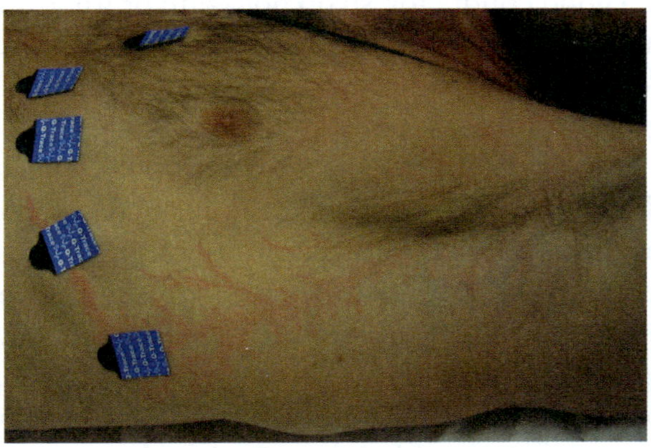

This rash, called Lichtenberg flowers, or ferning, is caused by lightning current passing through the dermis. The rash faded within hours.

A direct hit where the patient becomes part of the main path to ground is likely to be the most devastating but accounts for only 3–5% of lightning deaths because it is so rare. A person is more likely to be injured or killed by ground current that spreads out through the earth, rock, or water from the point of contact with the lightning column. It can follow underground roots, pipes, wires, and water courses. Because the energy is diffused, this form of indirect exposure is generally less devastating than a direct hit, but much more common. Ground current accounts for 50–55% of lightning fatalities.

Side flash occurs when a tall tree or structure is struck and some of the current arcs onto other nearby objects on its path to ground. This explains why seeking shelter near a tall object is not necessarily safe. Side flash causes 30–35% of lightning fatalities.

The term touch voltage describes contact with lightning current through an object like a wire fence or mast shroud and contributes to 15–20% of lightning fatalities. The remaining 10–15% of deaths are caused by contact with an upward streamer.

The extent of injury from current is related to the path the current takes over and through the body. If you are holding onto the mast of your sailboat when the masthead is struck, the current may pass through your arm and chest and out your feet. The vital organs of the critical body systems can become part of the path, producing serious critical system problems. If you are standing, ground current usually passes into one foot and out the other, leaving the vital organs outside the path.

Scene Safety

In responding to a lightning injury, the scene size-up for dangers is particularly important. If the storm continues, it may be very dangerous to approach the scene on a hilltop or cliff face. Look for more than one patient; about 10% of lightning injuries involve two or more people.

Lightning Injuries

Scene Size-up:

- Scene is unsafe if storm continues.
- Multiple victims are likely.

Mechanisms:

- Concussive force
- Shrapnel and splinters
- Electrical injury

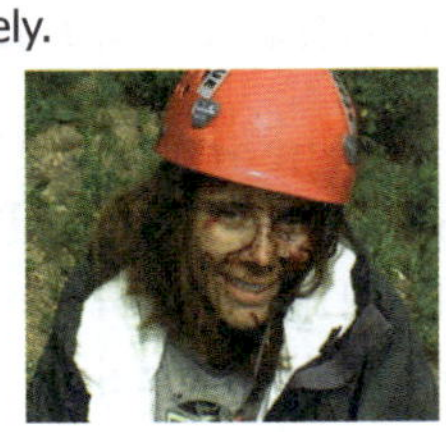

Although it is rare, the explosive force in a direct strike or near miss can cause significant blunt trauma, including ruptured organs and broken bones. Burns caused by lightning are generally superficial, with more serious deep burns occurring in less than 5% of patients. Nervous system injury, including noncontact traumatic brain injury, is common, with many patients experiencing loss of consciousness, amnesia, numbness, tingling, and weakness.

Treatment of Lightning Injury

Treat what you see. Lightning can induce cardiac arrest. If heart damage is minimal, the pulse often returns spontaneously. Lightning-induced respiratory arrest may not spontaneously resolve, even when the respiratory system is relatively intact. In these cases, the prompt initiation of cardiopulmonary resuscitation (CPR) or positive pressure ventilation (PPV) can be lifesaving. Burns, shock, brain injury, and musculoskeletal trauma are all treated as you would with any other patient. It is interesting to note that about 25% of survivors develop significant long-term physical or psychological problems, such as chronic pain or depression.

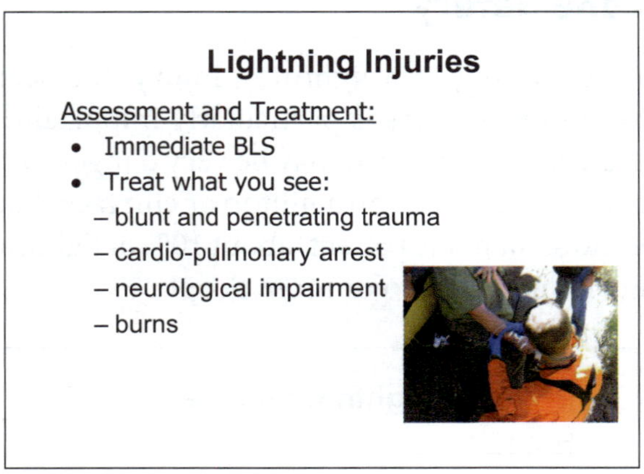

Prevention of Lightning Injury

The height and isolation of an object are the only two factors that predict the likelihood of a direct strike. The type of material has no influence of the probability of being struck. Metal, however, will do a much better job of conducting the current to ground than wood or plastic. As a result, side flash will be more common from a tree than from a metal tower. Lightning rods projecting above the top of a building increase the probability of a strike, but the heavy grounding cables to which they are attached reduce the risk of damage by offering a low-resistance pathway to ground. Trees and rocks, by contrast, offer higher resistance to the flow of current and will become hot, burn, and may explode as the moisture in the wood or rock instantly vaporizes.

In the field, the best tactic to avoid a lightning injury is to get away from the places most likely to be hit. Drop off the ridgeline or mountain top and into the forest. If continued travel takes you lower, keep moving. When travel is no longer possible or will not reduce your risk, stop and squat or sit as low as you can on your foam pad or backpack, which may help insulate you from ground current. Avoid being near the tallest trees or rock outcrops. A group should be well spread out, so that a strike will not incapacitate everybody at once. If you are onboard a larger boat, avoid having the whole crew clustered in the cockpit. Water is a good conductor, so do not swim or wade during a thunderstorm. If you are in a tent, sit up or squat to reduce the exposure of vital organs to ground current.

The inside of a vehicle is a relatively safe place during a lightning storm. The insulating value of the tires offers protection only from ground current, but the metal shell tends to conduct the energy of a direct strike around the occupants and into the ground. The metal shrouds and stays supporting the mast of a sailing vessel may have the same effect, provided there is a good grounding system and you are not leaning on them.

On a cliff, lightning current follows the cliff face, especially where it is wet. Wet climbing ropes may also become conductors. Hollows and caves may seem attractive as shelter, but current can jump across the opening and include you in the path. The same effect can occur between an object like an airplane wing or vehicle and the ground. No matter where you are during a lightning storm, always keep fundamental avoidance guidelines in mind.

Useful Information

- Isolation and height determine the likelihood of being struck.
- Enclosed, grounded structures or vehicles are protective (surface effect).
- Ground current is the most common source of injury.
- Metal and water can conduct current great distances.
- Leader strokes travel about 30–50 meters.

Because lightning can travel considerable distance, you should evacuate hazardous areas as soon as thunder is heard, or lightning is seen. The rapid development of cumulonimbus clouds is an early warning, although orographic convection (air passing over high terrain) can cause lightning from a clear sky in dry climates. Lightning also can strike during snowfall in higher elevations.

Risk Versus Benefit

Although there are ways to reduce the probability of being struck by lightning, as indicated in this chapter, there is no truly safe place during a thunderstorm. The physics of lightning have, so far, defied complete understanding and predictability. Fortunately, the overall probability of being struck is low, even if you do everything wrong.

Some lightning myths have been successfully debunked. For example, the fear that carrying metal objects or using a cell phone attracts lightning has been proven to be unfounded. Your trekking pole or ice axe will not increase your probability of being struck unless you pack it so that it projects above your head, making you taller. Devices marketed as lightning repellents or ion diffusers to reduce strikes do not work and will actually increase the probability of a strike if they project above the masthead or building. Unfortunately, the incidence of side flash renders the "cone of protection" concept unreliable for humans seeking shelter near tall trees or structures.

Risk Management

- Sit on an insulator to reduce contact with ground current
- Spread your group out to avoid a multiple casualty strike
- Inside a vehicle is best, on or under a vehicle is bad.
- If moving toward safety; keep moving
- Don't lean on a wire fence
- Lower is safer

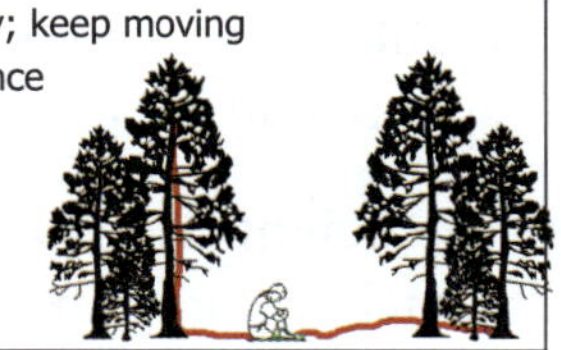

For raft guides, the perennial question is whether to stay in the raft on the river or to go ashore. Going ashore makes you higher, but if it allows for a large crew to spread out it might be worth it. If you choose to stay on the river, being close to the bank may reduce your isolation.

There are few options for boats on open water. The only way to reduce your probability of being struck is to reduce the time of exposure. If the storm cannot be avoided, at least set a course to take you clear of the storm as quickly as possible.

Chapter 22 Review: Lightning Injuries

- Lightning equalizes the difference in electrostatic charge that develops between regions of the atmosphere and between the atmosphere and the earth's surface during violent weather.
- The height and isolation of an object are the only two factors that predict the likelihood of being struck by lightning.
- Reducing the probability of lightning injury includes moving to a lower and less isolated position or inside a metal car, building, or ship.
- Fewer than 20% of lightning victims die of their injuries. Most of the current passes over the skin surface on its way to the ground.
- A lightning strike can disrupt the electrochemical function of the nervous system (causing respiratory and cardiac arrest), cause superficial burns on the skin, and can create enough explosive force to break bones and damage internal organs.
- Lightning injuries require no specialized field treatment. In the field, treat what you see.
- Even without obvious injury, lightning exposure can cause long-term medical and psychiatric problems.

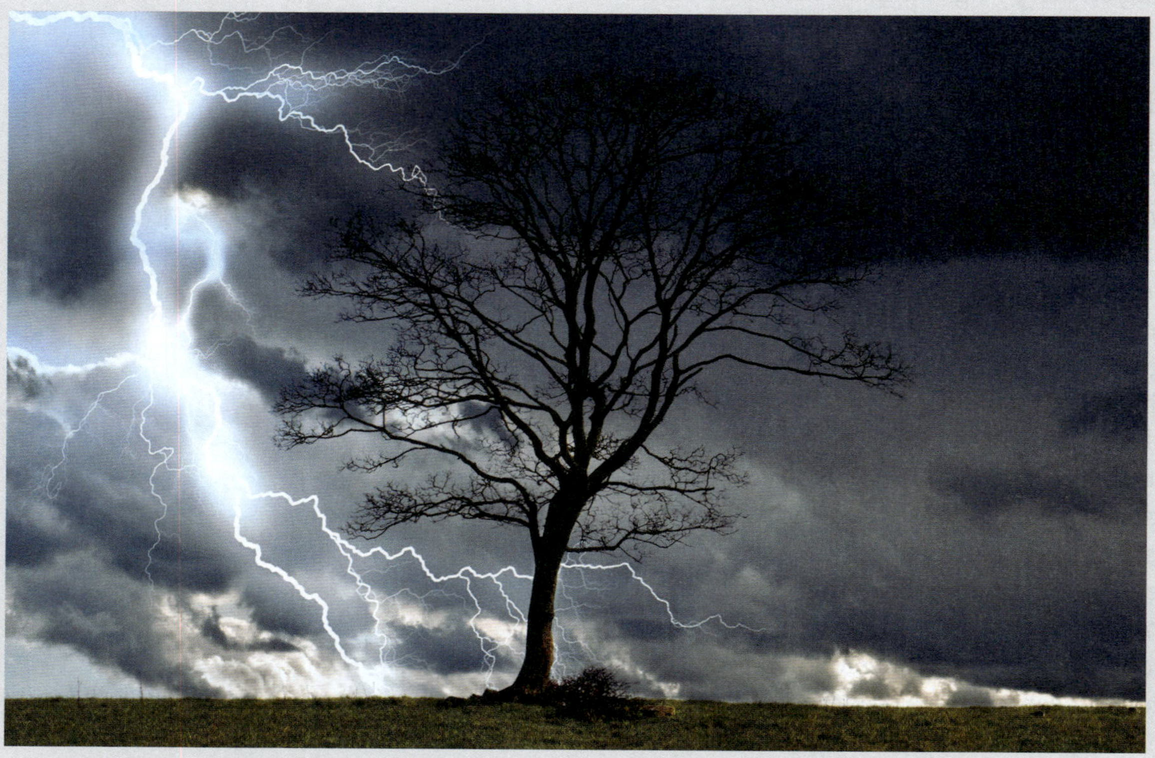

Because lightning can travel considerable distance, you should evacuate hazardous areas as soon as thunder is heard, or lightning is seen.

Chapter 23: Toxins, Envenomation, and Disease Vectors

Toxic substances can produce systemic effects, local effects, or both. Toxins, like trauma, can cause simultaneous involvement of more than one body system. The cause-and-effect relationship may be fairly obvious or quite confusing. Fortunately for field medicine, generic diagnoses and general principles work well.

A toxin can also be an allergen causing a release of histamine in addition to its toxic effects. A hornet sting producing anaphylaxis is an example of a substance that can do both. Fortunately, a toxic reaction is not often mixed with allergy, even though the type of exposure and symptoms may be similar.

Systemic toxins are those that affect the body as a whole. They may be ingested, injected, inhaled, or absorbed through the skin. Some common examples include mushrooms, organophosphate pesticides, and carbon monoxide. These toxins can represent an immediate threat to the function of the critical body systems.

Local toxins affect only the immediate area of contact. The toxin in a tarantula bite does not significantly affect critical body systems but may cause localized tissue swelling and pain. Some toxins have both systemic and local effects. An example would be an inhaled gas that irritates the respiratory system while being absorbed into the general circulation.

When you are not sure exactly what you are dealing with, base your initial treatment on the presenting signs and symptoms and the environmental conditions. In short, the generic response is to treat what you see.

Any toxin causing shock, respiratory distress, or brain failure represents an emergency in which urgent evacuation is indicated. Although you should try to obtain as much information from the scene as possible, the investigation should not delay appropriate evacuation and life support or increase the danger to rescuers.

Generic Treatment for Toxin Exposure:

- **Support** critical body systems.
- **Treat** what you see.
- **Treat** anaphylaxis if you see it.
- **Maintain** body core temperature.
- **Maintain** hydration.
- **Provide** pain relief.
- **Remove** or dilute the toxin, if possible.
- **Evacuate** (ALS intercept as needed).
- **Provide** antidote if available.

Ingested Toxins

A brief review of anatomy reminds us that our digestive system is essentially just a tube with the mouth at one end and the anus at the other. Whatever you swallow does not actually enter the body unless it is absorbed through the lining of the stomach or intestine. For example, a glass marble swallowed by a child will not be absorbed and will pass harmlessly through the gut. Although toxins are not inert like glass, we can try to keep more of the toxin in the gut with the marble, and speed its passage through, thereby reducing the amount absorbed by the intestinal lining.

To reduce absorption, the provider should attempt to dilute the toxin using water, which will also help move the substance through the gut more quickly on its way to excretion. Activated charcoal at a dose of 25 to 50 grams orally may bind some of the substances in the gut, helping to prevent absorption by the intestinal mucosa. Although this treatment may be helpful, remember that it is not definitive for high-risk toxins such as drug overdoses. Antidote and hospital care should be accessed urgently in these cases.

Unfortunately, effective antidotes to toxins are not always available. Additionally, their use is limited to cases where the toxin is known, such as certain drugs and plants. The availability of an antidote may influence your evacuation and destination. If possible, contact a poison control center (1-800-222-1222 in the United States) or local medical facility for specific treatments. In any case, most toxins are excreted or metabolized by the body over hours or days.

Drug Overdose

You should know the risks associated with overdose of any drug that you carry in quantity. The most likely source of a problem is overuse of over-the-counter pain medication, such as acetaminophen and ibuprofen, or prescription opioids like hydrocodone. Problems often occur when patients are confused about generic and trade names used for drugs. For example, a patient may take full doses of two different brands of pain reliever hoping for a better result, not realizing that both are brand names for the same acetaminophen. The effects of a mild unintentional overdose are usually limited to accentuated side effects like gastrointestinal (GI) upset or drowsiness. Discontinuing the medication usually solves the problem.

Intentional overdose is another matter. Even common over-the-counter medications like acetaminophen or iron tablets can be lethal in high doses. Immediate generic treatment followed by emergency evacuation is indicated. In opioid or antihistamine overdose, the anticipated problem is respiratory failure due to loss of respiratory drive. Oxygen and positive pressure ventilation (PPV) can be lifesaving. Naloxone, an opioid antagonist, given by intranasal or IM injection can reverse the effects of most opioid medications.

Ingested Toxins

Generic Treatment:

- BLS, PROP
- Remove and dilute: oral hydration
- Evacuate with ALS assistance as needed
- Contact poison control

American Association of Poison Control Centers
www.aapcc.org 800-222-1222
ASPCA – for pets
www.aspca.org/apcc 888-426-4435

Food Poisoning

Food poisoning is another form of accidental toxic ingestion. The toxin is produced by bacteria, such as staphylococci growing in poorly refrigerated food. There is usually no active infection because bacteria are destroyed by stomach acid, but the toxin survives to be absorbed by the gut. Symptoms are usually limited to GI upset, including cramps, diarrhea, and vomiting. The disease is self-limiting, and the most common anticipated problem is shock from dehydration. Hydration and easily-digested food are the primary treatment.

Food poisoning is differentiated from bacterial infection of the gut by the absence of fever or bloody or purulent diarrhea. Food poisoning is also very short-lived, usually resolving within 24 hours (an exception is Ciguatera, discussed below). You should suspect an active infection in any GI illness that lasts longer than a day. A bacterial infection of the gut should be considered serious and should be treated aggressively with antibiotics or evacuation.

It may be impossible to distinguish a mild gastroenteritis caused by a viral infection from food poisoning because the signs and symptoms are often the same. Your primary clue will be the mechanism of injury (MOI). You should suspect food poisoning when several people who ate the same meal develop the same symptoms at the same time. Identification and elimination of the contaminated food and thorough cleaning of dishware should be part of the plan.

Ingested Toxins

Food Poisoning:

- Preformed toxins like *Staph* enterotoxin, or ingested pathogens like Norovirus, *Clostridium*, or *E. coli*.
- Most cause nausea, vomiting, watery diarrhea, usually resolving within 72 hours.
- Most serious cause volume shock and/or inflammatory diarrhea with blood or pus, fever (e.g. *Salmonella*, *Campylobacter*).
- Treatment is generally supportive, with antibiotics for persistent or inflammatory diarrhea.

Viral gastroenteritis can affect a group in a similar way, but usually people will develop symptoms sequentially; early cases are improving while new cases are just developing. Thorough cleaning of dishware and hands is part of the plan, along with preventing symptomatic people from participating in food preparation or cleanup. Fortunately, in mild cases the field treatment of food poisoning and viral gastroenteritis is the same: hydration, easily digested foods, and time.

Ciguatera, scombroid, and paralytic shellfish poisoning are foodborne toxins worthy of special mention for the marine environment. Ciguatoxin is produced by a reef-dwelling dinoflagellate that is consumed by coral and other reef animals. It is concentrated up the food chain, reaching dangerous levels in larger predatory fish. It cannot be reliably detected and is not destroyed by cooking. Ciguatoxin produces GI and systemic neurologic symptoms, such as numbness, tingling, cramping, and reversal of hot and cold sensation that may persist for weeks. Ciguatera toxin can be avoided by restricting the diet to fish smaller than about one kilogram.

Ingested Toxins

Ciguatera:

- Neurotoxin from reef dwelling dinoflagellates concentrated in larger predatory fish
- Not destroyed by cooking or freezing
- Symptoms include vomiting, diarrhea, abdominal cramping, paresthesia, dysuria, metallic taste, temperature-related sensory defects.
- Generic treatment is symptomatic, including volume replacement.
- There are no proven specific treatments.

Scombroid toxin is a histamine-like substance produced by bacteria growing on the surface of dead fish in storage. Scombroid produces a histamine-like response including hives, itching, and flushed skin. It can be difficult to distinguish from an allergic reaction. Fortunately, the treatment is the same.

Ingested Toxins

Scombroid:

- Histidine in fish flesh converted by histamine by bacteria in fish stored in temps >4°C.
- Not destroyed by cooking or subsequent freezing or refrigeration.
- Symptoms generally develop with an hour. Flushing of the face, urticarial rash, diarrhea, headache are common.
- Sx rapidly improve with administration of antihistamine.

Paralytic shellfish poisoning occurs with consumption of clams or oysters that have concentrated an algae-produced neurotoxin. It is not destroyed by cooking. Symptoms include nausea, vomiting, diarrhea, abdominal pain, and tingling and burning sensations of the mucous membranes and skin. Respiratory paralysis can develop in severe cases. Treatment is primarily hydration and monitoring, with respiratory support in severe cases.

Symptoms developing after consumption of fish and shellfish should be treated like any other ingested toxin. Water and activated charcoal help dilute and remove the toxin, minimizing absorption by the gut. Hives and itching can be effectively treated with an antihistamine (e.g. diphenhydramine/Benadryl or ranitidine/Zantac). Persistent, progressive, or severe neurologic symptoms should be evacuated to medical care.

Ingested Toxins

Paralytic and Neurotoxic Shellfish Poisoning:

- Neurotoxin produced by algae concentrated in filter feeding shellfish (e.g., Red Tide)
- Not destroyed by cooking
- Symptoms include vomiting, diarrhea, neurologic symptoms, seizure, respiratory distress.
- Generic treatment is symptomatic, including volume replacement and antiemetics.
- Evacuate to medical care if possible.

Topical Toxins

Topical exposure can inflame the skin surface at the site of contact, causing open wounds at risk for infection. Toxins can also be absorbed through the skin, causing systemic effects. In the backcountry, most topical toxins come from plants like daphne and poison ivy that cause localized allergic reactions and inflammation. A few animals like the bufo toad excrete a toxin that causes primarily local effects on the skin of humans but can severely injure dogs and predators.

For treatment, clean the exposed area as you would for any skin wound. Irrigate copiously with water. Removal of some substances, such as manchineel sap (Hippomane mancinella) may require a different solvent capable of dissolving waxy or oily compounds. Alcohol, vinegar, and even WD-40 have found a place in initial treatment. Check with local medical facilities for recommendations on treating exposure to poisonous plants, preferably before the exposure occurs. Blisters caused by toxins should be left intact. Topical steroid creams may be helpful for superficial inflammation. Antibiotic ointment may help prevent infection.

Remember that the toxin may still be present on clothing and equipment that could come in contact with the patient or other members of the group. Examples of toxins that continue to spread on fingers and clothing include poison ivy (an allergen) and manchineel sap. Clean your gear thoroughly with an oil-dissolving soap or solvent to avoid perpetuating the problem.

Surface Absorbed

Treatment:

- BLS, PROP
- Remove and dilute: brush off or irrigate with water.
- Dress open wounds, burns, and blisters. BSA >10% is high risk.
- Evacuate with ALS assistance as needed.
- Contact poison control.

Eg: Manchineeal sap, organophosphate fertilizers.

High-Risk Topical Exposure

As with large burns or abrasions, the surface area involved in topical toxin exposure can lead to serious problems with even superficial injury. Anticipated problems in large surface area inflammation include dehydration, infection, and hypothermia. Any inflammatory process occupying more than about 10% of the body's surface area should be considered high risk. Be alert to respiratory involvement that carries the anticipated problem of respiratory distress and failure.

Inhaled Toxins

Toxic inhalation can cause problems through two distinct mechanisms. Inhaled substances can either be absorbed through the respiratory system into the systemic circulation or cause direct respiratory system injury. Carbon monoxide poisoning from using a heater or stove inside a poorly vented snow cave is an example of the former, and chlorine gas is an example of the latter.

Inhaled Toxins

Treatment:

- BLS, PROP
- Remove and dilute: PPV, fresh air and oxygen
- Respiratory system injury is high risk
- Evacuate with ALS assistance as needed
- Contact poison control

E.g.: Carbon monoxide, cooking and heating gas, volcanic gases.

Carbon monoxide gas causes no direct respiratory system injury but impairs oxygenation by displacing oxygen from receptor sites on hemoglobin molecules in red blood cells. Symptoms include headache, altered mental status, and nausea as the patient quietly asphyxiates at the cellular level. The problem may go unnoticed until it is too late. Like most inhaled toxins, the treatment is ventilation and fresh air. If instituted soon enough, there should be no lasting damage to critical body systems.

Direct injury can be caused by the inhalation of caustic substances. Chlorine gas directly damages the respiratory system. Symptoms include inflammation around the nose and mouth, coughing, wheezing, burning chest pain, and respiratory distress. Early recognition and treatment of respiratory distress is the key to survival. Identifying the causative agent in these cases is not as important as emergency field treatment and evacuation.

Injected Toxins

Although toxins can be injected by humans using needles, in the wilderness and marine setting we are more concerned about envenomation (toxins injected via animal stings and bites). Toxins used by organisms in the process of feeding or defense come in two basic types: neurotoxins and tissue toxins.

Neurotoxins interfere with the function of the nervous system, causing muscle spasm, paralysis, and altered sensation. When symptoms suggest a neurotoxin, you will need to include respiratory distress on your anticipated problem list. In the rare cases of fatal neurotoxin envenomation, the cause of death is usually respiratory failure due to paralysis of the diaphragm and chest wall musculature.

Tissue toxins destroy body cells, causing inflammation, pain, and swelling. Damage is usually localized, with distal ischemia and infection as anticipated problems. Severe envenomation can also produce systemic effects and multi-organ failure and volume shock.

Many organisms use a combination of tissue toxin and neurotoxin to subdue their prey. Antidotes are available to the toxins of some specific organisms and to some groups of similar species. It is well worth research into toxic species and the availability and location of antivenom before traveling to a new environment.

Injected Toxins

Tissue Toxins:

- Damage and destroy tissue cells
- Swelling, discoloration, pain
- Volume shock, multi-organ failure
- Coagulopathy

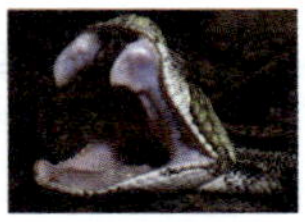

Neurotoxins:

- Inhibits function of nerve cells
- Numbness, cramping, paralysis, spasm
- Respiratory failure

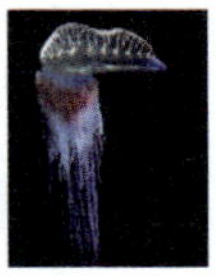

The vast majority of stings and bites are no more significant than the minimal discomfort they cause. The few that are significant are easily identified by severe pain, swelling, or the progression of neurologic symptoms. The important principle of field treatment for significant envenomation is to provide good basic life support while moving toward the appropriate definitive medical care. Identification of the specific species encountered can be valuable in planning treatment if medical facilities are accessible but should not delay evacuation.

Snakebite

Pit Vipers

The pit vipers (family Viperidae) in North America include rattlesnakes, copperheads, and cottonmouths. Viper venom is primarily a tissue toxin that causes local swelling and tissue damage. Systemic effects include problems with blood coagulation and shock caused by leakage of fluid from the circulatory system into the interstitial space (between the cells in body tissues). Some pit viper venom, notably the Mojave rattlesnake, also contains a systemic neurotoxin. The degree of systemic effect depends on the dose injected and the size and general health of the patient. Fatalities are extremely rare in North America but are more common in other parts of the world.

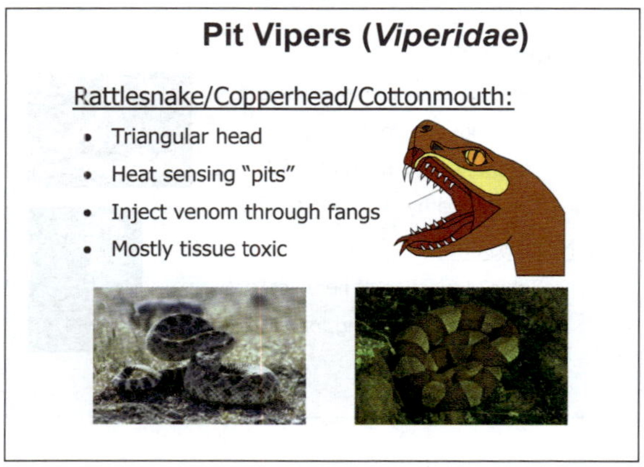

Treatment of Pit Viper Envenomation

The ideal treatment for a poisonous snakebite is antivenom. Evacuation to medical care should be started without delay by the fastest means available. Walking your patient out may be the quickest way to go, and this is fine unless prevented by severe symptoms. If possible, alert the receiving facility to expect your patient so antivenom can be acquired and prepared.

The use of antivenom is restricted to the hospital because it can cause life-threatening allergic reactions in rare cases. It is also extremely expensive and needs to be prepared carefully prior to use. It is most effective in the first 4 hours but can be given a day or more following the bite and still have some benefit.

Antivenom can be either monovalent (effective against the toxin of only one species) or polyvalent (covering several species). In North America, pit viper antivenom is the same for all the members of that family of snakes. It is not necessary to know the difference between a rattlesnake, copperhead, or cottonmouth. The presence of fang marks is enough. Specific antivenom may be used for species in other parts of the world.

Splinting the bitten extremity may help reduce pain and tissue damage, but it is an unproven treatment and should not delay evacuation. If ALS is easily available, IV hydration with isotonic saline should be initiated. Do not apply ice or arterial or venous tourniquets. Do not apply suction or incise the wound. Suction devices, even the more modern versions, have been shown to be ineffective and possibly harmful.

In anticipation of swelling, remove constricting items such as rings, bracelets, and tight clothing to prevent ischemia. Closely monitor any splint. If you can, mark the progression of swelling up the extremity. Make a line and write the time on the skin with a pen. This information will be helpful in the decision to use antivenom, and in deciding how much will be necessary.

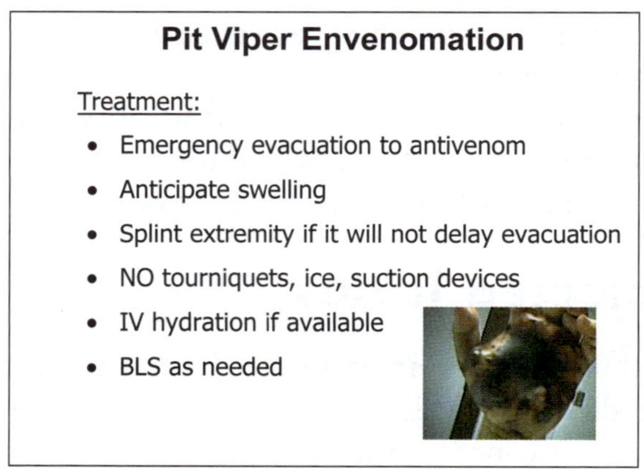

The amount of venom injected varies with the size and condition of the snake. Symptoms can range from mild to severe. A small number of strikes are dry bites in which no venom is injected at all. This is worth remembering if emergency evacuation will be a high-risk operation. In these situations, evacuation to medical care can be less emergent if no symptoms (e.g., pain, bleeding, or swelling) develop within 3 hours.

Coral Snakes

While many countries around the world have several examples of neurotoxic snakes, the US has only one, the coral snake (family Elapidae). Fortunately for humans, the fangs of the coral snake are quite small, and the snake must chew its way into your skin to inject venom successfully. Coral snakes do not bite unless they are handled, resulting in fewer than 25 envenomations per year in the United States. The venom's effects may be delayed for several hours.

Coral Snake Envenomation

S/Sx:

- Indistinct teeth marks, no discrete fangs
- Delayed onset of neurotoxic symptoms
- Numbness, tingling, cramping, respiratory paralysis

Treatment:

- Evacuate to medical care
- BLS / PROP

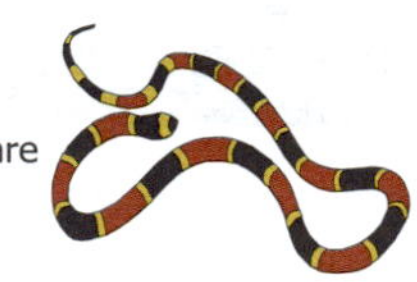

Symptoms of coral snake bite include tingling of the extremity, possibly progressing to the whole body. Fatalities are exceedingly rare, but when they occur they are usually due to respiratory failure. Treatment is symptomatic and supportive. The production of a specific coral snake antivenom has been discontinued in the United States and all remaining stock has had its expiration date extended by the USFDA. Antivenom is still produced in other countries but has yet to be approved by the United States Food and Drug Administration.

In parts of the world outside of North America, fang-bearing snakes possess more destructive forms of venom. A lymphatic compression bandage is sometimes employed in the field treatment of envenomation known to involve potent neurotoxins. It is worth research into the types of snakes, recommended treatments, and location of antivenom for the region in which you will be traveling. You may find, for example, that the nearest antivenom for the Fer de Lance in Trinidad is actually in Miami. Check before you need it.

Marine Toxins

In the marine environment, toxins are most commonly infiltrated by spines or injected by nematocysts. They range in potency from the merely annoying to the rapidly fatal. Again, the recognition of species is not as important as the recognition and treatment of a critical system problem.

Spiny Injury

Spines are used for defense and some are coated with toxins. Examples of marine life with spines include stingrays, scorpion fish, catfish, lion fish, and some sea urchins. The species found in waters around North America generally produce only localized pain and swelling from tissue toxins. In Indo-Pacific waters, the organisms can be more dangerous, carrying significant neurotoxic effects as well.

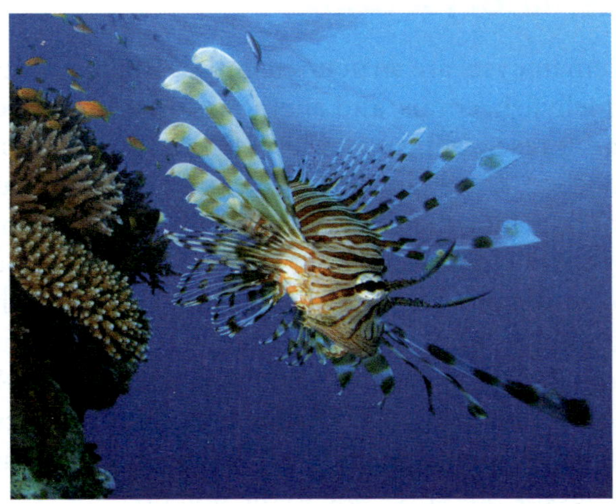

The lion fish is a rapidly spreading invasive species in the Atlantic basin. The toxin on its defensive barbs is painful but not lethal.

The sting of a poisonous ray, urchin, or fish is easy to distinguish from a nontoxic puncture. The pain caused by the wound itself is minimal compared to the quickly increasing discomfort caused by the toxin, which may possess both tissue toxic and neurotoxic characteristics. The barbed stinger or spine will often remain in the wound.

Because the spine is coated with a sheath of tissue that contaminates the wound, infection is likely. Treatment includes spine or stinger removal and aggressive wound debridement.

Most types of spiny toxins are inactivated by heat. Immerse the affected part in water as hot as the patient can tolerate until pain is relieved. Often this will be within a few minutes, but treatment may need to be continued for an hour or more.

Spiny Injury

Treatment:

- Immerse extremity in hot water up to 90 minutes
- High-risk wound care, anticipate infection
- BLS/ALS and immediate evacuation for progressive neurologic symptoms (lionfish, stonefish, cone shell)
- Pain control

Typically tissue toxin, sometimes combined with neurotoxin

Nematocyst Sting

Nematocysts are structures in the stinging parts of jellyfish, corals, and anemones, that fire something resembling a microscopic harpoon when touched. These harpoons then inject a potent neurotoxin into the skin. Individually, the amount of toxin is miniscule, but the toxin load can be considerable when the patient has contact with thousands of nematocysts at once. Of particular concern are stings from the Indo-Pacific box jellyfish (Chironex fleckeri), due to the high potency of the venom, and the Portuguese man-of-war (Physalia physalis), due to the potential for large surface area exposure.

The field treatment for stinging jellyfish includes removing tentacles by flushing with seawater and picking off any remaining tentacles with forceps or gloved fingers. Seawater is considered by some authorities to be preferable to fresh water because the osmotic difference of fresh water may stimulate more nematocysts to fire. Flushing and soaking the skin with vinegar will inactivate the nematocysts of some species and is specifically recommended for box jellyfish, fire worm, and sponge stings. There is also evidence that hot water soaks, as with spiny envenomation, or even a hot shower may reduce the pain immediately after the sting, although the mechanism is not well understood. Ice applications may help relieve persistent pain later. The use of alcohol, meat tenderizer, urine, or other chemicals to flush the skin is not helpful, and possibly harmful.

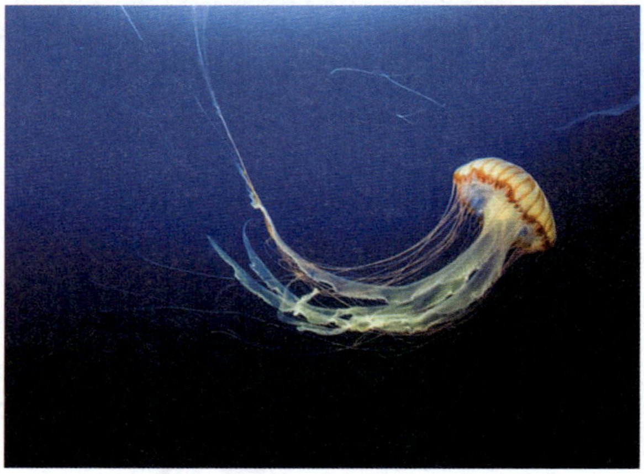

The long tentacles on jellyfish carry the potential for large surface area stings.

Persistent skin inflammation can be treated for several days with twice daily applications of a steroid cream or ointment (e.g., hydrocortisone). Antihistamines may also help because a local allergic reaction may be part of the patient's discomfort. As with any open wound, infection is an anticipated problem.

Nematocyst Injury

Treatment:

- Rinse with salt water, remove tentacles
- Hot water soaks
- General wound care, topical corticosteroids and topical anesthetics
- BLS/ALS and immediate evacuation for progressive neurologic symptoms (box jelly, man-of-war)
- Pain control

Systemic effects from large or potent exposure to nematocyst-borne neurotoxins include pain, spasm, and cramping. An exposure occupying more than 50% of a limb should be considered potentially serious with anticipated systemic neurotoxic effects. Truly life-threatening symptoms are generally limited to Portuguese man-of-war and the Indo-Pacific box jellyfish stings. Medical follow-up is recommended for any exposure that produces significant systemic symptoms.

The box jellyfish venom can produce cardiac arrhythmia, respiratory paralysis, and a dangerous elevation of blood pressure. For this reason, antivenom to this toxin is carried and administered in the field by rescue personnel in high-incidence areas of Australia and Southeast Asia. BLS and immediate evacuation are indicated. Consult local authorities about the area where you plan to operate.

There is no antivenom for the Portuguese man-of-war. Fortunately, fatalities from exposure are very rare. Symptoms include severe burning sensations and skin redness that tend to disappear within an hour. Initial treatment includes only flushing with water, removal of tentacles, and treatment for pain. In the case of Portuguese man-of-war stings, vinegar is not recommended.

More significant exposure can cause muscle cramping, temporary numbness and weakness in the area, and lymph node swelling. Allergic reactions are uncommon, but the practitioner should be alert to the signs and symptoms of anaphylaxis mixed with the toxic effects. Any persistent or severe symptoms require follow-up medical care.

Insects and Arachnids

Insect and arachnid venom are injected by a stinger or specialized mouthparts as the animal attempts to defend itself or warn you away from a nest. It is meant to hurt, and it usually does. This is typical of wasps, fire ants, spiders, and scorpions. More commonly, your skin reacts to the irritation of substances used by a feeding insect to prevent clotting of your blood. Many of them also inject a local anesthetic to reduce the pain caused by the bite, at least for as long as they're feeding. Examples of these insects include black flies, deer flies, moose flies, mosquitoes, and no-see-ums.

Local reaction to toxins can be severe but involve only the extremity or immediate area of the bite or sting. There may be some degree of acute stress reaction (ASR) that must be distinguished from systemic effects. Local reactions are treated for comfort. Use cool soaks, elevation, and rest. Aspirin, ibuprofen, or other anti-inflammatory pain medications help, as do diphenhydramine or other antihistamines.

Toxin load is the term applied to the cumulative effects of multiple stings or bites. The effects can be immediate (as with a large number of bee stings) or delayed up to 24 hours. Delayed reactions are common in black fly country in the spring and early summer. Symptoms include fever, fatigue, headache, and nausea. This is not an allergic reaction if the generalized swelling, respiratory distress, and other signs of anaphylaxis are absent.

Toxin load does not usually cause a serious critical system problem. Observe the patient for 24 hours. Give aspirin, ibuprofen, or other anti-inflammatory pain reliever for comfort. Watch for signs of infection at the site of insect bites. Keep the patient well hydrated and protected from excessive cooling or heating.

Black Widow

The black widow spider (Latrodectus mactans), found in the warmer parts of the United States and further south, uses a potent neurotoxin to immobilize prey and as a defense mechanism. This spider prefers dark and quiet places to feed and nest. People are bitten most often when reaching into confined spaces or sitting on an outhouse seat. The bite itself is mildly uncomfortable or painless.

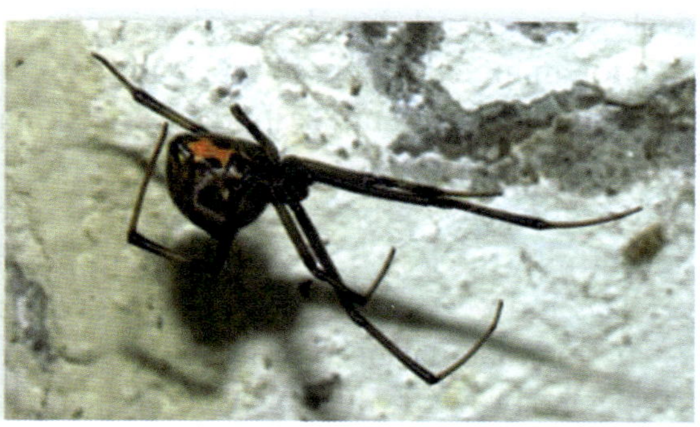

Black widow (Latrodectus mactans)

There are a variety of widow spiders found around the world. The systemic symptoms of widow envenomation include muscle cramping (especially in the abdomen), severe pain, numbness, and tingling. The development of these symptoms shortly after being in a likely habitat should raise the suspicion of a black widow bite. Treatment includes evacuation to medical care if your patient shows signs of critical system involvement or needs medication to reduce muscle spasm. Antivenom is available but may carry more risk than the venom itself. Symptoms usually resolve over several days but may persist for weeks. Despite its ominous name, death from the bite of a black widow in North America is extremely rare.

Brown Recluse

The brown recluse is a large spider found in the south-central United States that injects a long-acting tissue toxin causing localized tissue inflammation and necrosis.

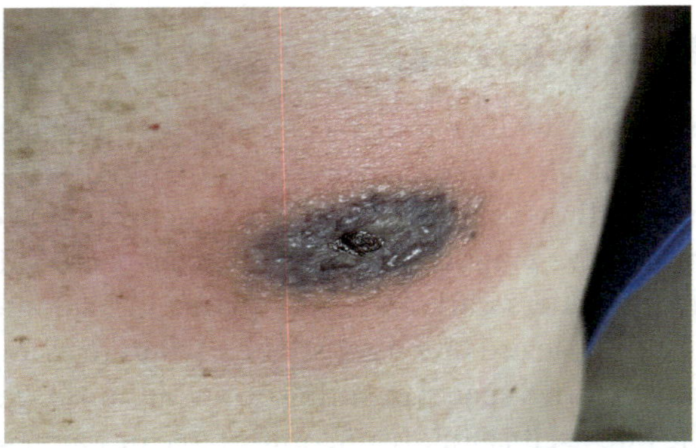

The initial bite may go unnoticed, with a pustule developing several days later. This is often mistaken for an infection caused by a splinter or other foreign body. It does not respond to incision and drainage or to antibiotics.

Although many of these envenomations resolve uneventfully, the lesion can continue to progress over days and weeks to involve a large area of tissue destruction that may become secondarily infected. A suspected brown recluse bite should be referred to a surgeon. Many lesions believed to be caused by a brown recluse turn out to be other problems.

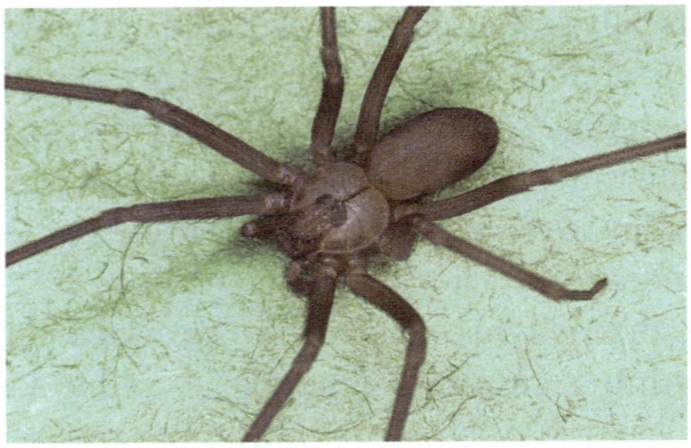

Brown recluse (Loxosceles reclusa)

Scorpions

Scorpions have a wide distribution around the world, but very few species are dangerous. Most scorpion stings are described as similar to, or a bit worse than, your average wasp. Most bothersome in North America is the bark scorpion (Centruroidies sp.), which employs a potent neurotoxin. Pain may last for hours or days. There is no specific field treatment beyond pain medication. Ice is not indicated. Significant systemic symptoms are rare and include agitation and respiratory paralysis; these should prompt an evacuation to medical care. An antivenom is available, but it is a high-risk treatment owing to the incidence of serum sickness and anaphylaxis. No fatalities from Centruroidies stings have been reported in the United States, and very rarely elsewhere.

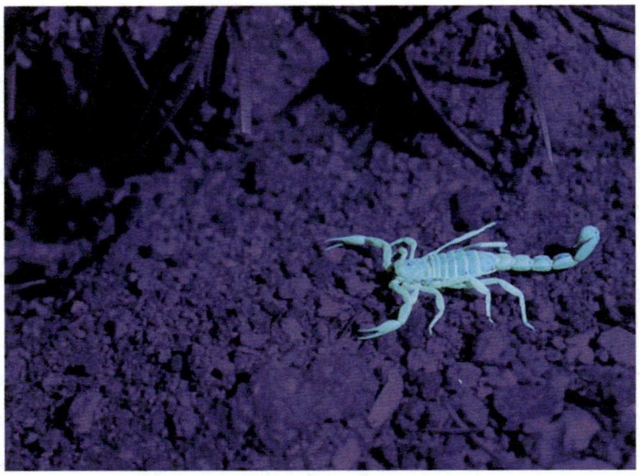

Arizona Bark Scorpion under blacklight

Tick Paralysis

The saliva of some species of ticks contains a neurotoxin capable of causing symptoms in humans, most commonly in children. Tick paralysis can develop after 4 or more days of attachment and is characterized by numbness and paralysis progressing up the legs and arms. The patient may exhibit ataxia (stumbling gait), restlessness, or irritability. The diagnosis is suspected by finding an engorged tick and confirmed by rapid improvement following its removal.

Tick paralysis is rare but can cause fatal respiratory paralysis if the tick is not found and removed. Ticks are more commonly implicated as vectors of bacterial and parasitic disease. Prevention of tick paralysis and tick-borne disease depends on avoiding bites and early removal of attached ticks.

Arthropod Disease Vectors

The phylum Arthropoda includes insects, spiders, crustaceans, and others that comprise over 80% of known animal species. Since many arthropods feed on humans, they are a significant disease vector. Some arthropods merely transmit viruses or bacteria from person to person. Others serve as a host for one stage of the parasite life cycle with humans hosting another. In either case, illness is often, but not always, the result.

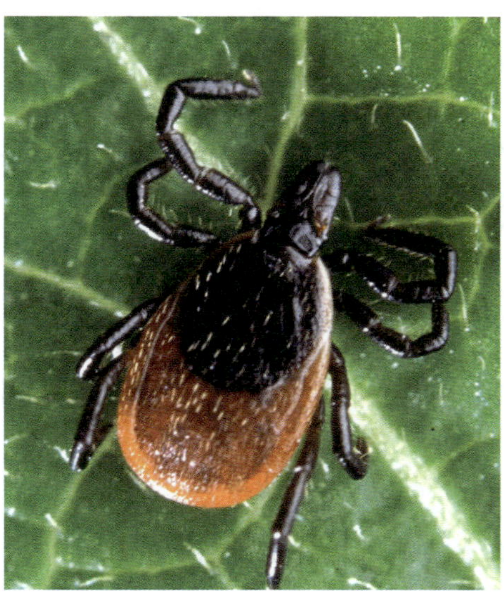

Adult deer tick

Ticks serve as a vector for diseases from anaplasmosis to ehrlichiosis and varieties of spotted fevers and encephalitides worldwide. One tick can carry multiple diseases. Fortunately for the medic on a short expedition, most of these conditions manifest themselves many days to weeks after exposure. Unfortunately for the patient and their doctor, these diseases present with a constellation of confusing symptoms making a definitive diagnosis difficult. The primary work of the practitioner in the field is prevention and education.

Inform your teammates or expedition members of the risks involved in hosting ticks. Instruct them to wear long-sleeved shirts with long pants tucked into high socks, and a bandanna high on the neck under a low hat. Encourage the use of repellent on clothing, especially around cuff and neck openings. Following these recommendations, your team members may look silly, but they will substantially reduce the chance of feeding a tick and acquiring a tick-borne disease.

It is also important to check for ticks frequently on your skin and clothing. Wearing light-colored clothing will help. They usually crawl around for a while before settling in to feed. Frequent inspections will get rid of most of them before they attach.

Tick-borne Disease

Prevention:

- DEET, Picaridin, or IR 3535 on skin
- Permethrin on clothing
- Tight weave clothing
- Frequent tick checks
- Prompt removal of attached ticks
- Post-Exposure Prophylaxis in Lyme endemic regions

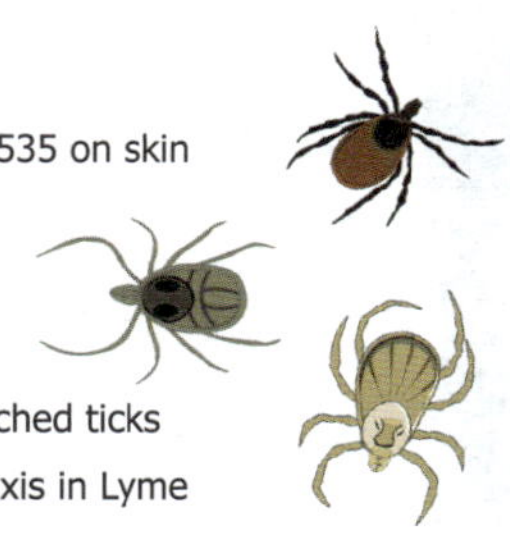

"Tick country" is vegetated: woods, grass, and brush. Tick season is spring, summer, and fall."

Ticks that are attached can be most safely removed by grasping them at the skin surface and gently pulling them off with tweezers. Sometimes, the mouth-parts break off and remain in the skin. Try to scrape these out with a sharp blade or needle.

The host should not attempt removal by burning the tick, or by suffocating or poisoning it with

Vaseline, alcohol, gasoline, or mineral oil. These tactics may cause the tick to regurgitate infectious material into the bite. Do not handle the tick without gloves or other protection.

Prompt removal of ticks can also help reduce the transmission of disease. Lyme disease, for example, is not effectively transmitted until the tick has been in place for a day or so. Rocky Mountain spotted fever can be transmitted in just a few hours. In regions where Lyme disease is endemic, medical practitioners will often prescribe a single-dose treatment of doxycycline or other antibiotic to patients who have suffered a prolonged tick attachment.

Tick country is vegetated with woods, grass, and brush. Tick season is spring, summer, and fall. Adult ticks are eight-legged arthropods ranging in size from nearly microscopic to a centimeter in diameter. The ticks of greatest concern, for Lyme disease at least, are two to four millimeters in diameter, and before they begin to feed are not easily recognized as a foreign creature on your skin.

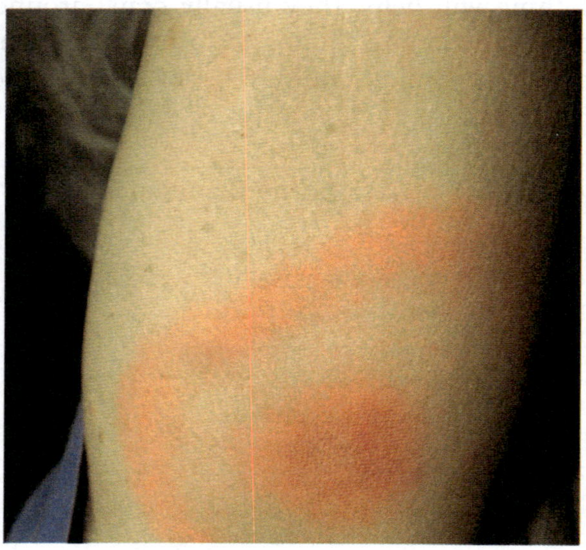

Lyme disease rash

Once attached and engorged with blood, ticks look more like a wart, mole, or other skin part, and may be missed by someone who does not know your body as well as you do. The appearance of flu-like symptoms, severe headaches, fever, rash, and muscular aches and pains several days to weeks after a confirmed long-term tick attachment or travel in a tick-infested area is worth immediate medical evaluation for several tick-borne illnesses.

Mosquitoes

The list of diseases transmitted by mosquitoes includes malaria, filariasis, West Nile virus, equine encephalitis, dengue fever, and a host of others. The key to avoiding these infections is to avoid being a host to mosquitoes. Like ticks, they can be deterred by insect repellent and tight-weave clothing. Unlike ticks, they can transmit disease in less than a minute.

Prophylactic medication with atovaquone/proguanil, doxycycline or others can help prevent malaria infection. However, some diseases, such as filariasis, have no definitive cure and no effective prophylactic medication. The fewer mosquitoes you feed, the less your chance of becoming ill.

Mosquito-borne Disease

Prevention:

- DEET, Picaridin, IR3535 or Lemon/Eucalyptus* on skin
- Permethrin on clothing
- Tight-weave clothing
- Avoid feeding time
- Pre- or post-exposure prophylaxis in Malaria endemic regions**

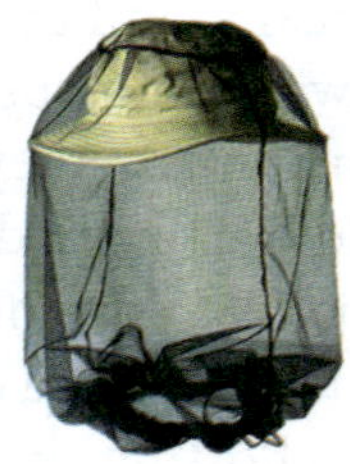

* not against malaria
** see www.cdc.gov

The same clothing and repellent tactics used with ticks apply well here. In addition, avoid being exposed during the times of day when vector mosquitoes feed. This is typically dawn and dusk but may be a few hours during the middle of the night depending on location. Permethrin-impregnated bed nets have been very successful in some places, but some mosquito populations have changed their feeding time behavior, possibly in response to the nighttime use of bed nets. Local knowledge may help with your prevention plan.

Fleas, Lice, and Mites

Sometimes the adult insect is easily seen, such as lice in the hairline or a flea in your bedding. More often, the infestation is suspected by the sudden appearance of itchy bites following a night in a strange bed or interaction with a pet. A careful inspection of hair, bedding, or clothing will usually identify the offending organism.

Only about 5% of a given flea population is actively feeding on blood. The rest are at various stages of development as eggs, pupae, and larvae. Adult fleas can hibernate for up to 2 years waiting for a blood meal.

The worst place to sleep is on that old mattress in the trekking hut that was last occupied 6 weeks ago. The eggs, pupae, and larvae have matured and are waiting for you. Only a few of them need to be carrying the bacteria Yersinia pestis to give you bubonic plague. Fleas can be killed or deterred by insect repellents and insecticides. Your own sleeping bag, frequently washed, is another good defense.

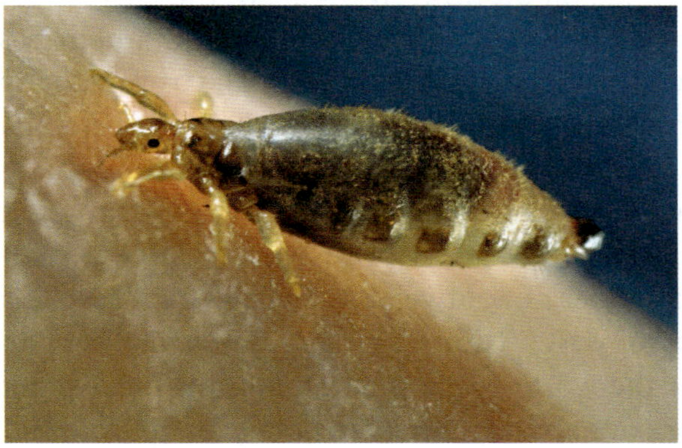

Human louse

Lice are easily transmitted between people sharing clothing and furniture. They tend to limit their range to groin or head hair. The adults are easily killed with permethrin or malathion. Reapplication may be necessary in 10 days to kill the newly hatched larvae. In the absence of permethrin shampoo, lice can also be smothered with a layer of any viscous substance such as Vaseline or mayonnaise. It may not be pretty, but it can solve your problem.

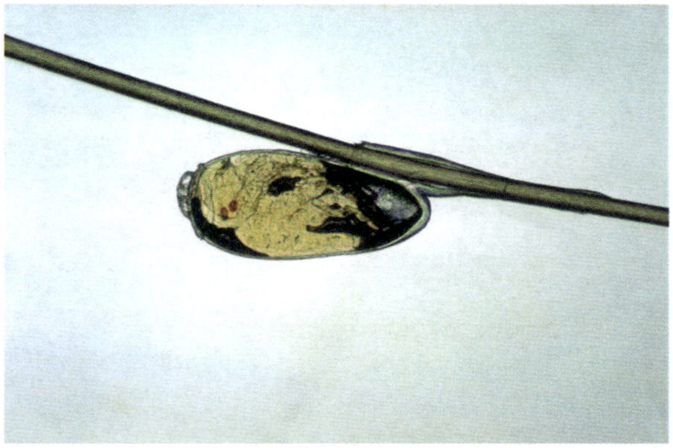

Nit of a louse on a hair

Mites can be a bit more difficult to identify and treat. Most are too small for the naked eye to see and can cause a variety of rashes. Most mite infestations are self-limiting because the human is not the normal host. The mite may feed temporarily and drop off without burrowing or reproducing. The rash disappears when contact with the host organism is discontinued.

The most common and troubling mite infestation is scabies (Sarcoptes scabiei). Humans are the normal host where the mite enjoys a full life cycle in the outer layers of the skin. Scabies is usually passed between people by skin-to-skin contact. The symptoms begin with a few small and intensely itchy red spots that slowly spread over days or weeks to involve other body areas, especially where the host human can scratch and spread eggs from one site to another. Epidemics within close groups or families is common. A host can begin to spread scabies before symptoms become apparent. Secondary bacterial infection is an anticipated problem.

Treating scabies requires application of 5% permethrin cream or other topical scabicide that is left on the skin for several hours. Bedding and clothing can be treated with a hot dryer. Preferably the patient, clothing, and bedding are treated simultaneously to prevent repeat infestation.

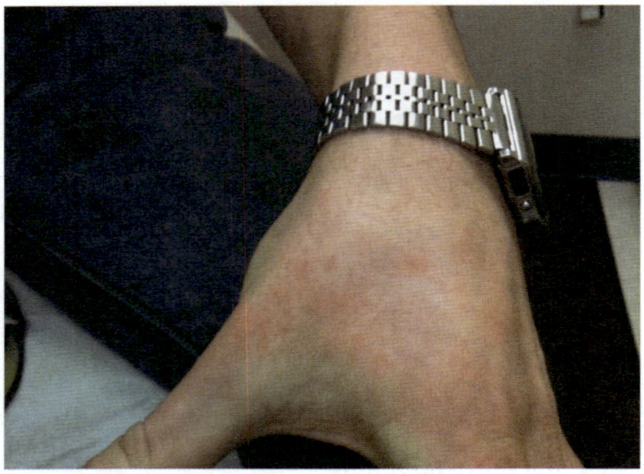

Scabies often appears first on the hands

Insect Repellents

The best insect repellents currently available include DEET, permethrin, picaridin, and IR3535. DEET and permethrin are both extensively studied and are considered safe and effective. DEET can be used on the exposed skin of hands, ankles, and the face. There is no advantage to using a formulation greater than 30% DEET. Permethrin is recommended for clothing and has been shown to remain effective after 20 or more washings.

Both DEET and IR3535 can damage plastics and irritate the eyes. Lotion formulations of either can minimize these problems and prolong the duration of effectiveness. Neither permethrin nor picaridin has the same affinity for synthetics and can be used safely around nylon sleeping bags and tent screens. Permethrin is typically used only on clothing and equipment, not directly on the skin.

Although there are numerous other products and claims on the market, there really are no other agents effective enough to recommend in the prevention of disease. Lemon eucalyptus is another popular insect repellant, but it does not enjoy the same effectiveness against mosquitos and sand flies as the other four. The various herbs and odors like citronella and garlic are significantly less effective.

Risk Versus Benefit

If a toxin is known to be particularly dangerous, early evacuation to medical care can be lifesaving. Examples include acetaminophen in toxic doses and several common mushroom species. In the remote setting where evacuation will be delayed or impossible, it is well worth reminding expedition members of the extreme consequence of a medication or culinary mistake.

In years past, the induction of vomiting was considered an emergency treatment for drug overdose and ingested toxins. We now recognize that vomiting is a high-risk activity in any environment and the benefit is questionable, even where evacuation is not an option. Preservation of the airway takes priority.

Some authorities are recommending the application of a pressure bandage for North American snake envenomation on extremities. The idea is to reduce the systemic spread of the toxin through lymphatic drainage without obstructing arterial or venous blood flow. In the field, the correct pressure is difficult to achieve and maintain, increasing the risk of local tissue damage from ischemia and sequestration of the toxin. Because fewer than 1 in 1,000 people die of pit viper envenomation in North America, and all but zero from coral snakes, the benefit of restricting systemic dilution does not outweigh the risk of increased local tissue destruction in the extremity. In other parts of the world where snake venom is more potent or contains a greater percentage of neurotoxin, a pressure bandage is more clearly worth the associated risks.

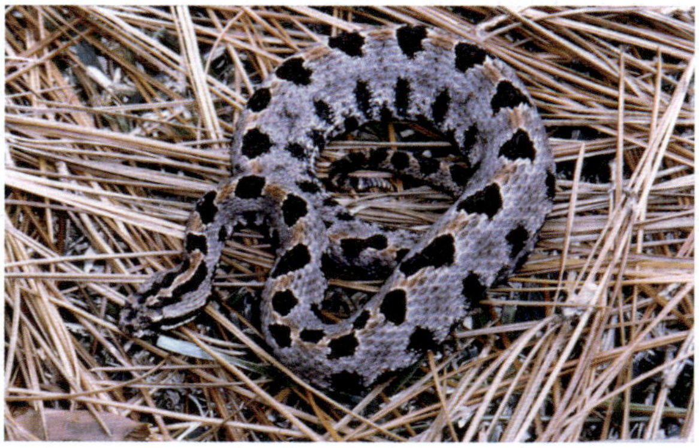

Pigmy Rattlesnake

When discussing arthropod disease vectors, many people express concern about the possible toxic side effects of DEET as an insect repellent. It should be reassuring that DEET has been extensively studied and found to be remarkably safe and effective in concentrations to the low 30% range. Some formulations use vehicles that are more resilient to the environment and allow for release over time, thus less likely to be absorbed and requiring fewer applications. The minimal risk in its use is well outweighed by the benefit of avoiding devastating diseases like filariasis, malaria, Lyme, babesiosis, West Nile, and dozens of others.

Toxins and Envenomations

High-Risk Problem:

- Persistent shock, respiratory distress, altered mental status
- Known dangerous exposure
- High-risk wounds or burns
- Cannot maintain body core temperature
- Cannot maintain hydration and calories
- The patient is getting worse

The same endorsement is warranted for Picaridin, which has been used extensively and safely throughout the world for the past three decades and is as effective as DEET in similar concentrations. Lemon/eucalyptus is listed by the United States CDC as an alternative, but is much less effective against mosquitoes, not proven against malaria vectors, and not effective against ticks.

Chapter 23 Review:
Toxins, Envenomation, and Disease Vectors

- Toxic substances can produce systemic effects, local effects, or both.
- A toxin can also be an allergen, causing a release of histamine in addition to its toxic effects.
- Toxins that produce significant systemic effects are serious and require emergency evacuation.
- High-risk ingestions like drug overdoses warrant immediate evacuation to medical care and, if available, an antidote.
- Toxic inhalation can injure the respiratory system. The anticipated problems include respiratory distress.
- Toxins injected by snakebite or other envenomation come in two basic forms: tissue toxins and neurotoxins. Pit viper envenomation is mostly tissue toxin.
- The anticipated problems with pit viper envenomation include swelling, pain, shock, organ failure, and infection. Aggressive hydration and urgent evacuation to antivenom is the ideal treatment.
- Coral snake envenomation is neurotoxic. Anticipated problems include numbness, cramping, and respiratory paralysis. Evacuation to a hospital is the ideal treatment. Antivenom may not be available.
- Nematocyst envenomation (jellyfish, man-of-war) is primarily neurotoxic. The treatment is removal of the nematocyst-bearing tentacle with sea water or vinegar and symptomatic treatment of pain and inflammation. Fatalities are limited to massive man-of-war stings or indopacific box jellyfish.
- Marine spiny envenomation is treated with hot water immersion to inactivate the toxin. The anticipated problem is infection from a high-risk puncture wound.
- Arthropod envenomation is generally more painful than serious (except for anaphylaxis). Treatment is symptomatic with pain medication and topical or systemic antihistamines.
- Prolonged, systemic, or progressive symptoms deserve medical evaluation.
- Toxic loading is the cumulative effect of many bites or stings, such as several hundred black fly bites. Treatment is symptomatic with NSAIDs and antihistamines.
- Tick paralysis is caused by a neurotoxin. Removal of the tick cures it.
- Many serious diseases are transmitted by arthropod vectors like mosquitoes and ticks. Diagnosis and treatment may be difficult. Avoidance and using protective clothing, nets, and repellent is the ideal field treatment.

Case Study 10: College Trip

SCENE

A college vacation trip to the shores of Lake Powel in Utah. It is early evening, the sky is clear, and the temperature is about 20°C with winds of 25 knots from the south. The camp is located approximately 7 miles by water from the marina at Bullfrog.

S: An 18-year-old man was bitten on the left forearm by a 4-foot snake that he was attempting to capture and bring back to camp. In the ensuing confusion, the snake escapes. The man is unable to describe it other than being dark in color and very fast. He complains of pain in the mid left forearm and of feeling very faint.

Despite a stiff headwind on the lake, the patient is carried to a canoe for evacuation to the marina. Unfortunately, the paddlers are intoxicated and become lost in the darkness. They return to camp two hours later, unsure of where they had been.

The patient is reevaluated by a Wilderness First Responder who had remained sober. The patient, now calm and alert, reports no allergies and is not taking any medication. He has no history of significant medical problems and had eaten dinner 4 hours ago, which included a six-pack of beer. There was no other recent trauma or illness.

O: The patient is awake but subdued, with normal mental status. He has two small puncture wounds on his left forearm. There is minimal swelling extending 7 cm proximal to the bite, but no discoloration. The area is mildly tender to the touch. Distal CSM is intact. There are no other injuries. Vital signs at 10:15 pm: BP: unavailable, Pulse: 80, Resp: 16, Temp: appears normal, Skin W/D/P, C: awake and oriented.

A:

1. Pit viper strike
   A': Local and systemic effects of the toxin
2. Dark, windy
   A': Hazardous evacuation

P:

1. Rings and watch removed from the arm. Continued monitoring.
2. Keep overnight in camp, evacuate in daylight

Discussion:

The decision to stay in camp was based on the low risk of serious problems from the snakebite and the high risk of waterborne evacuation in the dark. Proceeding with evacuation in the morning was appropriate, even though symptoms had not progressed. Problems with blood coagulation and compartment syndrome can develop later and should be monitored. A bite is also considered a high-risk wound.

Case Study 11: Ocean Voyage

SCENE
Transpacific voyage aboard a 135-foot sailing school vessel 500 miles northeast of Midway Island. The weather has been cold, wet, and windy for the past 24 hours.

S: A 20-year-old student is found huddled at the base of the foremast at dawn. He was last seen at watch change at 23:00 the previous day. He appears to be unconscious. The watch officer is summoned.

O: The student is responsive to painful stimuli. His foul weather gear is open in front, and he is soaked to the waist. A bruise is noted below his left eye. There is no other obvious injury. Vital signs at 05:30: BP: 110/70, Pulse: 60, Resp: 10, C: P on AVPU, Temp: felt cool, Skin: pale. An empty bottle of Dramamine tablets was found in his jacket pocket. According to his medical screening form, the student has no known allergies, he is not on medication, and he has no history of significant medical problems. His last meal would have been a snack at 21:00 the previous day.

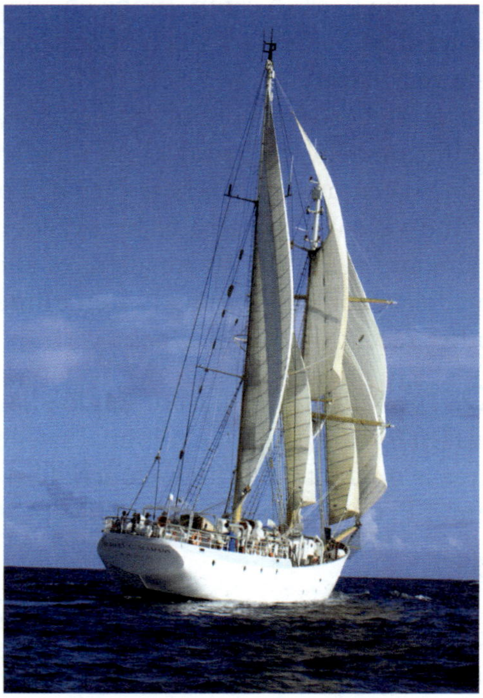

A:

1. P on AVPU. Consider low blood sugar, hypothermia, traumatic brain injury, toxins.
2. Spine cannot be cleared

P:

1. Hypothermia package, external rewarming
2. Monitor AVPU and airway
3. Monitor respiration
4. Sugar orally when airway can be protected
5. Spine protection until cleared

Discussion:

Wet clothing was removed, and the patient was wrapped in a sleeping bag. Hot water bottles were rotated into the package. Although the patient was breathing, ventilations were assisted by mouth to mask. A rectal temperature of 31°C was measured, confirming the suspicion of severe hypothermia. The patient responded to treatment, improved to V on AVPU, and began to shiver. As soon as he was able to take liquids safely, he was given warm tea and honey. After 3 hours, he was A on AVPU with normal mental status and a normal core temperature. He was able to explain what happened.

There had been no trauma. He had not been climbing the mast. The bruise below his eye had developed after being struck in the face by a flailing jib sheet two days before. He had taken twice the normal dose of Dramamine to treat his sea sickness and had fallen asleep in the location where he had been found.

Although this problem could have been avoided, it was handled appropriately once discovered. The watch officer's plan initially considered all the possible causes of reduced level of consciousness, including severe hypothermia. As the patient responded to treatment, the other causes could be ruled out by exam and history leaving only the hypothermia and successful recovery.

Section VI: Backcountry Medicine

Chapter 24: An Approach to Illness

The nonspecific symptoms typical of many illnesses can generate a long list of possible diagnoses. Even in the emergency department it can be difficult to determine exactly what you're dealing with. In the backcountry it can be impossible. There is little value in working through lists of symptoms and descriptions of diseases just so you can put a name on your patient's problem. The laboratory and CT scanner aren't available to confirm your suspicions anyway. Your working diagnosis may remain as generic as "serious," "not serious," or "I don't know."

As you evaluate an illness be sure to consider signs and symptoms in the context of the patient's behavior. The simple presence of a fever, for example, will alarm most people. But, you should worry more about a confused and lethargic person with a normal temperature of 37°C than about an active and oriented patient with a fever of 39°C. How the body and brain are working overall is more important than any specific sign or complaint.

Generic Assessment of the Ill Patient

A few quick observations and questions can help you make that important generic assessment: Serious or Not Serious? Your generic worry list for an ill patient is essentially the same as that for trauma: Any pattern that suggests shock, respiratory failure, or brain failure needs immediate attention. The rate of progression of the problem can help determine the urgency of treatment or evacuation. A patient who has become gradually worse over the past five days is usually less worrisome than the one who has become dramatically worse over the last five hours. A patient who is improving (or at least is not getting any worse) gives you more time to evaluate the illness and

1. Is there a critical system problem indicated by persistent respiratory distress, tachycardia, or altered mental status?
2. Is the patient responding appropriately to their situation?
3. Is the patient able to eat, drink, pee, and poop normally?
4. Is the patient in significant pain?
5. Are the symptoms getting better or worse?

the effect of treatment, or to initiate a less urgent evacuation.

If no serious problems exist right now, you will still want to observe and measure the function of the three critical systems to detect any anticipated problems that may become serious. A patient with a cough, for example, may have a respiratory infection with the anticipated problem of respiratory distress. A complaint of diarrhea carries the anticipated problem of dehydration and volume shock. A person with a headache may be on the way toward elevated ICP.

A person who is sick, but not serious, may be uncomfortable but will continue to think, eat, drink, pee, and poop more or less normally. These normal body functions are reassuring, and your primary job will be to keep them comfortable and to monitor for change. It is when your patient stops eating and drinking, loses interest in their surroundings, and is unable to take care of themselves that you should consider the situation serious regardless of the diagnosis.

Persistent pain is another complaint worth careful investigation. The location and character of the pain will sometimes lead you to a more specific diagnosis. Any pain out of proportion to the apparent problem should be taken as a serious sign until proven otherwise.

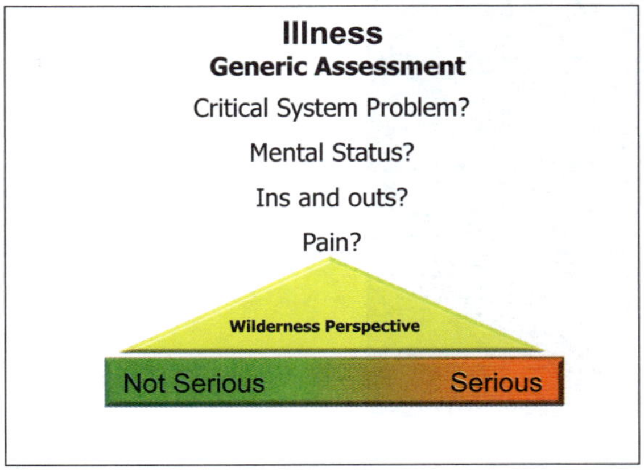

Your primary assessment of the ill patient begins with an evaluation of the circulatory, respiratory, and nervous systems looking for existing or anticipated problems. Your history evaluates the patient's regular functions of food and fluid intake and the output of urine and feces. Finally, investigate any complaint of pain. This process should detect the presence of any serious condition and the need for basic life support (BLS) and urgent evacuation. Or, the primary assessment may reassure you that the patient is okay, at least for now, and guide your secondary assessment toward a specific problem list and plan.

Risk Versus Benefit

Deciding what to do about serious illness is easy: BLS and evacuation. If you cannot evacuate, you need to bring medical care to the patient, or at least get expert advice. The obviously benign problems are easy too: treat the symptoms and observe. It is the illness in between, where you are not sure if it is serious or not serious, that presents the greatest challenge.

Unless your patient needs immediate life-saving treatment, there is little risk in taking the time to perform a thorough and thoughtful evaluation of an illness. You do not need to be an experienced clinician to perform a basic assessment of critical system and normal body function or to listen carefully to what your patient is telling you. The questions outlined above, along with the rest of the SAMPLE history, will usually point you in the right direction.

When an experienced practitioner makes an incorrect or incomplete diagnosis, it is often not by failure to ask the right questions, but by failure to listen to the answers and to examine the patient thoroughly. There is also danger in assuming too quickly that you know what the problem is. This can lead to grievous errors, especially when dealing with patients who are thought to be malingering, deceptive, or dramatic.

Remember the Generic to Specific Principle and the three critical systems. Take any complaint as legitimate until proven otherwise. Never be afraid to reevaluate and change your assessment.

Chapter 24 Review:
An Approach to Illness

- Careful evaluation and application of the Generic to Specific Principle is crucial in the field evaluation of illness.
- Any illness that includes a major problem with a critical system is serious. BLS and emergency evacuation to definitive care is the ideal treatment.
- Illness that does not interfere significantly with critical systems, normal body functions, and mental status is unlikely to be serious.
- Illness that begins to interfere with normal body functions and mental status may become serious.

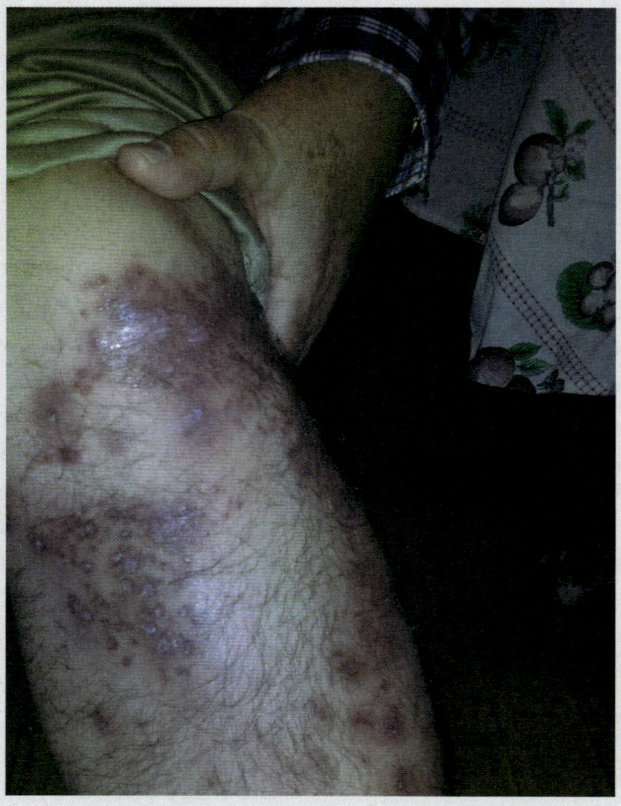

Illness can sometimes be confusing and frightening, but the most essential diagnosis remains: Serious or Not Serious. The rash on the leg of this fishing guide has developed slowly over several weeks. Since he is otherwise healthy, it would be considered Not Serious for field assessment and evacuation purposes. However, treatment for this Mycobacterium marinum infection is certainly important to this patient's long term health.

Chapter 25: Head, Eyes, Ears, Nose, and Throat

This chapter will discuss some of the common problems with ears, eyes, nose, throat, and teeth. Although critical system problems may be anticipated, the chief complaint is usually more bothersome and painful than life-threatening. Like everything else in wilderness and rescue medicine, the most generic and important diagnosis remains: is the problem serious or not serious?

Some facial problems are best treated with antibiotics and other prescription medications. For the basic rescuer this usually means that the patient needs to be evacuated to medical care. Practitioners with training and authorization to use prescription medications may be able to treat the problem effectively in the field. This could include emergency medical services (EMS) and search and rescue (SAR) personnel with a scope of practice extended by medical control, or the captain of a ship in communication with a medical advisory service.

Red Eye

The most common cause of red eye is conjunctivitis, sometimes called pink eye. This refers to inflammation of the thin membranous lining of the eye and the inside of the eye lids (conjunctiva). Like any other "itis" there are a number of possible causes including just about any eye problem. Conjunctivitis is most frequently caused by a viral infection but can be the result of sunburn, foreign body, trauma, chemical irritation, or fatigue. A red eye can also be one of the symptoms of a more serious but less common condition like glaucoma, iritis, or serious bacterial infection.

All the various causes of conjunctivitis produce similar symptoms. The patient will complain of an itching or burning sensation, tearing, and the eye will appear red as conjunctival blood vessels dilate in response to inflammation. There may be a small amount of eyelid swelling.

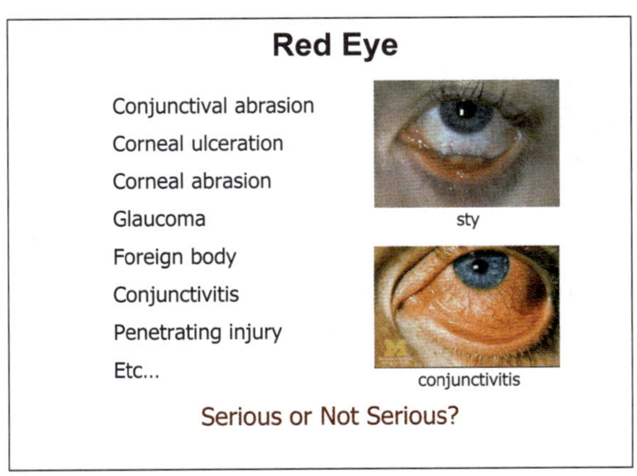

In cases of red eye that are not serious the cornea will remain clear, the pupil will continue to react to light and vision will be unaffected except for transient blurring caused by tears or exudate. Normal eye movements, called extraocular movements, might be uncomfortable, but are fully intact. There will be no evidence of blood behind the cornea (hyphema), and the patient will not report a headache.

Signs and symptoms indicating a more serious condition include clouding of the cornea, persistent visual disturbances, severe headache, or hyphema. Extraocular movements (EOMs) may be inhibited or very painful. The pupils may not react equally to light. Lid swelling may be severe. These signs and symptoms should prompt emergency evacuation.

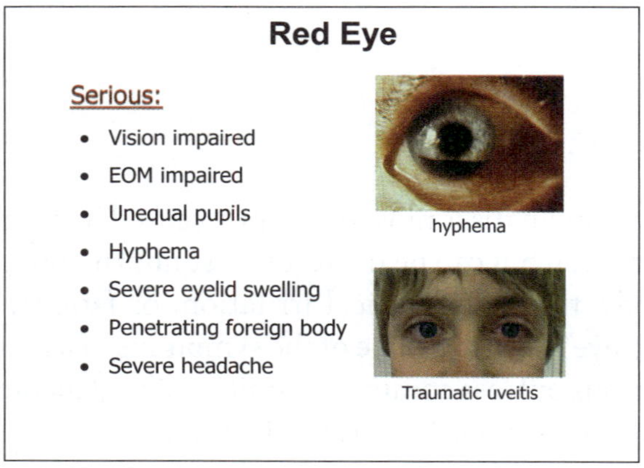

Treatment of Red Eye

The generic treatment for conjunctival irritation includes systemic pain medications, lubricating eye drops, and protective glasses or goggles. Antibiotic eye drops or ointment is applied when infection is present or anticipated. An eye patch is used only when extraoccular movements will cause further harm, such as with a penetrating foreign body.

A topical anesthetic, such as tetracaine or lidocaine, can be used by trained practitioners during eye examinations and foreign body removal. One or two drops will numb the conjunctiva and cornea for up to an hour. These anesthetics should not be used for routine pain relief or treatment. They could mask the development of a severe condition or allow the patient to cause further injury without realizing it.

Foreign Body Injury

Sand or other debris that contacts the conjunctiva causes immediate irritation, redness, and tearing. Onset is usually abrupt and the cause is often obvious. The easiest and least traumatic way to remove something from the eye is by irrigation with water. The simplest methods are to have the patient immerse their face in clean water and blink the eye, or to irrigate with your water bottle.

If the patient continues to have the foreign body sensation, you will need to examine the conjunctiva. Gently pull the lids away from the eye and use a bright light while the patient looks in all directions. The most common location of a foreign body is under the upper lid. If you find something, use a wet cotton swab or corner of a gauze pad to lift it off the membrane. If the object is imbedded in the conjunctiva or cornea, and resists your efforts to remove it, leave it alone.

Imbedded foreign bodies require medical attention. Patch the eye if safe to do so, and plan to walk out. Beware of using a patch in situations where impaired vision could be dangerous, and don't leave it on for more than 24 hours.

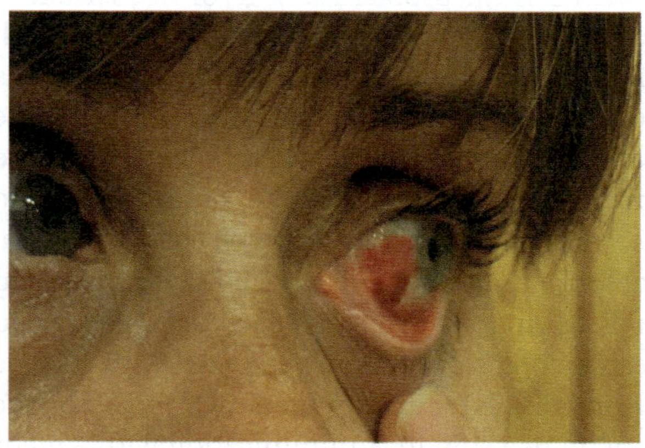

A subconjunctival hematoma is blood trapped under the conjunctival membrane on the surface of the eye. It is usually not serious.

The cornea is surprisingly tough but neurologically sensitive. Its outer surface can be scratched by a foreign body, branch, fingernail, or windblown ice crystals. Corneal abrasion can cause considerable pain and inflammation, making the patient feel like something is in the eye.

Sometimes the abrasion can be seen by shining a flashlight across the eye from the side. Corneal abrasions are usually more annoying than serious. If no serious signs are present, treatment may be generic and symptomatic. Healing usually occurs within 72 hours.

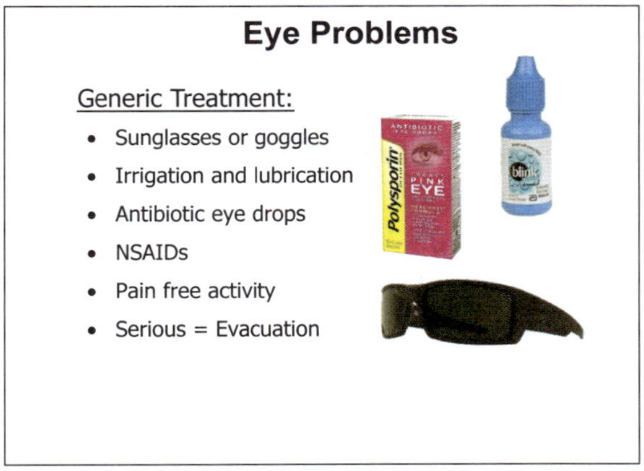

Sunburn

Your first clue in making this diagnosis is a lot of sun exposure without adequate eye protection. Your second is that the inflammation is limited to the sun-exposed part of the eye leaving the conjunctiva under the lids unaffected. In severe cases, the cornea may become pitted and cloudy in appearance causing the condition known as snow blindness. Fortunately, UV rays do not penetrate deeply so the damage is usually superficial. Symptomatic treatment with lubricating drops, pain medication, and protective glasses or goggles should allow healing within several days. Contact lenses should be removed and not reused until symptoms are completely clear.

Infection

A viral or bacterial infection of the conjunctiva is what most people mean by the term conjunctivitis or pink eye. The typical signs and symptoms include a yellow or green discharge that can stick the eyelids together during sleep. The eyelids themselves may appear slightly puffy and reddened. The conjunctiva appears red with inflammation. The patient complains of an itching or burning sensation that may resemble a foreign body.

A mild superficial infection will not cause symptoms such as a headache or severe eyelid edema. Vision is blurred when tears or pus pass over the cornea, but it is otherwise unaffected. Pain is bothersome but not severe. The cornea remains clear, pupils respond normally to light, and extraoccular movements are intact.

Most mild bacterial and viral conjunctivitis resolves spontaneously. Contact lenses in use should be discarded. Allow the eyes to drain and do not use a patch. Field treatment using frequent irrigation and warm soaks may improve the symptoms.

Treatment with antibiotics, either taken orally or instilled as an ointment or eye drops, is the preferred treatment, especially if symptoms are getting worse rather than stabilizing or improving. Serious infection is evidenced by severe pain, headache, and eyelid swelling and warrants an emergency evacuation along with antibiotic treatment.

Note that an eye infection can be quite contagious. Instruct your group to avoid sharing towels, goggles, or face masks. Insist on frequent hand washing and discourage infected people from handling dishes and other objects that are used by other people. Antibiotic drops or ointment should be used in both eyes even if only one eye is inflamed.

Chemical Exposure

Irritants like soap and caustic plant juices cause chemical conjunctivitis. In mild cases, the cornea remains clear. In severe cases, it may be pitted or cloudy in appearance. The treatment for chemical exposure is copious irrigation with water or saline solution. Expect mild redness following prolonged irrigation, but it should begin to resolve within several hours following treatment. If it gets worse, you should assume that the chemical may still be present. Irrigation should be repeated and evacuation should be considered.

Contact Lenses

Contact lenses are another frequent cause of inflammation, especially at altitude. Dry air and reduced oxygen availability can cause corneal damage. Affected patients should use lubricating eye drops and allow their eyes as many lens-free hours per day as possible.

Nosebleed

Most nosebleeds occur in an area of the anterior nostril called Kesselbach's plexus. Bleeding from this area drains out of the nose if the patient is positioned upright with the head forward. When the bleed starts spontaneously, or because of nose picking, the problem is generally not serious. Bleeding stops quickly with direct pressure. However, if the bleeding is the result of facial trauma you should consider the possibility of facial bone fracture and other more significant injuries.

In rare cases bleeding can originate in the posterior nasopharynx. Applying direct pressure to the bleeding site without a nasal tampon or other device can be impossible. If a patient is using anticoagulant medications, or even aspirin, bleeding can become serious.

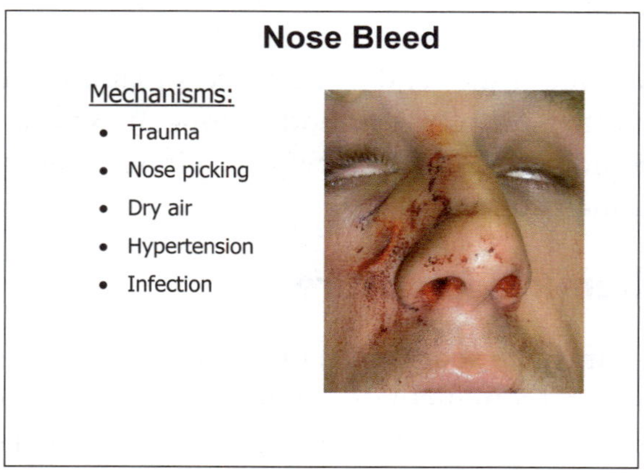

Treatment of Nosebleed

Position the patient sitting forward or lying face down to allow for drainage out of the nose rather than down the throat. Instruct the patient to blow out any clots, then pinch the nostrils together and hold firmly for 15 minutes. This applies simple direct pressure to the most likely bleeding source. Like any bleeding, it is essential to hold enough pressure for a long enough time. This will stop most nosebleeds that you are likely to see.

Persistent bleeds can be treated with nasal packing. A light-flow (small size) tampon can be gently inserted into the nostril for several hours. Soaking the tampon with a few drops of a decongestant nasal spray like oxymetazoline (the vasoconstrictor in Afrin) reduces bleeding by constricting blood vessels in the nasal mucosa. The packing should be removed within four hours unless the patient can also be treated with prophylactic antibiotics.

The frequency of nosebleeds from dry air and high altitude can be reduced by coating the inside of the nostril with Vaseline, antibiotic ointment, or a saline spray like Ayr Gel. Powdered clot-enhancers are available over the counter for nuisance bleeding, including nosebleeds.

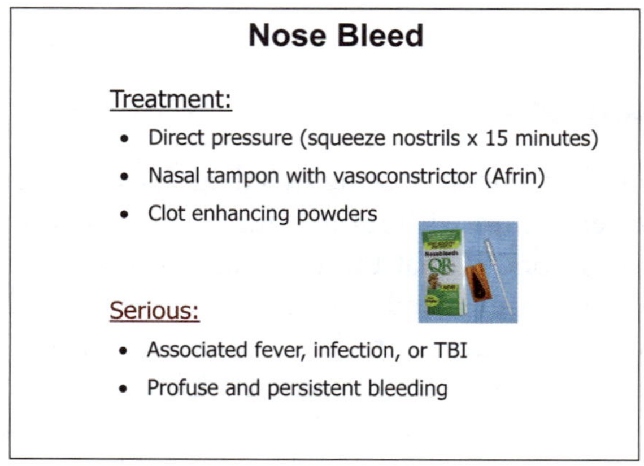

A nosebleed becomes serious when volume shock or airway obstruction is anticipated. If you cannot control a severe nosebleed in the field, make the patient as comfortable as possible and prepare for an emergency evacuation. If the patient needs to lie down, protect the airway by positioning the patient face down or on their side with the chest and head supported to allow for drainage from the nose and mouth.

Dental Problems

Dental Trauma

Loose teeth, tooth fragments, blood, and swollen tissues can result in airway obstruction. The mechanism of injury can be associated with brain and spine injury. Pain can produce acute stress reaction (ASR). Swallowing blood can cause vomiting. The primary assessment of dental trauma is directed at ensuring that critical body system problems are considered and stabilized. Beyond that, broken teeth do not represent a medical emergency.

Dental Trauma

Anticipate:

- Airway obstruction
- Infection
- Pain

Treatment:

- Recover tooth
- Replace and splint
- Pain medication
- See dentist ASAP

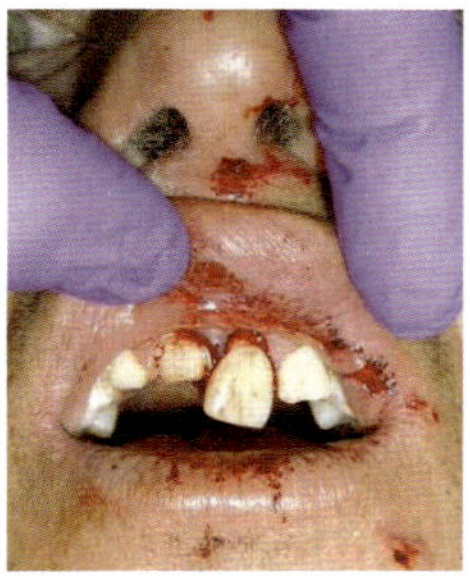

Treatment of Dental Trauma

Position the patient to allow drainage of blood and debris out of the mouth, rather than down the throat. Instruct the patient to rinse the mouth with cool water. This cleans out blood clots and loose teeth and helps stop bleeding. Examine the mouth with a good light. Look for teeth that are loose or fractured but still in the socket. Look for empty sockets that could match any avulsed teeth you have found.

Teeth that have been cleanly avulsed have a fair chance of reattaching if returned to their socket within a few hours. Handle the tooth only by the enamel, not by its root. Rinse the tooth in clean water and push it gently all the way into its socket. You can splint the tooth to a healthy one adjacent to it by tying it with dental floss or fishing line, or by constructing a bridge from dental wax or Cavit. Any teeth that are loose, but still in the socket, may be splinted in this manner as well.

Fractured teeth that are still in place may be extremely sensitive on exposure to air if the nerve is still alive. The fracture site can be anesthetized with topical oral pain relievers (e.g., oil of cloves or viscous lidocaine) and covered with temporary filling material or dental wax. The loss of a filling can be treated the same way, using wax or filling material to protect the sensitive nerve tissue that is exposed when the filling falls out. Loose fillings or crowns can also be temporarily glued back in place with toothpaste. The patient should eat only soft foods and cool liquids.

Fractured Teeth

Anticipate:

- Infection
- Pain

Treatment:

- Pain medication
- Clean and cover with dental wax
- See dentist ASAP

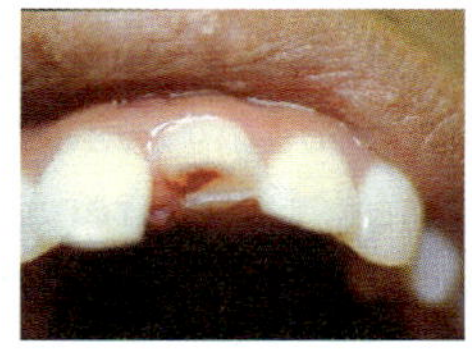

Referral of trauma or lost fillings to dental follow-up may be non-emergent if infection does not develop. In significant trauma where teeth have been avulsed or fractured, prophylactic antibiotics are indicated. Pain medication and a soft diet may also be required.

Dental Infection

Infection and swelling within the confined space at the base of a tooth or in the gum can be excruciatingly painful. Eating and drinking will be difficult or impossible. If the infection penetrates the soft tissues of the head and neck, it can become dangerous. Both the infection and the pain it causes will be difficult to manage in the field.

Bacteria usually enter through a break in the enamel caused by trauma, or through a cavity, and form an abscess with the typical swelling, pressure, and pain. Swelling of the gum on the affected side may be evident, as well as the tenderness of one or more teeth when tapped with a finger or stick. A patient with a more serious infection will show facial swelling and fever.

Treatment of Dental Infection

Evacuation to dental care is indicated if swelling, fever, or severe pain is present. The ideal treatment includes drainage, antibiotics, and pain relief. The usual method is drilling and cleaning the inside of the tooth and installing a filling.

In the field, temporary pain relief may be obtained with topical pain relievers like Orabase or oil of cloves, and with oral or injectable pain medication. If immediate evacuation is not possible begin high-dose antibiotics and warm compresses. This may reduce the severity of the infection pending evacuation to dental care. In a worst-case scenario remember that up until quite recently in dental history pulling the tooth was the definitive treatment for dental infection.

Dental Abscess

Anticipate:

- Systemic infection
- Impaired food and fluid intake
- Pain

Treatment:

- Pain medication
- Urgent evacuation
- Antibiotics

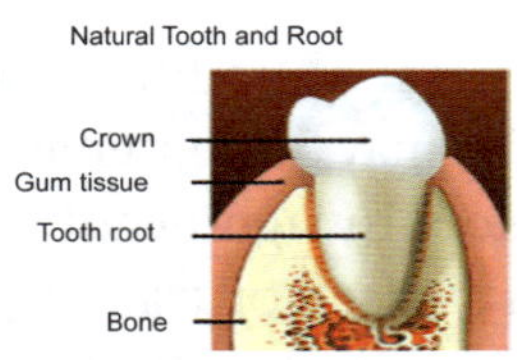

External Ear Infection

External ear infection, sometimes called swimmer's ear or external otitis, is a superficial bacterial infection of the external auditory canal. It develops when prolonged exposure to water leads to breakdown of the protective skin barrier. The signs and symptoms are not difficult to distinguish from middle ear infection.

Like any infection, swimmer's ear is characterized by redness, warmth, swelling, and pain. The external structures of the ear and surrounding area are tender to pressure and manipulation. The external ear canal may be swollen and obstructed.

Treatment of Swimmer's Ear

Using mineral oil drops before swimming reduces maceration of the skin and the incidence of infection. A few drops of vinegar combined with alcohol instilled into the ear canal after swimming is a good preventive treatment. There are also commercial preparations, such as SwimEar, available over the counter to help prevent external otitis. Do not use dry cotton swabs, such as Q-tips, because they will further irritate the ear canal. Once the ear canal is infected, the ideal treatment is antibiotic eardrops, available in the United States only by prescription.

External Ear Infection

Mechanism:

- Skin maceration and bacterial invasion

Signs and Symptoms:

- Ear canal red and swollen
- External ear is tender and painful

Treatment:

- Antibiotic ear drops
- Dilute vinegar drops
- Oral antibiotics

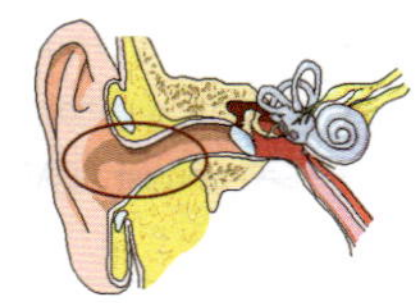

Middle Ear Infection and Sinusitis

The sinus cavity referred to as the middle ear lies behind the ear drum and extends through a narrow opening into the nasopharynx. Like the other sinus cavities inside the skull, the middle ear is lined with mucous membrane and drains through one small opening. In the healthy individual, mucous is continuously produced and drained through the eustachian tube into the throat where it is swallowed. Problems begin when the tube becomes obstructed by swelling and inflammation from a viral infection or as the result of irritation by seawater or smoke. The trapped mucous provides a growth medium for bacteria, and a middle ear infection develops.

The typical symptom of middle ear infection is pain. Bending over at the waist increases pressure in the affected ear and increases the pain. Middle ear infection can be differentiated from swimmer's ear by the fact that, although the ear hurts, the external ear structures and ear canal are not red, swollen, or tender to touch.

The problem called sinusitis develops by the same mechanism in the frontal, maxillary, or ethmoid sinuses in the skull. Typical non-serious symptoms include sinus pressure, a stuffy nose, and a clear, green or yellow nasal discharge. These are almost always a viral infection (common cold) or a local allergic reaction to something in the environment. Decongestants and antihistamines may offer some relief. Antibiotics are not helpful or necessary.

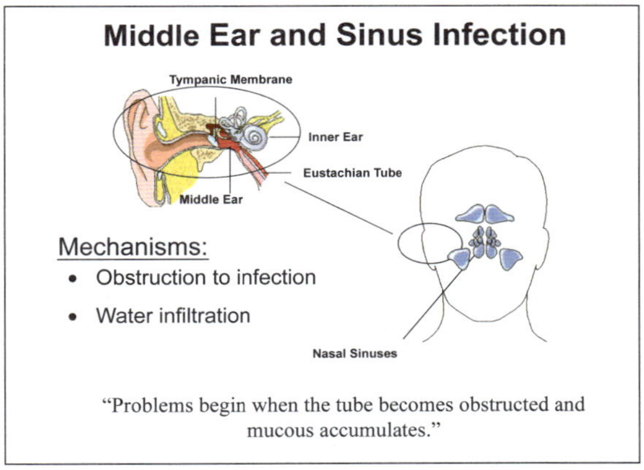

A more serious bacterial infection will cause severe pain, fever, and a bloody green nasal discharge. Involvement of the maxillary sinus in the face can feel like a dental infection in the upper teeth, but you won't find one specific tooth that is tender to percussion. Serious middle ear and sinus infection carries the anticipated problem of spread to adjacent structures like the skull, inner ear, and brain.

Treatment of Middle Ear Infection and Sinusitis

As with any obstructed organ, the situation can be improved with drainage. Try to reduce the swelling and obstruction of the eustachian tube and sinus passages with decongestant nasal spray or by having the patient breathe steam from a pot of hot water. Keeping your patient well hydrated is important. This will keep mucous from drying and becoming too thick to drain.

Antibiotics are sometimes necessary for complete treatment of more serious middle ear and sinus infections if the patient is not responding to decongestion and hydration. A middle ear infection may ultimately perforate the eardrum and drain spontaneously through the external ear canal. Pain is almost immediately relieved as the pressure is released but hearing may be temporarily impaired. If no fever or other adverse symptoms develop, there is no emergency. Avoid swimming and diving and see a medical practitioner when possible.

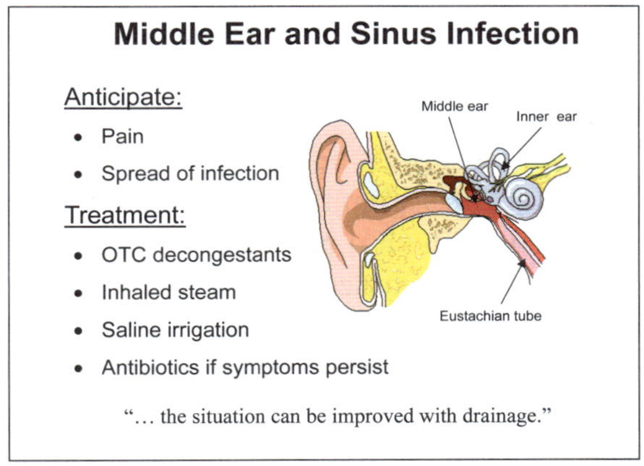

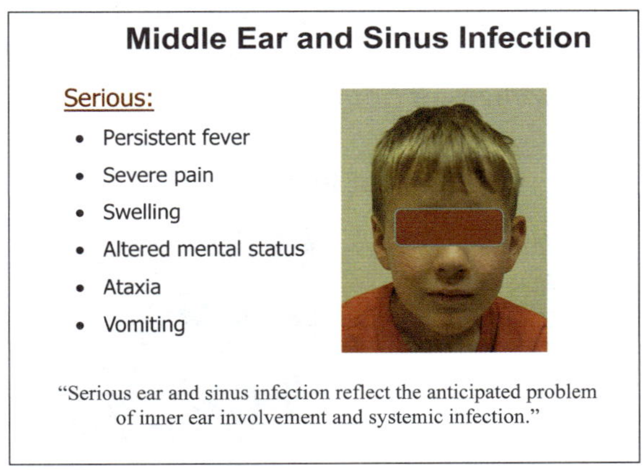

Treating infection of the other sinus cavities is similar except that there is no safety valve like the eardrum for perforation and drainage if necessary. Aggressive decongestion and hydration to promote drainage through the sinus passages may improve symptoms and cure the infection. Sinus infection not responding to field treatment is best evacuated to medical care, especially if moderate pain or fever is present. Steroid and other decongestant nasal sprays may be prescribed to reduce inflammation and swelling. Antibiotic therapy, sometimes for several weeks, is indicated in resistant cases.

Sore Throat

Most sore throats are caused by viral infection and occur as part of a constellation of symptoms related to a cold or flu. These are self-limiting and require only treatment to relieve symptoms. However, you must monitor for the development of severe infection where swelling of the tonsils, epiglottis, and uvula have the potential to cause airway obstruction.

This will most often be the result of a bacterial infection such as strep throat or epiglottitis, but it can occur with viral mononucleosis. Bacterial infection is characterized by persistent pain, difficulty swallowing, and obvious edema of pharyngeal structures. Pus is white patches on the throat and tonsils. Fever tends to be persistent. Suspected bacterial infection should be seen by a medical practitioner. Mild pharyngitis can be effectively treated with ibuprofen and acetaminophen, cool liquids, and topical medication like throat lozenges or honey.

Throat Infection

Serious:

- Respiratory distress
- Impaired food/fluid intake
- Persistent fever
- Persistent severe pain
- Coughing blood
- Getting worse

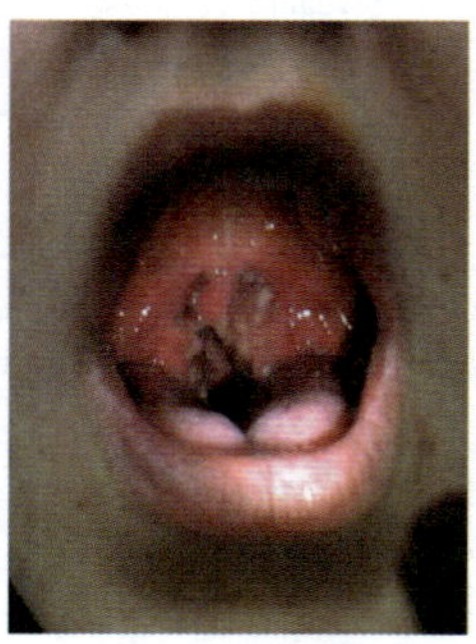

Strep pharyngitis

Impending airway obstruction is suggested by the patient's inability to swallow secretions or water. The patient may position themself in a chin thrust to keep the airway open. Stridor may be noted. This is a serious respiratory problem for which emergency evacuation and advanced life support is indicated. In a desperate situation, inhaled epinephrine and steroids may be used by advanced providers to temporarily reduce swelling and keep the airway open.

Risk Versus Benefit

Antibiotics are listed as part of the temporary or definitive treatment for many illnesses but are controversial in others. The use of antibiotics to prevent wound infection is also controversial. However, in the wilderness setting where a specific diagnosis is often unavailable or high-risk infection is an anticipated problem, the threshold for the use of antibiotics is lower. The primary goal is to reduce the need for an emergency evacuation from a remote setting.

The appropriate use of antibiotics by SAR personnel, expedition medics, wilderness guides, voyaging sailors, and some rural EMS units should be considered part of the overall effort at risk reduction. The common bacterial infections contracted by otherwise healthy people generally respond to well-known oral and topical antibiotics with an acceptable side effects profile. Medical directors will need to provide instructions and precautions as well as authorization and protocol.

Chapter 25 Review:
Head, Eyes, Ears, Nose, and Throat

- In facial injury and infection the most important initial diagnosis is: serious or not serious?
- Significantly impaired eye function or associated severe pain indicates a serious problem. These issues include persistent visual changes, impaired EOM, impaired pupil dilation and constriction, severe lid swelling, hyphema, and headache.
- The generic treatment for eye problems includes protective lenses, lubricating eye drops, irrigation as needed, and oral or topical antibiotics. Emergency evacuation is indicated for serious problems.
- Nosebleed is usually easy to treat with direct pressure. A nosebleed that cannot be controlled carries the anticipated problem of volume shock.
- Avulsed or fractured teeth are not a serious problem. Treatment includes replacing the tooth in the socket or cleaning and covering the fracture site. Infection is anticipated and antibiotics and non-urgent evacuation to dental care is warranted.
- Dental infection is a serious problem. Field treatment includes pain relief, antibiotics, and evacuation to dental care.
- External otitis is a superficial skin infection of the ear canal and effectively treated with vinegar and alcohol or antibiotic ear drops. It becomes serious when it produces swelling and fever.
- Middle ear and sinus infection is an obstruction-to-infection problem. It becomes serious when it produces persistent fever and severe pain and interferes with normal body function. The ideal treatment is drainage and antibiotics.
- The use of antibiotics, where appropriate, in the treatment of injury and infection requires authorization and medical direction and is part of the overall risk reduction effort in the remote setting.

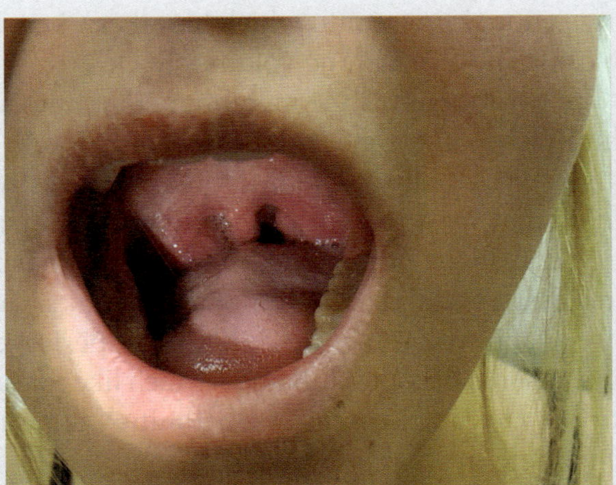

This peritonsillar abscess carries the serious anticipated problems of airway obstruction, aspiration, and sepsis.

Chapter 26: Abdominal Pain

The differential diagnosis of abdominal pain is extensive. Making a specific diagnosis can be a challenge for experienced clinicians even when using laboratory data and sophisticated imaging equipment. The wilderness medical practitioner must usually be satisfied with the generic assessment: Serious or Not Serious? Because the treatment of a serious intra-abdominal problem requires hospital and surgical care anyway, the specific diagnosis can usually wait.

Abdominal Pain

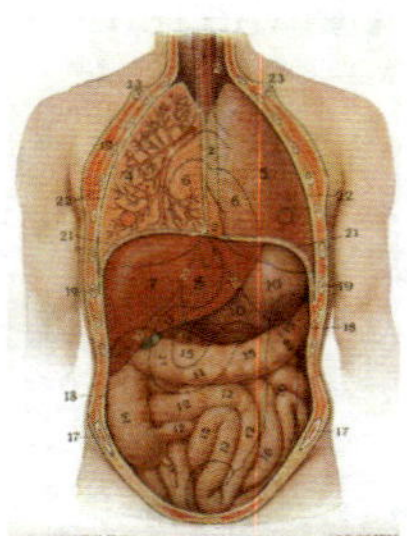

Gastroenteritis
Ectopic pregnancy
Appendicitis
Cholecystitis
Diverticulitis
Perforating ulcer
Pancreatitis
Internal Bleeding...

Serious or Not Serious?

Practical Abdominal Anatomy

For field purposes, we can consider the contents and structure of the abdomen to consist of four major components: hollow organs, solid organs, the peritoneal lining, and the muscular abdominal wall. Hollow structures such as the stomach, intestines, and gall bladder are muscular organs that excrete and move fluids and food through the digestive system using rhythmic muscle contractions called peristalsis. The ureters and urinary bladder are of similar structure and function to contain and excrete urine.

Solid organs within the abdomen have a variety of functions and associated diseases, but we worry most about their potential for rupture in abdominal trauma. The liver, spleen, pancreas, and kidneys are part of the body core and are richly supplied with blood. Solid organs can fracture and bleed on impact. The abdomen offers a large enough space into which blood can be lost to cause life-threatening volume shock.

The peritoneum is the membrane that lines all the abdominal organs and the abdominal wall. It is easily irritated by bacteria, blood, and digestive fluids that have leaked into the abdominal cavity. Because the peritoneum represents a surface area greater than that of your patient's skin, it can lose a large volume of fluid in a short period of time when it becomes inflamed. Much like a large surface area burn, extensive peritonitis will result in volume shock.

The muscular wall of the abdomen lies outside the peritoneum, and therefore it is not within the abdominal cavity. These skeletal muscles provide protection and support for the abdominal contents. They contract in response to both the commands associated with voluntary movement and the involuntary need for abdominal protection. The muscles themselves can also be a source of pain that can be difficult to distinguish from intra-abdominal problems.

Assessment of Abdominal Pain

Your assessment of abdominal pain will go much better with a basic understanding of the structure, function, and nerve supply of the abdominal organs. The nerve cells in hollow organs transmit pain sensations primarily when stretched, like when your stomach is distended by a big meal. Stretching a hollow organ stimulates muscular contraction, causing the pain of distention to become worse temporarily. We usually call this a cramp.

It is also useful to note that the pain of a distended hollow organ tends to be poorly localized to the general level that the associated nerves enter the spinal cord rather than identified as a specific spot. Because peristalsis increases the pain in waves, the discomfort tends to be intermittent. The mechanism is usually gas, fluid, and spasm created by a viral illness, food intolerance, or constipation. This type of poorly localized and intermittent pain is less likely to be serious.

The patient with non-serious abdominal pain may tighten the abdominal wall muscles in response to the pressure of your abdominal palpation but can voluntarily relax them when encouraged to do so. This is known as voluntary guarding. Tenderness elicited on examination tends to be nonspecific and relatively mild. Bowel sounds are usually normal to hyperactive. This kind of abdominal pain is usually associated with conditions that are well contained within the gut, not affecting the abdominal cavity itself.

If the condition progresses to a more serious problem, you may begin to see the signs and symptoms of peritoneal irritation inside the abdominal cavity. Unlike the hollow organs, the peritoneum is specifically innervated like your skin surface. An inflamed peritoneum causes pain localized to the site of irritation and aggravated by movement as the inflamed membranes rub against each other. The pain tends to be better localized and more constant than crampy. Bowel sounds may be reduced or absent.

Hollow Organ Problems

In a textbook case of appendicitis, for example, the problem usually begins with obstruction. The appendix is a hollow organ connected to the large intestine in the lower-right quadrant of the abdomen. Obstruction of the appendix ultimately leads to infection and swelling. The early symptoms are often the generalized cramp-like discomfort typical of intestinal distention. Because the appendix and first few centimeters of the large intestine are innervated with the small intestine, the pain is felt around the umbilicus. It would be impossible to distinguish this from mild gas pains and you would not label it as serious.

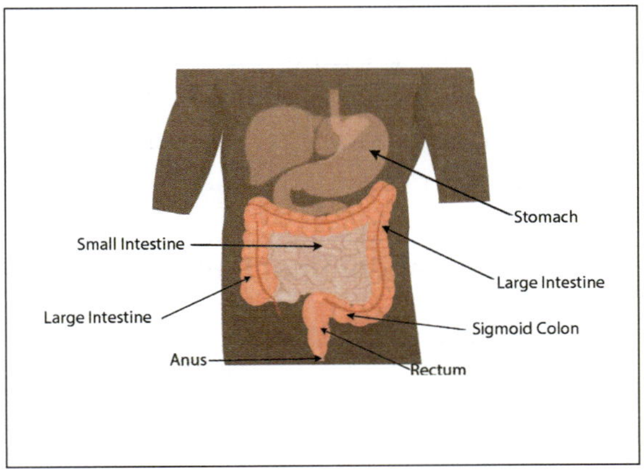

The hollow organs including the stomach, intestines, appendix, and gall bladder are prone to obstruction, infection, and rupture due to trauma.

As the infection progresses, the swollen and inflamed appendix begins to irritate the peritoneal lining of the intestine and abdominal cavity. The symptoms begin to change from poorly localized intermittent cramping to a well localized constant pain in the lower-right quadrant. Abdominal wall muscle spasm causes involuntary guarding as the body protects the abdominal contents from movement. Palpation elicits tenderness that tends to be specific to the problem area. Jostling or walking the patient produces pain in the same location. Peristalsis slows or stops so bowel sounds diminish dramatically. These are called peritoneal signs and indicate a serious problem within the abdomen.

If appendicitis is allowed to progress, the organ may burst spilling digestive enzymes and pus into the abdominal cavity and peritoneal lining. Pain is severe, constant, and will spread throughout the abdomen. Shock and death are often the result.

The key to early recognition of appendicitis, or any other serious hollow organ problem, is the change in the character of pain from the cramp-like and generalized pain of hollow organ distention to the constant and localized pain of peritoneal inflammation. Other, less specific signs and symptoms like fever, diarrhea, vomiting, and tachycardia all add to your concern.

The same progression of signs and symptoms can develop with other serious hollow organ problems and may present anywhere in the abdomen. It is not necessary to know exactly what you're dealing with to know that it needs a surgeon and an operating room. Peritoneal signs indicate a serious abdominal problem regardless of the location or cause.

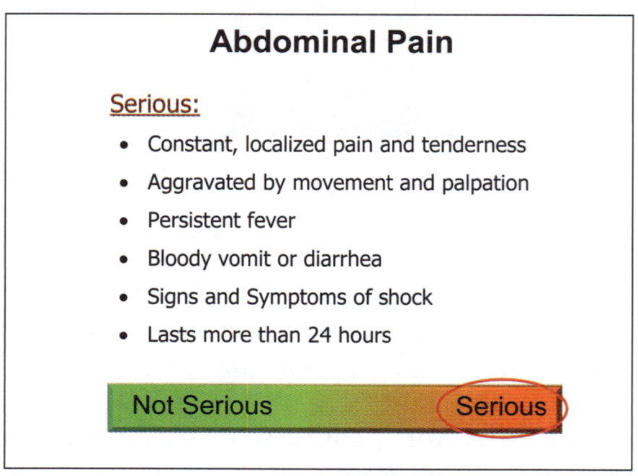

Other Abdominal Problems

Solid organ rupture and bleeding can also cause irritation of the peritoneal lining. The wilderness medical practitioner should be alert to the development of peritoneal signs following significant blunt trauma to the abdomen. With constant pain and localized tenderness, volume shock from internal bleeding is the anticipated problem.

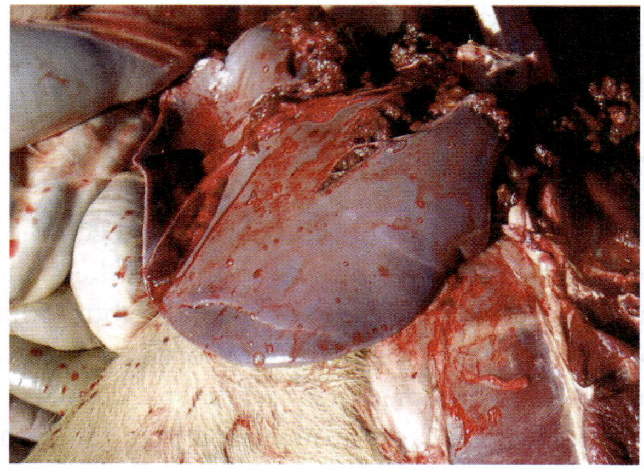

This elk viscera demonstrates the membranous peritoneum, intestines, and a fractured liver.

A similar type of pain can be caused by muscle contusion or strain of the abdominal wall. This may not be associated with any internal organs and is not serious but it can be difficult to distinguish from peritoneal irritation. This type of pain is usually relieved by rest and made worse specifically by use of the injured muscles.

Even if the abdominal pain itself is identified as not serious, an illness with vomiting and diarrhea may lead you to anticipate volume shock from dehydration. The presence of blood or pus in the stool or vomit, or a persistent fever, could indicate a serious bacterial or viral infection within the gut that, like any other local infection, can become a serious systemic infection. If rehydration and definitive treatment in the field are not possible evacuation is indicated even if surgery is not.

Treatment of Abdominal Pain

If an evacuation will exceed two hours, give fluids and calories to make up for normal and abnormal losses. This should be restricted to water, rehydration solutions, and easily absorbed simple sugars.

Oral pain medication should be restricted to acetaminophen because nonsteroidal anti-inflammatory drugs (NSAIDs), like ibuprofen and aspirin, can irritate the gut. If opioids are available the injectable forms are preferred. Pain medication should not be withheld in the belief that it will mask serious symptoms or inhibit diagnosis in the emergency room.

Abdominal pain labeled as not serious can be treated symptomatically with the appropriate attention to hydration and calories. To avoid further irritating the gut, the patient should still avoid NSAIDs. Acetaminophen would be a better choice. Gut soothers like bismuth subsalicylate and antacids are generally safe. Food should be restricted to easily digested carbohydrates and sugars. Vomiting and diarrhea can be treated with antiemetics like ondansetron/Zofran, meclizine/Antivert, or diphenhydramine/Benadryl and with mild opioid antispasmodics like loperamide/Imodium, provided there are no signs of bacterial infection. The patient should be frequently monitored for the development of peritoneal signs or dehydration.

Serious Abdominal Pain

Anticipate:

- Volume shock
- Systemic infection

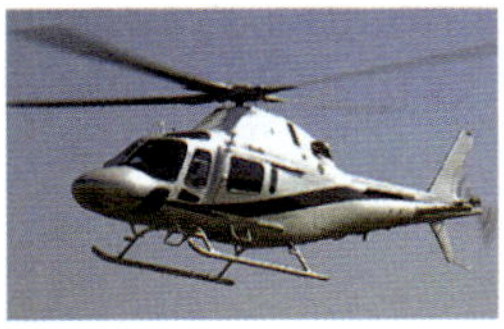

Treatment:

- Maintain hydration
- Maintain body core temperature
- Restrict foods to easily absorbed sugars
- Emergency evacuation

Risk Versus Benefit

Although the evolution of CT, MRI, and ultrasound has vastly improved the diagnosis of abdominal problems in the hospital setting, little has changed for the practitioner in the field. Assessment still depends on a good history, careful exam, and a few simple diagnostic tools like a stethoscope and thermometer. Fortunately, peritoneal signs are relatively easy to identify and generally become steadily worse as you monitor your patient. The outcome is usually poor and probably worth an emergency evacuation if you cannot treat the cause.

If evacuation is unavailable or exceptionally dangerous you can take some comfort in what has been learned by the use of sophisticated imaging over the past three decades: a lot of people survive serious abdominal injury and illness without surgery. Doctors have been able to monitor a bleeding spleen or liver and operate only if necessary to save the patient's life. Infections, like appendicitis, can be evaluated and monitored for response to antibiotics before surgery is performed. To those of us in the field this means that a patient with a serious condition may well survive if we pay attention to good basic life support (BLS), hydration, and calories.

Remote expeditions and offshore sailors should carry antibiotics useful in intra-abdominal infection as well as tools for hydration and pain control. The benefit of good basic treatment on site may well outweigh the risk associated with a desperate evacuation to what may be inadequate medical care somewhere else.

Chapter 26 Review: Abdominal Pain

- Abdominal pain can be caused by a wide variety of problems. The mechanism may be trauma, obstruction, infection, or ischemia to infarction.
- A specific diagnosis in the field is rarely possible. The generic diagnosis of serious or not serious is sufficient to initiate treatment and evacuation if necessary.
- The signs and symptoms of serious abdominal pain include localized and constant pain, pain aggravated by movement, persistent fever, persistent tachycardia, and blood or pus in stool or vomit.
- For field purposes, we can consider the abdomen to consist of four types of organs: hollow organs, solid organs, the peritoneal lining, and the muscular abdominal wall.
- A problem within a hollow organ generally results in cramp-like pain as the organ is distended and is stimulated to contract. Problems that remain within the hollow organ are generally not serious.
- A problem within the abdominal cavity will irritate the peritoneum, causing localized, constant pain aggravated by movement. Problems that involve the peritoneum should be considered serious.
- A problem originating within the gut or another hollow or solid organ may progress to involve the peritoneum. Pain often evolves from generalized and cramp-like to localized and constant.
- Serious abdominal pain requires emergency evacuation to a hospital. Field treatment includes maintaining hydration, calories, and normal body core temperature. Preferred analgesics include acetaminophen and opioids. NSAIDs should be avoided. Antibiotics may be used to temporarily treat a suspected intraabdominal infection pending evacuation to definitive medical care.

Chapter 27: Chest Pain

As with the abdomen, there are a number of possible causes of chest pain including heart attack, muscle spasm, and respiratory problems. Again, the diagnosis is often limited to the generic assessment: Serious or Not Serious? With a history of significant trauma, any persistent chest pain should be considered serious.

Chest Pain

Myocardial ischemia
Stable angina
Respiratory infection
Chest wall muscle strain
Chest wall contusion
Esophageal spasm
Pulmonary embolus
Etc.

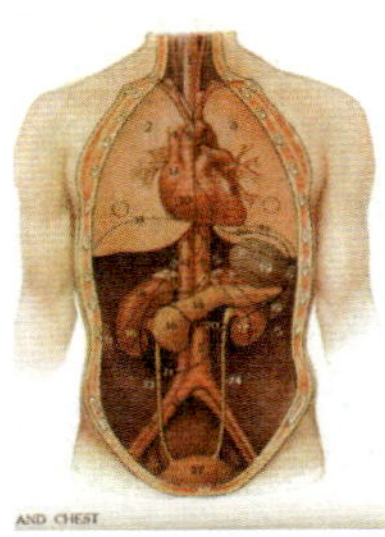

Serious or Not Serious?

Myocardial Ischemia

In the absence of trauma, the type of chest pain that is most worrisome is the pain of myocardial ischemia. The mechanism for myocardial ischemia may be an acute clot or spasm in a coronary artery or it may be a chronic coronary artery constriction that prevents adequate blood flow to the heart muscle when oxygen demand is increased. Either way, the heart muscle is ischemic and not getting enough oxygen. If the condition persists, infarction will result.

If the area of the heart that is ischemic includes a major branch of the electrical conduction system, a cardiac dysrhythmia may develop. Whether you refer to it as myocardial ischemia or heart attack, it is a major circulatory system problem with the anticipated problem of cardiogenic shock and death.

The pain of myocardial ischemia can present in a variety of ways from the classic substernal pain radiating to the jaw and left arm to back or abdominal pain. The patient may also experience shortness of breath, sweating, and nausea. These symptoms can be caused by the parasympathetic and sympathetic acute stress response to pain or to the effects of early cardiogenic shock. Of these, the most predictive sign and symptom for myocardial ischemia are sweating and radiation of pain to either arm. Of course, these same symptoms can be caused by indigestion, chest wall muscle spasm, altitude adjustment, respiratory infection, and a host of other less serious problems.

Myocardial Ischemia

Signs and Symptoms:

- Chest pain with radiation
- Shell/core effect, sweating
- Elevated respiratory rate
- Pulse may be variable

Anticipate:

- Myocardial infarction
- Dysrhythmia
- Cardiogenic shock

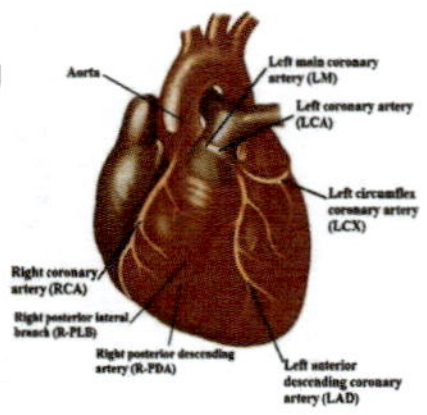

Risk Factors

Where evacuation to medical care will be a high-risk operation, you need to be able to decide whether the complaint of chest pain indicates a truly serious problem. To help with this decision, you can evaluate the patient's risk factors for coronary artery disease.

Serious Chest Pain
Myocardial Ischemia

Risk Factors:

- Hypertension
- High blood cholesterol
- Age over 40 years
- Post menopausal
- Smoking, obesity, diabetes
- Family or personal history of heart disease
- Recreational use of amphetamines or cocaine

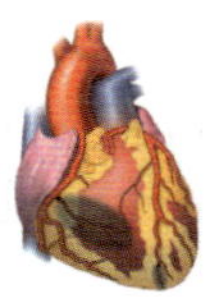

Any patient with chest pain and a collection of risk factors should be considered at elevated risk for myocardial infarction and cardiac arrhythmia. Risk factors include disease states, genetics, medications, and lifestyle factors that contribute to narrowing and inflammation of the arteries supplying the heart. The more risk factors that your patient has, the more worried about their chest pain you should be.

Treatment of Myocardial Ischemia

"Time is myocardium" is the mantra of treatment. The sooner the ischemia can be reversed, the less heart muscle will be damaged and the better the patient's chance for survival. This means an emergency evacuation even if the patient cannot present to definitive medical care within the 2-hour window for clot-dissolving treatment.

The ideal evacuation would not increase the stress or level of exertion for your patient. You may find yourself choosing between a walking evacuation that takes an hour and a carryout that may take several hours. You should favor the route that will access advanced life support (ALS) care as soon as possible while causing the least increase in activity and myocardial oxygen demand.

Myocardial Ischemia

Specific Treatment:

- Assist with nitroglycerin as prescribed
- Give one adult aspirin
- PROP
- Gentle but urgent evacuation:
  - Activity increases myocardial oxygen demand
  - Time increases infarction
- ALS care as soon as possible

"Time is myocardium…you should favor the route that will access ALS care as soon as possible…while causing the least increase in myocardial oxygen demand"

If your patient is not already taking it daily, give one adult aspirin tablet (325 mg) or four baby aspirin (81 mg) by mouth. This reduces the tendency of the blood to clot which may reduce ischemia in heart muscle. If the patient is currently taking other heart medication like nitroglycerin, assist them in taking it according to directions.

Stable Angina

Your patient may give a history of stable angina: chest pain with exertion that resolves with rest. This develops when physical exertion increases the myocardial oxygen demand beyond the ability of chronically narrowed coronary arteries to supply it. The relative ischemia is temporary, assuming that the patient can reduce activity and oxygen demand.

If the pain does not resolve with rest it may require that the patient use their sublingual nitroglycerin tablets or spray. Nitroglycerin relaxes the smooth muscle of blood vessels to reduce the resistance to flow and thus the work the heart must do to circulate blood. Usually, a maximum of three doses of nitroglycerin is taken before referral to medical care is considered necessary. Pain that does not resolve as expected should be considered a heart attack and treated as such.

Patients with angina are at increased risk of myocardial infarction. Increased exertion and unexpected crisis in the backcountry can create a situation in which rest is not possible. If persistent ischemia develops, definitive treatment is a long way off. This elevated level of risk should be discussed with any angina patient contemplating wilderness travel.

Stable Angina

- History of chronic coronary artery constriction with *transient* myocardial ischemia
- Oxygen demand exceeds supply *temporarily*
- Exacerbated by exertion
- Relieved by rest
- Treated with nitroglycerin and oxygen
- Not urgent if responds to normal treatment

"Increased exertion and unexpected crisis in the backcountry can create a situation where rest is not possible."

Risk Versus Benefit

Almost anyone who presents to a hospital emergency department with the complaint of chest pain is evaluated for heart attack even if the probability is low. The risk to patient and medical personnel is minimal and the benefit of detecting a heart attack is worth the trouble. The hospital has the equipment, personnel, and controlled environment necessary to make the specific diagnosis and begin the definitive treatment. Unfortunately, these resources are not available in the wilderness environment.

You will need to make the generic diagnosis, serious or not serious, without the benefit of lab tests and cardiology consults. Even if you have a high index of suspicion for myocardial ischemia, the evacuation may still represent the greater risk to the patient as well as add the risk to rescuers. On a good day with safe flying conditions, launching a helicopter is the right plan. On a bad day it is worth remembering that many people survive myocardial ischemia, but few people survive helicopter crashes.

Serious Chest Pain

Anticipate:

- Cardiogenic shock
- Respiratory failure

Treatment:

- PROP: specific treatments if MOI is known
- Pain medication
- Maintain hydration
- Maintain body core temperature
- Urgent evacuation

As with abdominal pain, there are times when you can give your patient a better chance of survival as well as protect the lives of others involved by performing good basic life support on scene rather than performing a complex and dangerous evacuation through an unstable environment. There are unfortunate examples of trained rescuers suspending or ignoring bleeding control, ventilation, or body core temperature in a desperate run for the trailhead or harbor. Remember, the goal is to deliver a living patient to the hospital. Quickly is ideal, but not always real.

Chapter 27 Review: Chest Pain

- Chest pain associated with shock, respiratory distress, or the risk factors for myocardial ischemia is serious.
- Persistent chest pain after trauma carries the anticipated problems of shock and respiratory distress.
- Risk factors for myocardial ischemia include being over 40 years old, post menopausal, obesity, diabetes, smoking, high blood pressure, high cholesterol, and a family history of heart disease.
- The field treatment of myocardial ischemia is to give one adult aspirin and oxygen and evacuate emergently. Assist the patient in using nitroglycerin if it has been prescribed for them.
- Prolonged ischemia will result in more heart muscle infarction. Emergency evacuation is ideal even if some exertion is required.
- Stable angina is the temporary pain of myocardial ischemia caused by increased demand not met by constricted coronary arteries. The pain resolves with rest. Stable angina is not an emergency if it resolves as expected.

Chapter 28: Gastrointestinal Problems

The gastrointestinal (GI) system, including the stomach and intestines, is responsible for the maceration and digestion of food and the excretion of waste. The process involves digestive acids and enzymes secreted by your stomach, liver, and pancreas and the action of what has been called your microbiologic organ: the billions of bacteria inhabiting your gut.

The digestive process can be disturbed by a variety of mechanisms, such as changes in diet, the introduction of foreign bacteria, or the elimination of normal and necessary bacteria as a side effect of antibiotic use. Problems with the digestive organs can result in inadequate or excessive secretion of digestive enzymes. Digestive organs are also subject to inflammation and obstruction. The patient experiences diarrhea, constipation, gas, vomiting, cramps, or other nonspecific pain.

A specific diagnosis for GI distress is rarely possible. Fortunately, most of these problems are mild and self-limiting. The worrisome ones present as a critical system problem or with the signs and symptoms of serious abdominal or chest pain.

Diarrhea

One of the functions of the large intestine is to absorb fluid from feces just before excretion. This serves to conserve the body's fluid balance and to allow some degree of control over when and where excretion occurs. Diarrhea develops when capillaries dilate and leak in the inner lining of the intestine. The usual cause is irritation by infection or toxins, but local or systemic allergy and even altitude illness can have the same effect. Like abdominal pain, we're usually left making the generic assessment: Serious or Not Serious?

Assessment of Diarrhea

Diarrhea that is a softer version of normal stool and relatively infrequent in an otherwise healthy individual is not considered serious if fluid losses can be replaced by oral intake. Pain is limited to cramping that is relieved by a bout of flatulence or diarrhea. Fever, if present, is low grade and intermittent.

Diarrhea can be a symptom of more serious problems when accompanied by the signs and symptoms of serious abdominal pain. Diarrhea itself becomes a critical system problem when fluid loss occurs so rapidly that it cannot be replaced. For example, the cause of death in cholera is volume shock from diarrhea.

Diarrhea

Serious:

- Associated with serious abdominal or chest pain
- Fluid losses exceed intake
- Persistent fever
- Bloody diarrhea
- Signs of shock

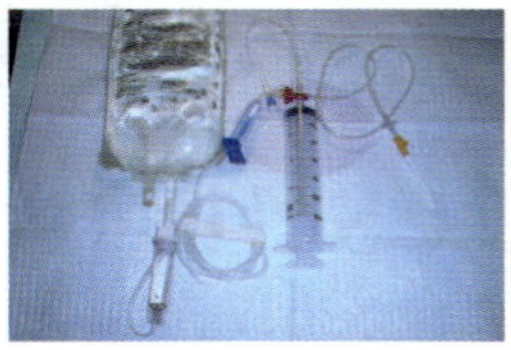

Treatment of Diarrhea

Mild diarrhea can be treated effectively with bismuth subsalicylate (Pepto-Bismol) or similar over-the-counter preparations. Opioid antispasmodic drugs, such as loperamide, inhibit intestinal motility, allowing more time for the absorption of fluid. Beware of using loperamide if the cause of the diarrhea is bacterial infection, evidenced by blood or pus in the stool or the presence of fever. Obstructing drainage can increase the severity of the infection.

Replace fluid losses with oral or intravenous (IV) electrolyte solutions. Time will usually correct the situation, but if the problem persists longer than a week, medical advice should be sought. If signs of volume shock are present, evacuation should be urgent if fluids cannot be replaced quickly in the field. During evacuation, oral fluids should be given as quickly as the patient can tolerate.

Diarrhea

Anticipate:

- Volume shock from dehydration

Treatment:

- Fluid and easily absorbed food
- Preserve body core temperature
- Loperamide (Imodium) if no serious S/Sx (4 mg x 1 dose, then 2 mg after each loose stool)
- Bismuth subsalicylate (Pepto-Bismol)
- Antibiotics for traveler's diarrhea (azithromycin, ciprofloxacin)

Constipation

The usual cause of constipation is dehydration. The large intestine absorbs fluid from feces, producing a hard stool that is difficult to excrete. The patient reports fullness, cramping, and intermittent pain in the lower abdomen and pelvis.

Constipation becomes bothersome when the patient feels uncomfortable and a problem when the rest of the body begins to suffer. Constipation becomes an emergency when associated with serious abdominal pain. The four most common causes of constipation are dehydration, lack of opportunity for bowel movement, a low-fiber diet, or a bowel obstruction.

Treatment of Constipation

Hydration is the best initial treatment and often relieves the problem. The next step is the use of a stool softener and mild stimulant such as Senna (Senokot) or docusate sodium (Colace). Mineral oil taken orally as an intestinal lubricant can reduce friction and allow stool to move. These treatments are very mild and generally safe.

Laxatives such as bisacodyl (Dulcolax) given orally or by suppository stimulate the bowel to contract. This is most effective and least painful after hydration and the administration of a stool softener. Laxatives can be dangerous if the patient has a bowel obstruction. Do not use these drugs in the presence of serious abdominal pain.

Constipation

Anticipate:

- Obstruction to infection
- Serious abdominal pain

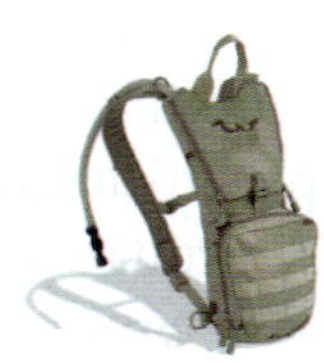

Treatment:

- Hydration
- Stool softeners; Colace, Senokot
- Laxatives*; Dulcolax, Ex-lax
- Enema*

* Not in the presence of serious abdominal pain.

An enema is viewed by most people as the treatment of last resort. Warm water is instilled into the rectum by gravity feed. A small amount may be all that is necessary to lubricate and soften stool. An enema is also contraindicated with serious abdominal pain.

Constipation can be prevented in the backcountry by staying well hydrated and adding fiber to the diet. Carrying dehydrated or high-protein food can make this a challenge. Consider using a bulk agent like psyllium capsules to supplement your diet. It is also important to take the time and find the privacy for a decent bowel movement.

Nausea and Vomiting

Like diarrhea, vomiting can be the result of a problem with the GI system or a symptom of other problems such as motion sickness, toxic ingestion, head injury, or infection. Finding and treating the primary cause is ideal. You must consider the additional problems that can be caused by severe fluid loss as well.

Vomiting

Serious:

- Cannot control airway
- Cannot replace fluids
- Cannot maintain calories and body core temp
- Associated with red flags for abdominal pain

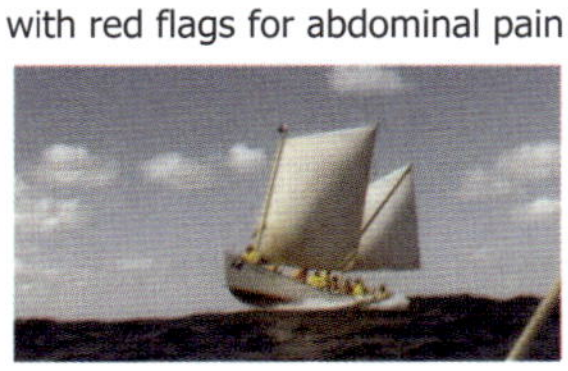

Treatment of Vomiting

Replacement of lost fluid is a priority. Because nausea inhibits oral intake, IV or subcutaneous rehydration may be necessary. Infusing fluid by periodic IV or subcutaneous bolus can be much easier than trying to maintain a continuous drip, especially during a carry out or aboard ship in heavy seas. Oral intake may be successful if the patient can take small amounts frequently enough to maintain hydration. Look for normal urine output as evidence of success.

Airway obstruction and aspiration is an anticipated problem in any vomiting patient. Positioning for drainage and constant monitoring is important if the patient is not A on the AVPU scale or is exhibiting altered mental status. Keep somebody nearby to assist when necessary.

Antiemetic drugs can be given by intramuscular (IM) or IV injection, by mouth, or by rectal suppository. The prescription drugs promethazine/Phergan, ondansetron/Zofran, and prochlorperazine/Compazine are examples. The over-the-counter antihistamines meclizine/Antivert and diphenhydramine/Benadryl can be effective. If the patient cannot swallow a pill, diphenhydramine can be delivered in the form of an oral dissolving strip and ondansetron comes in an oral dissolving tablet. Acetaminophen is preferred over nonsteroidal anti-inflammatory drugs (NSAIDs) or oral opioids for pain.

Vomiting

Anticipate:

- Airway obstruction and aspiration
- Volume shock from dehydration

Treatment:

- Airway control
- Hydration and calories
- Maintain body core temperature
- Antiemetic medication

Risk Versus Benefit

Although a number of drugs are mentioned here, it is worth noting that treating GI problems offers an easy opportunity to make things worse if you are not careful. A mildly annoying but otherwise functioning gut is often best left alone. The problem will usually resolve itself within 24 hours. Being too quick to add drugs can cause a resolving problem to swing too far the other way. You can easily turn diarrhea into constipation or vice versa. Antibiotics can do more harm than good by killing off beneficial bacteria along with the target organisms and should generally be reserved for serious infections. A day of clear liquids and easily digested foods in small amounts will often do more good with less risk than any medication.

Chapter 28 Review: Gastrointestinal Problems

- The GI system, including the stomach and intestines, is responsible for the maceration and digestion of food and excretion of waste.
- A specific diagnosis for GI distress is rarely possible. Most of these problems are mild and self-limiting; serious ones present as a critical system problem or with the signs and symptoms of serious abdominal pain.
- Diarrhea develops when the lining of the intestinal space is irritated by infection or toxins and fails to absorb fluid. The intestine can also leak more body fluid on its own, contributing to general fluid loss.
- Mild diarrhea can be treated effectively with bismuth subsalicylate (Pepto-Bismol) or similar over-the-counter preparations or with opioid antispasmodic drugs.
- The usual causes of constipation are dehydration and lack of opportunity. The patient reports fullness, cramping, and intermittent pain in the lower abdomen and pelvis.
- Hydration is the best initial treatment for constipation and often relieves the problem. The next step is the use of a stool softener and mild stimulant.
- Constipation can be prevented in the backcountry by staying well-hydrated and adding fiber to the diet.
- Vomiting can be the result of a problem with the GI system or a symptom of other problems such as motion sickness, toxic ingestion, head injury, or infection. Finding and treating the primary cause is ideal.
- Replacement of fluid loss is a priority with a vomiting patient. Because nausea inhibits oral intake, IV or subcutaneous rehydration may be necessary.
- Treating GI problems offers an easy opportunity to make things worse if you are not careful.

Chapter 29: Genitourinary Problems

As the name implies, the genitourinary (GU) system is really two systems sharing some common structures. It can be difficult to distinguish between problems that lie in reproductive organs and those affecting the urinary system. In the absence of a specific diagnosis, the generic assessment of serious or not serious is still possible. Anything that interferes significantly with the normal body functions of eating, drinking, and excretion can be considered serious. This includes any GU problem with significantly impaired urination.

Problems within the GU system are likely to be either obstruction to infection or ischemia to infarction. The common examples are urinary tract infection (UTI), vaginitis, and kidney stones. Often the patient will have a history of similar problems and will know what it is. Less common are urinary obstruction, testicular torsion, ovarian torsion, and ectopic pregnancy.

Vaginitis

Infection of the vagina occurs when something upsets the normal balance between yeast and bacteria, allowing one of the species to grow out of control. Antibiotics taken for a strep throat, for example, will kill many of the bacteria in the vagina allowing for an overgrowth of yeast. Changes in the vaginal environment can also be caused by clothing, sexual activity, stress, dehydration, and other factors.

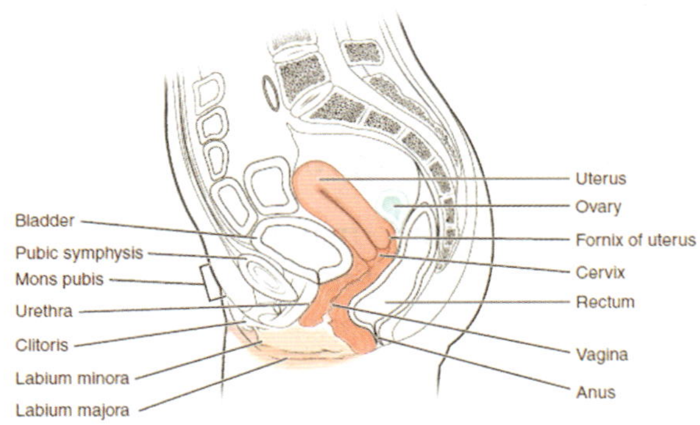

(a) Human female reproductive system: lateral view

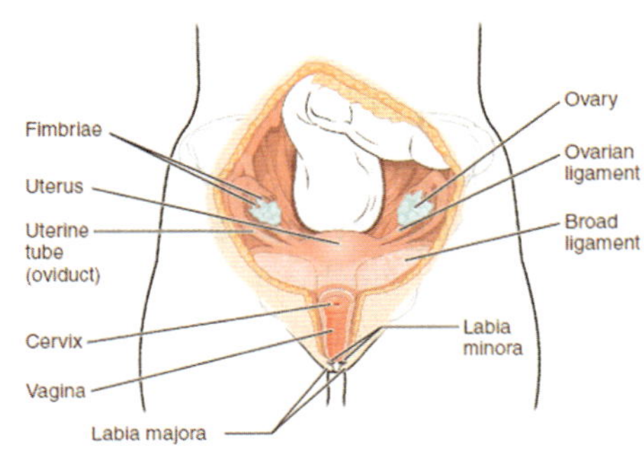

(b) Human female reproductive system: anterior view

Yeast infection is more common than bacterial infection. Signs and symptoms include itching or burning, and a whitish or "cheesy" vaginal discharge. There may also be tingling or burning as urine irritates inflamed tissues, causing some confusion with UTI. The practitioner will need to ask specific questions about the presence of discharge and the location of discomfort to make the distinction.

Many patients presenting with yeast vaginitis will have a previous history of similar symptoms and will recognize the problem and know the treatment. New onset cases with no previous history should be evaluated by a medical professional if possible.

Bacterial vaginitis also causes itching and burning, but the discharge is typically yellow or brown and malodorous. A lost tampon is a common cause. Medication use, diabetes, and other systemic problems can also contribute.

Vaginitis becomes serious when it migrates into the uterus and fallopian tubes causing the infection known as pelvic inflammatory disease (PID). The symptoms include the easily recognized signs and symptoms of serious abdominal pain. A strong suspicion of sexually transmitted disease should also be considered a serious condition.

Treatment of Vaginitis

Simple yeast vaginitis may respond to nonprescription treatment in the field. Medications like miconazole/Monistat suppositories and cream are available over the counter in most countries and should be carried on expedition. The manufacturers warn against relying on this treatment unless the patient is certain of the diagnosis through past experience.

Because yeast and bacteria grow well in a warm and moist environment, the situation can also be improved by staying dry and cool. This means wearing loose-fitting clothing and spending less time in a bathing or wet suit. Good hygiene is also important.

Bacterial vaginitis is best evaluated and treated in a medical facility. Practitioners will want to rule out sexually transmitted disease and treat with antibiotics. Evacuation need not be an emergency if symptoms are not progressing and no fever or pain is noted.

Vaginitis

Signs and Symptoms:

- Yeast - white, cheesy discharge
- Bacterial - yellow/brown, malodorous discharge
- Itchy, burning sensation on contact with urine

Serious (Red Flags):

- Associated with red flags for abdominal pain
- Pregnancy

"Many patients presenting with yeast vaginitis will have a previous history of similar symptoms and will recognize the problem and know the treatment."

Vaginitis

Treatment:

- Yeast Infection:
  - oral antifungal (fluconazole, Rx)
  - topical antifungal (miconazole, OTC)
- Bacterial Vaginitis:
  - oral or vaginal antibiotics
  - evacuation for medical evaluation

Urinary Tract Infection

Uncomplicated and easily treated UTIs are more common in people with vaginas because the associated urethra is usually shorter than that in people with penises. Also, because the urethra is located near the openings of the vagina and anus, it is easier for skin or intestinal bacteria to migrate from the outside into the bladder. Normal urination usually flushes bacteria out of the urethra preventing this from happening, but this system can be upset in several ways.

Perhaps the most common cause of UTI in wilderness travelers is urinary retention. This is usually due to dehydration or simply a lack of opportunity to urinate. Getting out of a warm sleeping bag, bracing yourself against the pitch and roll of a small boat at sea, or negotiating relief around a climbing harness on a big wall can inhibit frequent flushing. Any bacteria entering the bladder and urethra have a longer period of time in which to multiply and invade the mucosal lining.

Urinary Tract Infection

Mechanisms:

- Obstruction
- Dehydration
- Inadequate hygiene
- Localized trauma

Treatment:

- Hydration
- Antibiotics

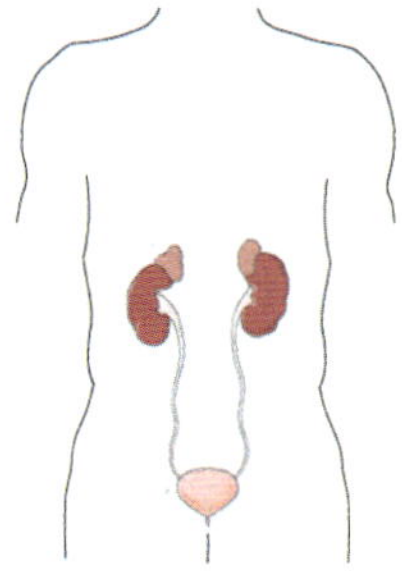

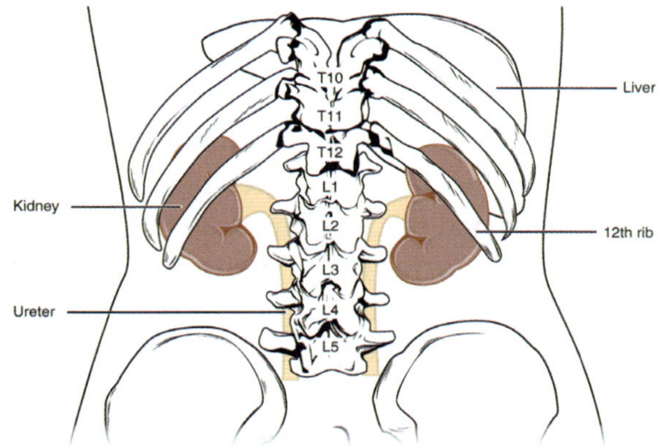

The urinary tract is normally sterile. Migration of bacteria from the urethral opening can result in an uncomplicated bladder infection, or a serious kidney infection.

Another predisposing factor for UTI is inadequate hygiene. Even though the urinary tract is normally sterile, in settings where bathing is difficult the number of bacteria on the outer surface of the skin increases dramatically making invasion and infection more likely. A third factor is direct trauma to the urethra. The usual culprit is frequent or vigorous sexual activity. The urethral opening becomes inflamed and is invaded by bacteria resulting in infection.

More complicated and serious infections can develop when the bacteria climb beyond the bladder to invade the ureters and kidneys. Sexually transmitted infections are also considered more dangerous because the bacteria or virus is foreign to the body and is more difficult to eradicate.

With a penis the urethra is much longer, acute infection of the urinary tract is unusual and may indicate a potentially serious condition. The most common cause is sexually transmitted infection. However, some patients may experience this occasionally as a result of urinary obstruction and retention.

The signs and symptoms of uncomplicated (not serious) UTI include low pelvic pain, frequent urination in small amounts, cloudy urine, and pain, tingling, or burning on urination. It is possible to confuse uncomplicated UTI with a vaginal infection because the inflamed vaginal mucosa and external genitalia may sting and itch on contact with urine.

Treatment of Urinary Tract Infection

The standard of care for uncomplicated UTI is oral antibiotics for three to ten days. Temporary measures pending access to medical care involve treating UTI with drainage and cleansing like any other soft tissue infection. Keep the external genitalia as clean as possible and drink plenty of fluids to promote frequent urination.

Signs and symptoms indicating that infection has progressed beyond the superficial lining of the urethra and bladder indicate a more serious condition. These include fever, back pain, and an ill-appearing patient. The possibility of sexually transmitted infection should also be considered an indication for early medical evaluation. Antibiotic therapy and evacuation are indicated.

Urinary Tract Infection

Serious:

- Longer urethra (penis)
- Back pain (kidney involvement)
- Fever (systemic infection)
- Serious abdominal pain
- Bloody urine
- Known sexually transmitted infection

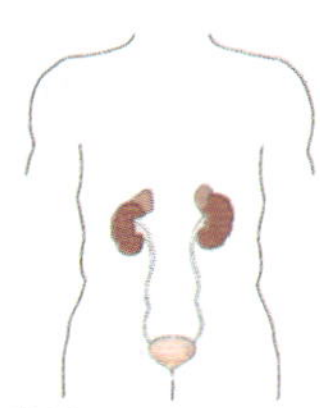

"Antibiotic therapy and urgent evacuation are indicated."

Urinary Tract Obstruction

The kidneys filter blood and produce the filtrate (urine) at a rate of about one milliliter a minute in a healthy and normally hydrated person. Urine is then transported through the ureters to the bladder. This transport is both passive due to gravity and active by peristaltic action of smooth muscle in the wall of the ureter. The bladder stores urine until you are ready to urinate. Sphincters at the bladder outlet allow you some degree of control over when and where you do so.

Loss of bladder control with involuntary urination can be a symptom of a serious problem like spinal cord injury or brain failure, or a less serious issue like uncomplicated urinary tract infection. While it is inconvenient or embarrassing, unplanned urination is rarely due to a serious problem within the urinary tract itself. Obstruction of urinary drainage, on the other hand, is serious.

Anything that blocks the normal flow of urine from the kidneys to the outside can cause kidney failure, infection, or rupture of the bladder or ureters. In an awake and responsive patient, the problem usually presents as increasing pain and agitation. In an unresponsive patient, failure of the bladder to empty may go unnoticed if you are not paying attention. In either case, a urinary tract that is not urinating regularly indicates a serious problem.

Bladder Outlet Obstruction

Bladder outlet obstruction usually affects people with penises because the associated prostate can become enlarged or infected causing a stricture in the urethra. This chronically constricted urethra can become an acutely obstructed one with just a little inflammation. Some drugs can contribute as well (e.g. diphenhydramine/Benadryl). The initial complaint of "I can't pee" will become serious abdominal pain as the bladder distends.

The usual treatment is to pass a catheter through the penis into the bladder. The sooner that you recognize the problem and catheterize the patient, the better. In extreme cases a suprapubic tap can be accomplished by inserting a long hypodermic needle through the abdominal wall into the bladder just above the pubic bone. Emergency evacuation is indicated if you have neither the equipment nor the training to perform these procedures.

Kidney Stone

Urine is a solution with various compounds (the solute) dissolved in water (the solvent). Under certain conditions, some of the solute can precipitate as crystals, some of which can become large enough to obstruct the transport of urine. These "stones" usually lodge in the ureter below the kidney.

Symptoms include increasing flank pain, nausea, and vomiting. Fever is rare until infection develops. The treatment for a known or suspected kidney stone is hydration and pain medication until the stone passes. Emergency evacuation should be considered if symptoms do not improve within 24 hours or anytime pain or disability is unmanageable.

Testicular Pain

Like any other organ, testicles can become obstructed, infected, or ischemic. A rare but dangerous cause of sudden onset pain is testicular torsion, where the testicle twists inside the scrotum, impinging its blood supply. Ischemia causes pain and will result in infarction of the testicle if not corrected. Testicular torsion can sometimes be relieved by gently elevating the scrotum and allowing the testicle to unwind spontaneously. Even if this maneuver is successful and pain is relieved, nonemergent medical follow-up is advised. Persistent pain unrelieved by this procedure should be considered an emergency. Persistent pain following trauma is also of concern, especially if swelling is severe. Immediate evacuation to surgical care is indicated.

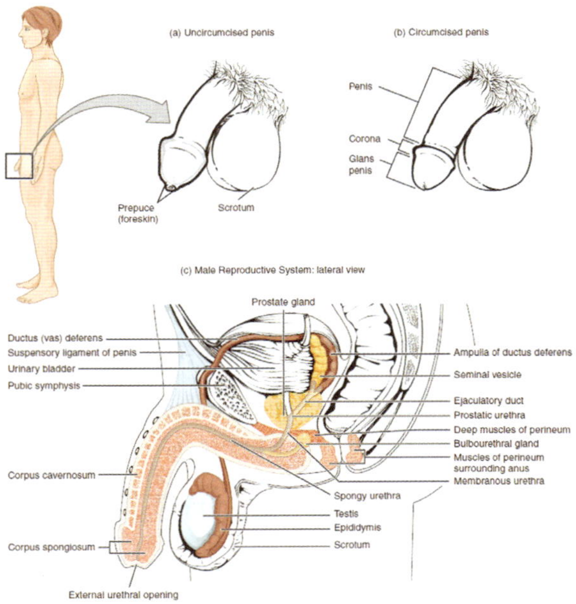

Bladder infection in people with penises is uncommon because of the length of the urethra. Infection and swelling of the prostate with severe pain and obstruction is possible.

Infection of the testes or epididymis is more common than torsion, but still unusual. It is extremely uncomfortable and potentially serious. Persistent testicular pain with or without swelling should motivate an early medical evaluation. Antibiotics can be used if evacuation is delayed or impossible. Epididymitis can be difficult to distinguish from testicular torsion.

Risk Versus Benefit

A mild UTI or vaginitis can often be treated in the field as a low-risk problem in cases where the patient has a previous history of similar symptoms and is confident in the diagnosis. You should see rapid response to medication and return to normal function within two days, or evacuation should be considered.

The urethra in the penis can become mildly irritated by dehydration or sexual activity, but persistent pain is not normal. If infection is suspected, evacuation for testing and diagnosis before treatment is ideal. In the remote setting, treatment with antibiotics under medical advice may be necessary before any testing can be accomplished. The risk of complications increases substantially with time. In any case, sexually transmitted disease should be suspected and medical follow-up sought as soon as practical.

Severe pain in the urinary tract from an infection, kidney stone, or bladder outlet obstruction will fit the criteria for serious abdominal pain. A specific diagnosis is not necessary. Evacuation is warranted.

Chapter 29 Review:
Genitourinary Problems

- It can be difficult to distinguish between problems that lie in reproductive organs and those affecting the urinary system. A careful history will help.
- Problems within the GU system are likely to be either obstruction to infection or ischemia to infarction.
- Infection of the vagina occurs when something upsets the normal balance between yeast and bacteria, allowing one of the species to grow out of control.
- Vaginitis becomes serious when it migrates into the uterus and fallopian tubes, causing the infection known as pelvic inflammatory disease.
- Simple yeast vaginitis may respond to nonprescription treatment in the field, including over-the-counter medications, staying dry and cool, and practicing good hygiene. Bacterial vaginitis is best evaluated and treated in a medical facility.
- Uncomplicated and easily treated UTIs generally limited to people with vaginas because of the short length of the associated urethra.
- One of the most common causes of UTI in wilderness travelers is urinary retention.
- The signs and symptoms of uncomplicated UTI include low pelvic pain; frequent urination in small amounts; cloudy urine; and pain, tingling, or burning on urination.
- The standard of care for uncomplicated UTI is oral antibiotics.
- Like any other organ, testicles can become obstructed, infected, or ischemic. A rare but dangerous cause of sudden onset pain is testicular torsion. Ischemia causes pain and will result in infarction of the testicle if not corrected.
- Persistent testicular pain with or without swelling should motivate an early referral for medical evaluation.
- A mild UTI or vaginitis can often be treated in the field as a low-risk problem in cases where the patient has a previous history of similar symptoms and is confident in the diagnosis.
- The urethra in the penis can become mildly irritated by dehydration or sexual activity, but persistent pain is not normal. If infection is suspected, evacuation for testing and diagnosis before treatment is ideal.

Chapter 30: Respiratory Infection

Like abdominal pain, respiratory infections have a variety of causes and effects. Pneumonia is an infection of lung tissue, resulting in the accumulation of pus or serous exudate in the alveoli. Bronchitis is an infection of the bronchial tubes of the lower airway causing lower airway constriction. Pharyngitis, tonsillitis, and epiglottitis are infections of the structures in the upper airway. Pleurisy involves the chest wall and outer surface of the lung. In the field it can be difficult to tell one respiratory infection from another. The diagnosis often remains generic: Serious or Not Serious?

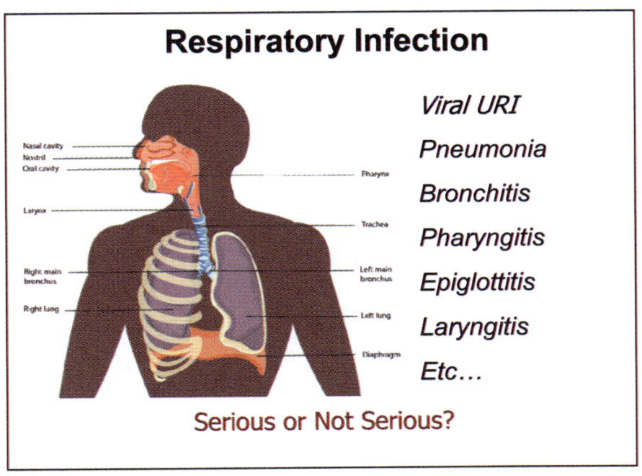

Respiratory Infection

Fortunately, most respiratory infections are caused by viruses and are relatively mild. They typically produce a constellation of symptoms such as runny nose, mild headache, sneezing, coughing, irritated eyes, sore throat, muscular aches, and intermittent fever. The patient is usually not impaired in their ability to perform normal tasks and continues to eat, drink, urinate, and produce stool more or less on schedule. Respiratory distress is not significant.

Problems develop when the virus is particularly virulent like COVID-19 and some strains of influenza, or the viral infection opens the way for a secondary bacterial infection. This is how patients who start with a cold can end up with a bacterial pneumonia, bronchitis, or strep throat. Bacterial infections are suspected when the cough is productive of thick yellow, green, or brown sputum. The patient may experience chills, shortness of breath, and chest pain on respiration. You may hear wheezing, or fine or coarse crackles, when listening to the chest with your stethoscope. Fever will be more persistent.

A viral or bacterial respiratory infection becomes serious when it causes respiratory distress, interferes significantly with eating and drinking, or shows signs of becoming systemic. Bacterial pneumonia, for example, is a frequent source for sepsis and dehydration in older people. Bronchitis can exacerbate asthma. A parapharyngeal abscess can cause airway obstruction.

Respiratory Infection

Serious:

- Respiratory distress
- Significant difficulty swallowing secretions
- Persistent fever
- Bloody sputum
- Tachycardia
- Persistent chest pain

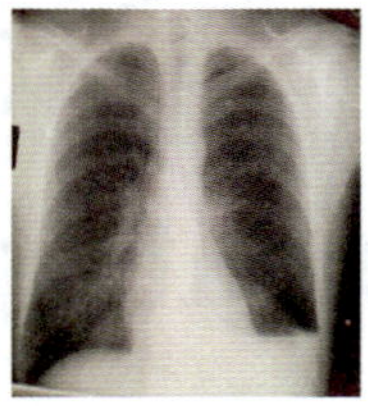

Treatment of Respiratory Infection

Although antiviral drugs may be used in the early stages of a cold or flu, eradication of the virus really depends on the body's immune system. A patient with a constellation of mild symptoms suggestive of viral infection should be made more comfortable while the body works to defeat the virus. Use whatever over-the-counter medications are available to make the patient feel better while not interfering with their ability to function. Local decongestants such as nasal sprays, systemic decongestants, and nonopioid cough medications can be very helpful at alleviating symptoms, as can anti-inflammatory medications like ibuprofen. Equally important is maintaining fluid balance, eating well, staying warm, and getting enough rest. This reduces the number of stressors that the body must deal with.

Respiratory Infection

Treatment:

- OTC NSAIDs and cough medication
- Maintain hydration and calories
- Bronchodilators for wheezing (Rx)
- Antibiotics for infection (Rx)
- PROP and evacuation for serious S/Sx

"The availability of antibiotics should not cause you to delay the evacuation of a patient in respiratory distress."

A patient with symptoms of bacterial infection may need antibiotics, especially if wheezing or crackles are detected on auscultation of the lungs. If you are authorized to use these drugs, the patient can safely be treated in the field if they are doing well otherwise. The availability of antibiotics should not cause you to delay the evacuation of a patient in respiratory distress.

Risk Versus Benefit

It is unusual for an otherwise healthy individual to develop a serious respiratory infection. Most cases are just annoying viral syndromes that do not respond to antibiotics. However, certain patients are at increased risk for complications in viral infections and more likely to develop serious bacterial infections. These include infants, the elderly, asthmatics, recently hospitalized patients, and people with impaired immunity.

Respiratory viruses and some bacteria are spread when mucous from an infected person contacts the next host's mucous membranes. This can occur by contact with mucous left on surfaces or more commonly by inhaling aerosolized droplets generated by sneezing and coughing. Public health warnings during epidemics call for the use of conscientious hand washing, wearing face masks, and isolating infected people from food preparation and other common areas as much as practical. These are good ways to reduce the risk of spreading any respiratory infection to other members of an expedition whether you are dealing with the common cold or a COVID-19 pandemic. Simple hand washing and the use of masks can greatly reduce the spread of respiratory infection even in the confined space of a voyaging sailboat or group tent.

Chapter 30 Review:
Respiratory Infection

- Respiratory infection in otherwise healthy people is usually caused by a virus, or less commonly, a bacterium.
- Respiratory infection can occur anywhere in the airway causing sore throat, bronchitis, or pneumonia.
- People at higher risk for complications and serious infection include infants, the elderly, asthmatics, and people with impaired immunity.
- A respiratory infection that causes airway obstruction or other respiratory distress is considered serious.
- Treatment of serious infection includes PROP, antibiotics, and emergency evacuation.
- Treatment of non-serious infection is directed at relieving symptoms and maintaining hydration and calories. Evacuation is non-urgent or deferred.

Chapter 31: Skin Rash

Determining the cause, significance, and treatment for skin rash can be a confusing exercise for both you and your patient. To the untrained observer most rashes look pretty much the same. However, the assessment of rash will be much easier when approached using the same principles that we apply to any other illness or injury starting with that most useful of diagnoses: Serious or Not Serious?

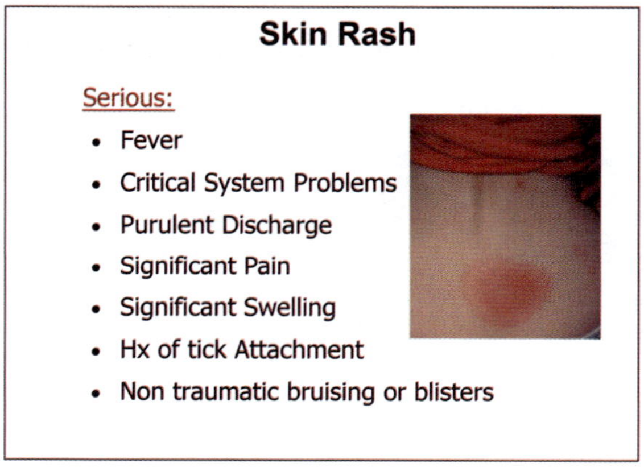

Serious or Not Serious?

First, look beyond the rash to the function of the three critical systems. Generalized hives and redness, for example, may be a symptom of anaphylaxis. Rash associated with a fever, shock, and altered mental status may be a symptom of a serious systemic infection. In these cases, the treatment will focus on supporting critical systems, not the rash itself.

If there is no evidence of shock, respiratory distress, or changes in brain function, you can assume that whatever is causing the rash is not serious, at least for now. You could probably ignore it, but your patient will be concerned and may be uncomfortable. In any case, you will want to be sure that there is nothing serious on your anticipated problem list.

Local or Systemic?

A rash is either a problem localized to the skin itself or the symptom of a systemic problem. A rash associated with a systemic illness will usually be bilateral and generalized. That is; appearing on both sides of the body and distributed over the whole body or large parts of it like the chest and abdomen. Generalized urticaria, as in mild allergic reaction, is one example (see Chapter 8: Allergy and Anaphylaxis). The rash associated with measles or chicken pox is another example. The presence of a fever and other changes in vital signs, like tachycardia, suggests local or systemic infection.

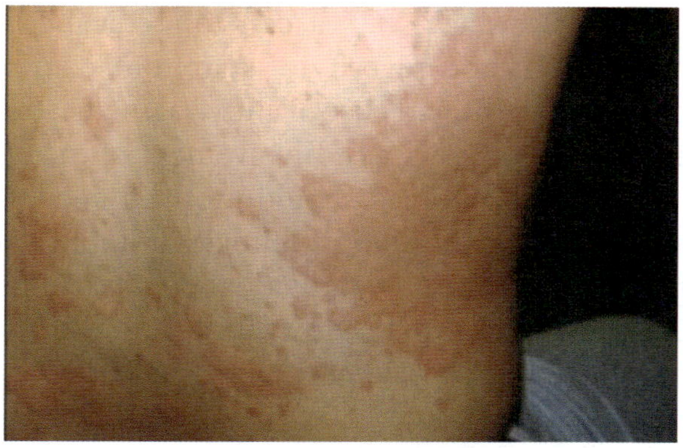

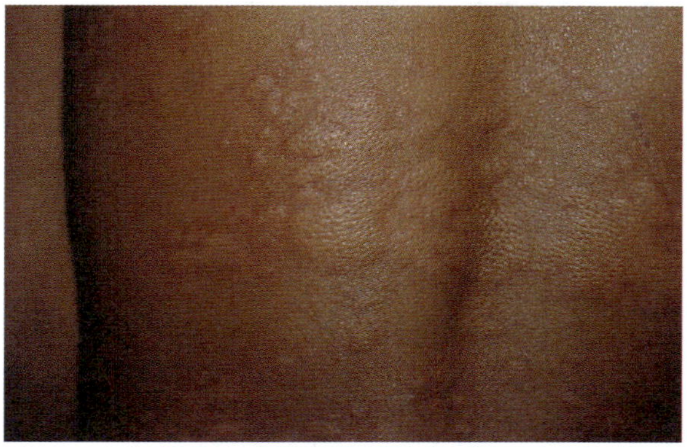

Generalized Urticaria (Hives)

Whatever the cause, a rash that appears as a symptom of systemic illness should prompt careful monitoring. Decay in critical system function would be an anticipated problem. Evacuation to a medical facility should be considered before the problem become an emergency. There is also the anticipated problem of the spread of infection to other team members.

A spreading bacterial infection of skin, called cellulitis, is typically red, hot, sore, and swollen. The presence of blisters, black or blue discoloration, and pain out of proportion to what you are seeing is also worrisome. It starts locally around a wound or abscess and can become quickly worse in just a few hours. A localized cellulitis can become a systemic infection with a full body red rash, fever, and swollen lymph nodes. Septic shock is the anticipated problem. In the field, aggressive and early antibiotic treatment of localized cellulitis may be warranted to prevent serious systemic illness.

Fortunately, the appearance of a generalized systemic rash is not always a symptom of a serious condition. If vital signs are normal and the patient feels otherwise healthy there is no emergency. You may never be able to make a diagnosis more specific than "little red skin bumps". It may disappear as quickly as it started or remain visible until a more specific diagnosis can be made. Medical follow up can be non-emergent.

The Not Serious Rash

A localized rash is unlikely to be caused by an acute systemic illness. This is a rash that appears in one spot or isolated area as the result of an infection, infestation, allergic reaction, or irritation from trauma, chemical exposure, or environmental conditions. If you can determine the cause, even generically, you can prescribe a treatment and relieve some of the annoying symptoms. As we have mentioned, there is also some value in preventing spread to other team members.

Skin Rash

Field Treatment:

- Clean and cover exudative rash and broken skin.
- Antihistamines for itching
- Topical steroids are generally safe for non-infective rashes.
- Antibiotic ointment is generally safe when you don't know.
- Avoid sun burning the affected area.

Generically, infections hurt and allergies itch. Trauma, and chemical and exposure are usually obvious based on location and history. Infections need cleaning and in some cases antibiotics. Allergies respond to antihistamines. Trauma needs to stop, and irritating chemicals need to be removed. Protection from the environment is part of basic life support. If generic diagnosis and treatment is as far as you get, you've done a good job and you could stop right there. However, if you have the time and inclination to be more specific you can do even better.

The process continues with a little amateur epidemiology. Where and when did the rash first appear? Is there an obvious or suspected mechanism? How is it spreading on the patient and/or to other people? What is the course of the illness in the people affected?

A rash that appears on everyone at the same time implies a common cause. Examples would include the heat rash that afflicts the whole crew of a sailing vessel in the heat and humidity of the tropics, or an outbreak of itchy red bumps on a group of trekkers after a night in a hut infested with bed bugs. Infections, allergies, and infestations typically don't present this way, but environmental insults do.

A rash that appears in one place on one person could be almost anything on the list. If it spreads to other people, you can rule out individual allergy, localized trauma, and usually toxic chemical exposure. A rash that spreads through a group over time suggests an infection like Methicillin Resistant Staphylococcus aureus (MRSA) or an infestation like scabies or lice. The characteristics of the rash can help make the distinction.

As with any other illness, a rash that is spreading through a group but beginning to resolve in the people first affected is somewhat reassuring. This is unlikely to be an infestation like scabies or an infection like MRSA. It is more likely to be a mild viral exanthem (widespread rash caused by a virus) that will probably resolve in everyone else, too. Further investigation is seldom needed.

Infection

A small bacterial infection without cellulitis can usually be managed with cleaning, warm soaks, and topical antibiotic ointment (e.g. mupirocin/Bactroban). Since some bacteria like MRSA can be spread to other parts of the body or other people, meticulous body substance isolation (BSI) is required.

Shingles is a rash caused by a Herpes virus that usually lies dormant in nerve tissue. When activated, a vesicular (small blisters) red rash breaks out in the local distribution of a nerve branch. Shingles can be painful, and the lesions can be an invitation to secondary bacterial infection, but the problem tends to remain localized and not serious. If you have easy access to medical care, the duration and severity of symptoms can be reduced with the early use of antiviral medication (e.g., acyclovir/Zovirax). Involvement of the eye in a shingles outbreak should motivate medical evacuation or consultation. Shingles is unlikely to spread to other healthy individuals, but transmission can be a risk to the very young or old, and to immunocompromised people.

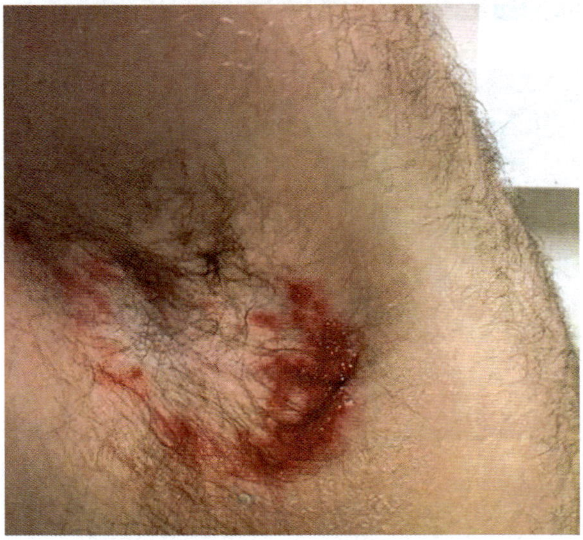

Shingles in the Axilla

A fungal infection like athlete's foot develops much more slowly and usually results in cracked and irritated skin with painful fissures. The usual cause is persistently moist conditions. The treatment is dry socks and antifungal cream or ointment (e.g., terbinafine/Lamisil) applied over several weeks. A similar condition can develop on the hands and scalp. These infections are seldom serious and will resolve when environmental conditions improve.

Infestation

The usual culprits are mites or lice living and feeding on the human body. The rash is a local allergic and irritant reaction to the substances produced or injected by the offending organism. Small red bumps and Itching is the usual symptom. This typically starts in one or two places and spreads all over the skin surface (scabies) or throughout the scalp or pubic region over time (lice).

Antihistamines can provide some relief from symptoms, but eradication using topical toxins is the definitive treatment (see Chapter 23: Toxins, Bites, and Stings).

Bed bugs, mosquitos, and black flies can produce a similar rash, but these are not infestations. The organism may be feeding on you, but it is not living on or in your body. The symptoms and the rash can also be reduced with antihistamines and NSAIDS.

Local Allergy

Most of the rash associated with insect and arachnid bites and stings are the cutaneous manifestation of a local reaction to the substance injected. These rashes are often mistaken for cellulitis and many people are treated with antibiotics unnecessarily. Remember, these local toxic and allergic reactions tend to itch whereas infections tend to hurt. The rash of a local allergy may be slightly warmer than the surrounding skin, but cellulitis tends to be hot. The rash of a local reaction will remain localized around the bite or sting, cellulitis tends to spread quickly. In a remote field setting you would be justified in treating with antibiotics if you are not sure which you are dealing with.

Poison ivy is another common rash that is also a localized allergic reaction. It responds to antihistamines and, if more bothersome, topical or systemic steroids. Removal of the allergen from the skin and clothing with soap that can break down plant oils will help reduce the duration of misery and the spread of the allergen to other places on the body.

Contact dermatitis is a generic term for inflammation from contact with an irritant or an allergen. The rash of Poison Ivy, for example, is a local allergy that develops after contact with the oils of the plant. Usually, the location of the rash and history of contact is sufficient to diagnose the rash. A reaction to the metal on the back of a wristwatch or earring is an example. Prolonged continuous contact is more likely to produce it.

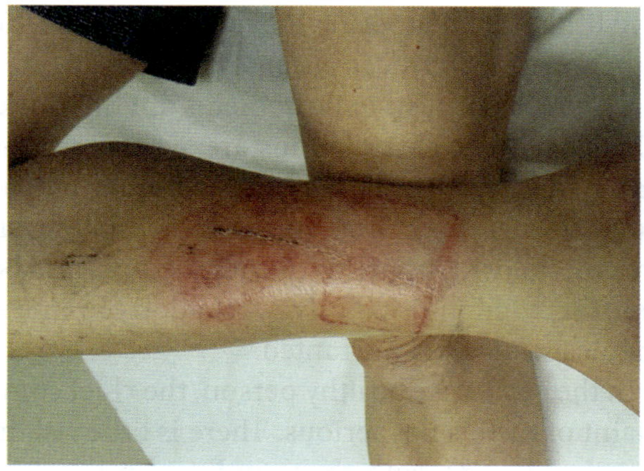

Contact Dermatitis from Tape

Trauma and Chemical Irritation

It would seem that a rash produced by trauma should be easy to figure out. Not always. The groin rash that develops after a day of hiking in wet shorts comes to mind. The chaffing occurs during the hike, the rash develops overnight. The patient may not make the connection. This is where your skills as an epidemiologist will come in handy.

Exposure to chemical irritants from plants and animals can be more difficult to diagnose. The exposure may be forgotten or unknown. The symptoms tend to itch less and burn more, suggesting something other than a local allergy. In either case, washing the area with soap and water can help remove toxins or allergens and reduce the chances of a secondary infection, especially if the skin surface is broken. Antihistamines may help with symptoms, but topical steroids are more likely to be effective.

Risk vs Benefit in Skin Rash

Rash is seldom the chief complaint in a serious illness. The patient is usually more concerned about the fever, respiratory distress, vomiting, or weakness than any rash that might go with it. The risk, of course, is that the practitioner will become more focused on the rash than the underlying critical system problems. There is great benefit, and little risk, in ignoring the rash to evaluate the function of the critical systems first.

Serious critical system problems are high risk. That's obvious. Less obvious are systemic signs and symptoms that should motivate you to anticipate critical system problems. A rash with a fever, weakness, loss of appetite, or cough should also be considered high risk. Early evacuation or remote medical consult is warranted.

In the otherwise healthy person, the chief complaint of rash is not serious. There is little risk in simply agreeing with them and recommending follow up with a dermatologist. However, your obligations as an expedition medical officer or your desire to relieve suffering may take you deeper into diagnosis and treatment. Now, you have an opportunity to increase the risk if you are not careful.

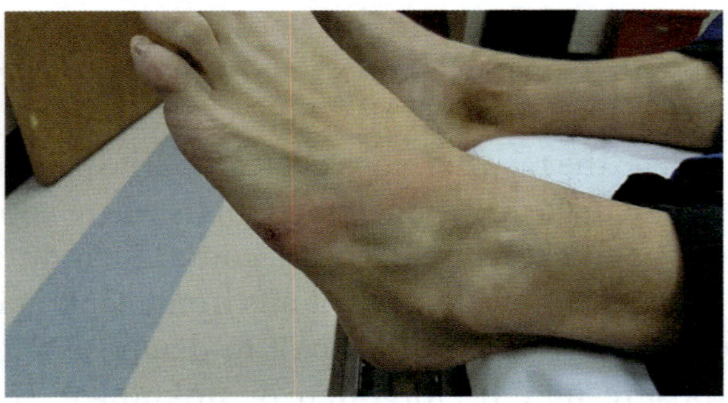

Cellulitis extending proximally from a small wound in the foot.

Generally, over the counter antihistamines, NSAIDS, topical steroid creams, and antibiotic ointments are safe and may even be effective. Choosing the wrong medication is unlikely to cause problems. It just won't help much. If you are contemplating systemic steroids or antibiotics, or high potency topical medication, you would be well advised to seek expert consultation if you are not an expert. You can end up causing more problems than you solve and chasing your tail trying to fix it.

Chapter 31 Review:
Skin Rash

- A rash can be a symptom of a serious critical system problem. Treatment is directed at supporting critical systems, not curing the rash itself.
- A rash can be a symptom of a systemic problem that is not serious but requires careful monitoring and possibly infection control measures to prevent spread to other group members.
- A localized rash is unlikely to be serious except in the case of cellulitis or other red flags.
- Serious or not serious is the most generic and important diagnosis in field medicine and is the beginning of risk vs benefit analysis. The only true emergency is the serious problem that you cannot fix in the field.
- Generally, over the counter medications for relief of symptoms are safe. Stronger medications, especially steroids, can cause more problems and should be used in consultation with a medical professional.

Chapter 32: Behavioral Issues

As with most other chapters in this book, the goal here is to frame a large and complex topic in terms that are simple and practical enough for field use. This is not intended to impart any psychological expertise or provide a substitute for training on the topic beyond patient and rescuer safety considerations. Those of you who are operating within programs specifically dedicated to mental health and rehabilitation will need significantly greater insight and education than we can provide here.

Unlike the topics of other chapters, primary behavioral problems do not come with a characteristic mechanism of injury or vital sign pattern. People are less likely to reveal a psychiatric history like depression or bipolar disorder than they would be to discuss a physiologic problem like hypertension or diabetes. The practitioner in the field is sometimes left with a confusing picture and little information to go on. Fortunately, general principles apply and a generic diagnosis is all that is necessary in most situations.

Unless you are dealing with a well-known preexisting condition, your first job is to exclude a metabolic or traumatic mechanism. Use the STOPEATS mnemonic; is there anything going on that could cause a change in brain function? Only after you have excluded an organic illness or injury can you attribute unusual or inexplicable behavior to a psychological problem. This is particularly important with outdoor programs working with youth at risk, PTSD patients, and others where behavioral issues are expected. In these situations you could be tempted to jump to a diagnosis like malingering, acting out, or attention seeking and miss the low blood sugar, stroke, sepsis, or toxin.

Assessment of Behavioral Problems

The list of available diagnoses is huge. Problems can range from situational anxiety reactions to personality disorders to severe psychoses. You are not going to make a specific diagnosis in the field. Keep it generic: Serious or Not Serious?

The patient may be unable or unwilling to care for and protect themselves. There may be talk or actions that suggest an intent to harm someone else or themselves. The patient may lose touch with reality to the point that they attempt to fly off a cliff or walk on water. Anything this severe is a backcountry emergency regardless of the specific diagnosis.

Milder cases tend to be more of a logistical and social dilemma than a medical emergency. Sometimes, what a patient says is alarming out of proportion to what they are actually doing. Inflammatory or uncooperative talk may be accompanied by actions that are quite the opposite. It may be more valuable to observe actions rather than react to words.

Many patients know their condition well and are aware of exacerbations as they happen. They may be able to reassure you, let you know what they need to feel better, or forewarn you of more serious problems to come. Don't be afraid to obtain a pertinent history, as you would with any other patient.

Field Treatment of Behavioral Problems

Provide reassurance and protection. Be vigilant for any threat of violence. Do not try to talk the patient out of their symptoms. Protect yourself, your crew, and the patient if possible. Call for help or initiate an evacuation if serious signs and symptoms develop.

Behavioral Issues

Serious:

- Verbal or physical threats to harm self or others
- Unwilling or unable to feed and protect self
- Delusions or hallucinations that could result in injury to self or others
- No obvious temporary or treatable cause
- The symptoms are getting worse

Unless you are a trained mental health provider working in a dedicated treatment program, it is not your job to provide specific treatment for a behavioral diagnosis. Allowing inconvenient but safe concessions may de-escalate an evolving confrontation while you work on evacuation or another solution. In most cases, everyone in your group who is affected should be aware of the plan. Beware of being manipulated by the patient or others in the group into an unsafe or overzealous response.

Physically restraining a patient who is violent or aggressive is a high-risk treatment for both patient and rescuers, even with the appropriate training. It would be far less dangerous to remove yourself and other from the scene. In fact, taking the pressure off may allow the patient to calm down. Early involvement of law enforcement personnel, if available, is ideal.

If you are authorized to carry medication, the judicious use of an anxiolytic like lorazepam can keep symptoms under control and reduce risk to the patient and other group members. Beware of combining this type of medication with other drugs like alcohol and opioids that are also respiratory depressants. Use the lowest effective dose.

Drug and Alcohol Overdose

One positive aspect of drug or alcohol overdose is that the substance will eventually wear off if the patient lives long enough. Treatment is focused on airway and ventilation, body core temperature, and hydration. Violent patients should be deflected and avoided with restraint as a last resort.

The use of naloxone/Narcan has become recognized as a first response emergency treatment for serious opioid overdose. It is given by intranasal spray or injection. If successful, you should anticipate potentially aggressive or violent behavior in the patient you have just resuscitated. Use naloxone in an uncontrolled setting only if absolutely necessary to reverse respiratory depression.

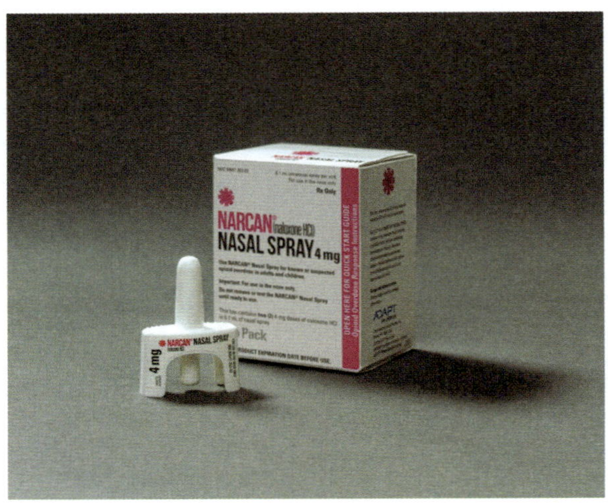

Naloxone nasal spray

Drug and Alcohol Withdrawal

Alcohol, opioid, or benzodiazepine withdrawal can present a diagnostic challenge on a backcountry trip. Some people will jump aboard an offshore boat delivery or sign up for a trek in the wilderness specifically in an attempt to beat their addiction. Symptoms of withdrawal can show up hours or days into a trip when return to port or retracing a route can be difficult or dangerous.

Unfortunately, the signs and symptoms of withdrawal can look a lot like heat exhaustion, sea sickness, sepsis, myocardial infarction, or a number of other conditions. A history of long-term use with recent discontinuation of an addictive substance is necessary to entertain the diagnosis. A rapid return to baseline when the substance is reintroduced will confirm it.

Outside of a specialized treatment program, it is unrealistic to expect to cure your patient's addiction while operating in a high-risk environment. The best emergency field treatment for alcohol withdrawal is to allow just enough alcohol consumption to stop the problem. For opioid withdrawal, administer enough opioid to keep symptoms under control. And, the same for benzodiazepine withdrawal. If symptoms are controlled and the scene is safe, evacuation can be accomplished on a non-emergent basis.

Chapter 32 Review:
Behavioral Issues

- Those of you who are operating within programs specifically dedicated to mental health and rehabilitation will need significantly greater insight and education than we can provide here.
- Only after you have excluded an organic illness or injury can you attribute unusual or inexplicable behavior to a psychological problem.
- You are not going to make a specific diagnosis in the field. Keep it generic: Serious or Not Serious?
- Provide reassurance and protection. Be vigilant for any threat of violence. Call for help or initiate an evacuation if serious signs and symptoms develop.
- Physically restraining a patient who is violent or aggressive is a high-risk treatment for both patient and rescuers, even with the appropriate training.
- The use of naloxone has become recognized as a first response emergency treatment for life-threatening opioid overdose.
- The best emergency field treatment for alcohol withdrawal is to allow just enough alcohol consumption to stop the problem. For opioid withdrawal, administer enough opioid to keep symptoms under control. And, the same for benzodiazepine withdrawal.

Case Study 12: High-Altitude Hunting

SCENE

A hunting camp in the western United States at 0830 on day four of a week-long horse pack trip into the high country. One of the parties, a 63-year-old man, complains of mild indigestion and shortness of breath. The camp is at 3200 meters in elevation and 9 kilometers from the trailhead over a single-track horse trail. The weather is cold with low overcast and visibility is restricted to 500 meters in moderate snow. The group is sheltered in a wall tent heated by a portable wood stove.

S: A 63-year-old man complains of pressure in the lower chest and upper abdomen, mild shortness of breath, and nausea since eating breakfast an hour ago. He denies any pain but describes the discomfort as radiating through to his back and slightly worse over the past 15 minutes.

Although he is certain that his symptoms are indigestion related to breakfast and that a good burp will fix it, he admits to not feeling well since arrival at camp last evening. He denies allergies and takes medication for high blood pressure and elevated cholesterol. His history is also significant for mild exercise-induced asthma and one episode of altitude illness on a hunting trip 12 years ago. He smoked a pack of cigarettes a day from age 16 to 55. He quit the day his father died of a heart attack. He underwent a cardiac evaluation after an episode of chest pain two years ago, but claims he was given a clean bill of health. None of the other members of the hunting party complain of similar symptoms.

O: Alert and oriented, sitting upright without obvious respiratory distress. The patient appears slightly pale and sweating. He is fit and muscular for his age. Auscultation of the chest reveals clear lungs without crackles or wheeze. The abdomen is not tender to palpation and not distended. Bowel sounds are normal. Vital signs: Pulse: 90 and regular, Resp: 24, Temp: 37°C, Skin: cool, moist, and pale, O2: 90%, C/MS: awake and oriented, BP: 162/98.

A:

1. Myocardial ischemia (heart attack)
   A': Cardiogenic shock
2. Remote location and adverse weather
   A': Prolonged evacuation
3. High elevation
   A': Decreased oxygenation

P:

1. One adult aspirin by mouth
2. Begin evacuation on horseback
3. Request Mountain Rescue to respond up the trail with oxygen and advanced life support capability to meet the evacuation in progress.

Discussion:

Given the disruption to the camp and crew, it would have been very tempting for the guide to accept the patient's diagnosis of indigestion, or at least wait to see if a burp solved the problem. However, there are enough concerning symptoms and risk factors in the patient profile and history for myocardial ischemia to be at the top of the problem list. Immediate evacuation to definitive care has the best chance of reducing infarction and preserving heart function. A helicopter evacuation would be ideal but would be a high-risk operation in the mountains with the current weather.

Allowing the patient to rest to reduce oxygen demand would be ideal as well but would significantly delay evacuation. It would take at least a day for a mountain rescue team to access the patient by foot and perform a 9-kilometer carry-out on a rough single-track trail. A horse can cover the distance in a few hours. The benefit of time saved would be worth the risk associated with the increased exertion required to ride.

If you wondered about possible carbon monoxide poisoning because of the wood stove in the tent, you should look for similar symptoms in the other people staying there. It would be unusual for only one person to show symptoms of such exposure. Another clue to CO inhalation would be an unusually high reading on a pulse oximeter. At 3200 meters elevation you would expect a reading of somewhere between 86 and 93%. A reading of 99 or 100 could indicate that the color of the carboxyhemoglobin molecule in the blood could be fooling the meter.

Case Study 13: Remote Canoe Trip

SCENE
At 1430 on day 5 of a month-long canoe trip in central Quebec, several students begin to complain of severe sore throat and pain on swallowing. One student admits to arriving with the illness on day one, but now seems to be improving. The group is now 75 kilometers downriver from the launching point. The only evacuation route is by float plane. The weather is overcast with light rain with a temperature of 12°C and light winds.

S: The most uncomfortable of the ill students reports the onset of pain two days ago with swallowing inhibited by the discomfort. He also reports a runny nose and intermittent mild ear pain and thinks he might have a fever. He gives no complaint of difficulty breathing, nausea, or dizziness. His tent mate has similar symptoms but not as severe. His last meal was at 1230 but "hurt a lot to eat." He has been able to drink well and reports that cold water makes his throat feel better. He has no other complaints and is normally healthy. He denies allergies and is not taking medication.

O: Alert, oriented, and appears mildly uncomfortable. No evidence of respiratory distress, shock from dehydration, or altered mental status. The throat looks inflamed but not swollen and there are no white patches visible. The patient's neck is mobile with mildly swollen glands. Clear nasal drainage is noted. The chest is clear to auscultation and the abdomen is not tender to palpation. Vital signs: Pulse: 64 and regular, Resp: 16 and easy, Temp: 37°C, Skin: warm, pink, and dry, O2: 98%, C/MS: awake and oriented.

A:

1. Sore throat, not serious
   A': Discomfort when eating
   A': Airway obstruction (unlikely)
2. Contagious illness spreading through the group

P:

1. Symptomatic treatment with ibuprofen and cool water. Encourage normal food and water intake. Monitor for any changes.
2. Enforce hand washing. Avoid sharing utensils and water bottles. Keep the remaining healthy crew in separate tents if possible.

Discussion:

There is no emergency here. The patient, like the others who share the illness, is uncomfortable but still performing normal body functions. There is no loss of appetite and no fever, which is a good sign. There is no evidence of airway obstruction and little reason to anticipate it, and the patient is normally healthy. The student who appears to have brought the virus to the group is recovering. Everyone else is expected to do the same.

Section VII: Roles, Responsibilities, and Technology

Chapter 33: The Expedition Medical Officer

The informal title "doc" is given to an army platoon's medic regardless of the level of the medic's training and certification. It recognizes the medic's special role as lifesaver, caregiver, and confidant to the soldiers to whom they are assigned. Whether in combat, civilian search and rescue operations, or on a sailing expedition the role of the medical officer is unique and demanding. In some circumstances, the task can be considerably more complex and challenging than that performed by an emergency physician in a hospital.

Expedition Medic

Planning:

- Anticipated problems
- Emergency communications
- Expectations and limitations
- Evacuation routes and methods
- Group medical supplies and equipment

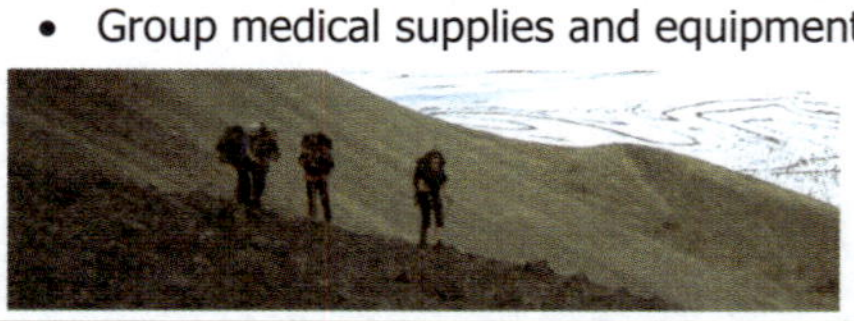

Responsibilities

In most situations, your role as an expedition medic becomes an educator and safety officer as well as a medical practitioner. It may be your job to brief your traveling companions on safety concerns, environmental threats, and preexisting conditions among those in your group. Also, by default or by design you may be the only one anticipating and planning for rescue and evacuation. The more you can anticipate and address problems before a crisis develops, the more time you will have to deal with the unexpected issues that inevitably arise.

Expedition Medic

Prevention and Early Intervention:

- Medical screening
- Hygiene protocols
- Basic medical skills training for the group
- Medical hazard assessment and briefing
- Personal medical equipment expectations

"You will need a working knowledge of local environmental conditions, medical resources, and the condition of your crew."

You need a working knowledge of local environmental conditions, medical resources, and the condition of your crew. You should also be intimately familiar with the equipment and medication you carry. Your confidence and competence are directly related to the quality of your preparation. Finally, the scope of your role and responsibilities, as well as your limitations, should be clearly understood by all concerned.

Medical Screening

Pre-trip screening discussions with clients and their medical advisors have also become a normal and expected part of the job. Recent trends in adventure travel and experiential education now require a greater understanding of chronic disease states and the ability to make reasonable risk/benefit decisions with your clients. People with angina, asthma, and diabetes are as interested in trekking and sailing as anyone else and it is no longer routine practice to exclude them.

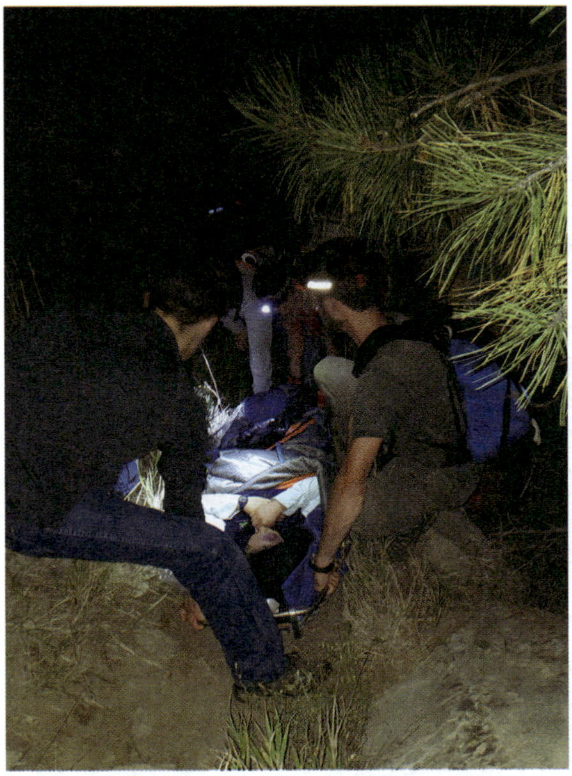

If an anticipated problem becomes an existing problem, you and your group will be the ones dealing with it. Be sure that you are able and willing to do so.

If you will be serving as the expedition medic or instructor who will be responsible for a client with a chronic condition, it may be appropriate (with the patient's permission) for you to have a direct discussion with their physician. Between your expertise in backcountry travel and wilderness medicine and the physician's clinical experience and knowledge of the patient, you should be able to assess the risk involved in the trip being contemplated.

A review of the medications people are taking is an important part of medical screening and your conversation with the treating physician. For you, it is more important to know what the consequences of overdose, withdrawal, and the drug's effect on thermoregulation than to know about specific therapeutic mechanism of a drug.

The patient can also be an excellent source of information about their condition and medications and the proper response to emergencies. People with diabetes, for example, are usually very well informed about their disease and can help to further your understanding of the condition.

Risk Versus Benefit

As a guide or medical officer, the final decision to accept responsibility for the care of a client with a preexisting and potentially dangerous medical condition should be yours. If the anticipated problem becomes real, you and your group will be the ones dealing with it. It is not practical or reasonable to defer this judgment solely to a physician who will not be traveling with you and who may not fully understand the environmental and logistical challenges that you will face. "Cleared by the doctor" is just useful information, not a dictum that you must live by.

Chapter 33 Review:
The Expedition Medical Officer

- The more you can anticipate and address problems before a crisis develops, the more time you will have to deal with the unexpected issues that inevitably arise.
- You should also be intimately familiar with the equipment and medication you carry.
- Pre-trip screening discussions with clients and their medical advisors have become a normal and expected part of the job.
- Between your expertise in backcountry travel and wilderness medicine and the physician's clinical experience and knowledge of the patient, you should be able to assess the risk involved in the trip being contemplated.
- "Cleared by the doctor" is just useful information, not a dictum that you must live by.

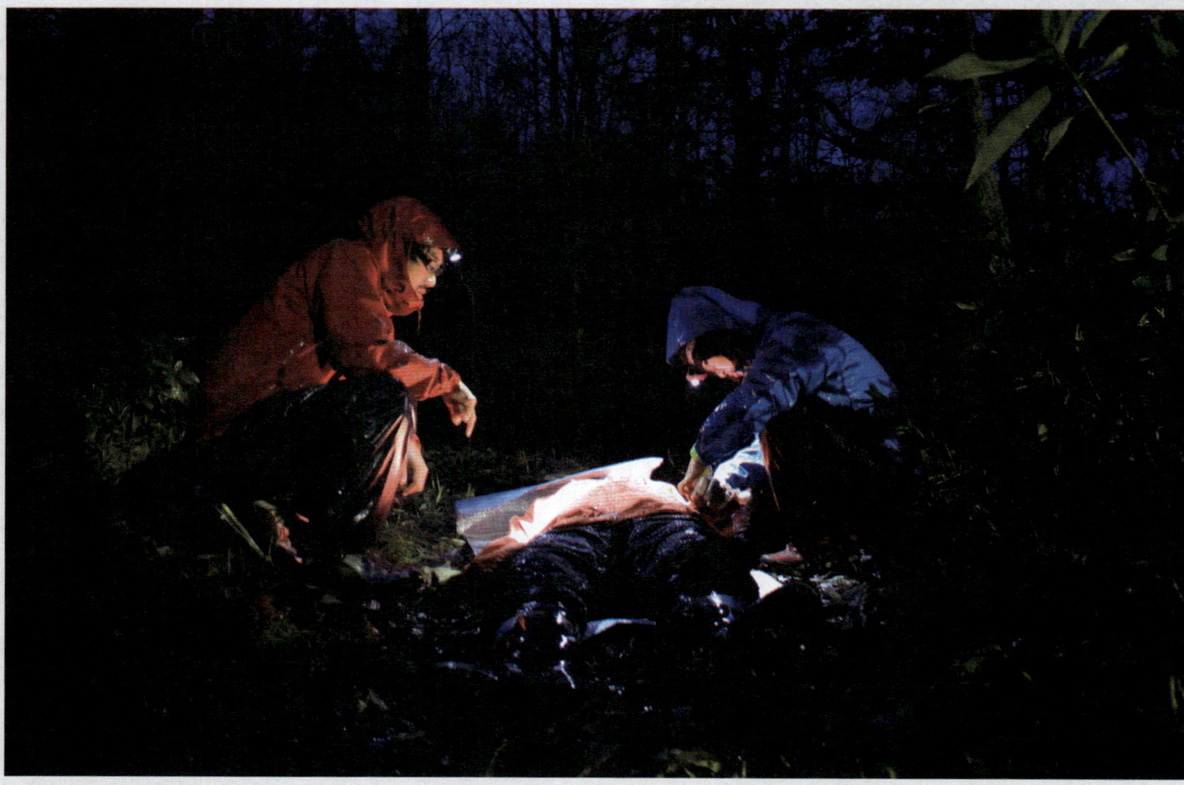

Chapter 34: The Medical Role in Search and Rescue

Worldwide most search and rescue missions are performed by volunteers. Teams range from loosely organized groups that come together only once or twice when needed, to highly skilled and well-disciplined teams that train regularly and run hundreds of missions a year. The work can be exciting, interesting, and rewarding. It can also be dirty, dangerous, and expensive.

If you choose to get involved you will need a fair degree of physical and mental fitness, self-discipline, and enough time to become proficient in the necessary skills. Functioning as a SAR medical officer requires solid field medical skills and a willingness and ability to act quickly and independently when needed. As we have emphasized throughout this text, it is often up to the medical officer to set the level of urgency and help develop a mission profile that keeps risk within the range of acceptable.

Medical Roles

In a large-scale disaster response or search and rescue operation, there will be several medical roles to fill, from field treatment to medical control. By contrast, a small team on a limited mission may field only one medical officer. Whatever the situation, and for any role to which you are assigned, you should know at a minimum who you are working for, who is working for you, what you are doing, and how long you are expected to do it.

Search and Rescue

Medical Roles:

- Medical leader
- Triage officer
- Hasty medical
- Patient leader
- Team "doc"

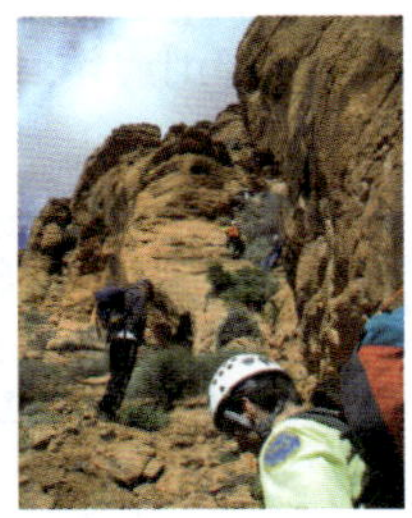

You should know:

- Who you're working for
- Who's working for you
- What you're doing
- How long you're expected to do it

Incident Management System

Knowing something about the National Incident Management System (NIMS) will help you understand your role in the field. The system is used in one form or another in most fire, rescue, and disaster situations in developed nations. The depth and complexity vary with the size and duration of the mission.

The incident commander (IC) has responsibility for the entire operation. Supervision of field operations, where most medical personnel are deployed, is usually delegated to an operations section chief, often stationed at or near the incident site. The section chief directs branch, division, or group leaders responsible for specific tasks or geographic areas.

NIMS and SAR management is beyond the scope of this text. However, if you choose to become involved in search and rescue it is certainly wise to become familiar with the system, how it might be used by any team with which you will deploy, and where you fit in as a medical provider. If you are responding to an unfamiliar operation, look for the incident commander (IC) or the command post (CP). In the field, look for the operations section chief or medical leader.

Recognize, however, that the typical top-down application of IMS may not be the best command and control structure for every situation. It tends to work best within a single agency dealing with a predictable problem, such as a fire department fighting a structure fire. It is less successful in managing unpredictable emergencies, situations that involve multiple agencies, or people who aren't as familiar with their roles or the IMS structure.

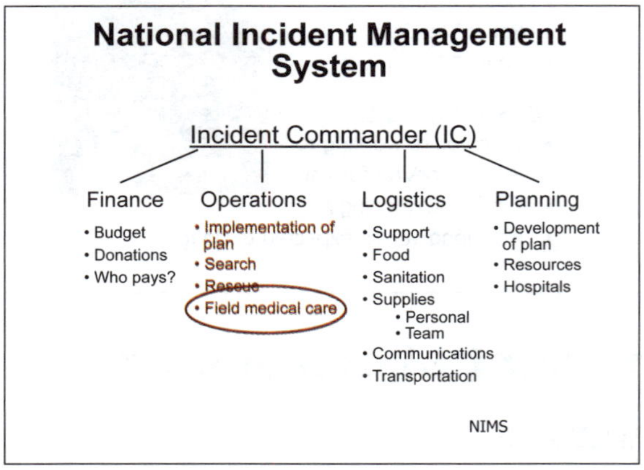
National Incident Management System
Incident Commander (IC)
Finance
• Budget
• Donations
• Who pays?
Operations
• Implementation of plan
• Search
• Rescue
• Field medical care
Logistics
• Support
• Food
• Sanitation
• Supplies
• Personal
• Team
• Communications
• Transportation
Planning
• Development of plan
• Resources
• Hospitals
NIMS

Rigid adherence to the IMS can hamper response in rapidly changing situations where quick decisions and reallocation of resources are needed. Usually, the rescuer on the scene has a much better grasp of the situation than the officer in the command post many miles away. In these cases, a more flexible bottom-up approach to emergency management is often more useful.

Response Preparation

Your preparation and response will be determined by the type of incident that is involved. A known medical problem at a known location allows you to be fairly specific in your choice of equipment and personnel. A search for a lost subject who may or may not have a medical problem, however, requires more generic medical preparation. This is basic information that the field medical officer should obtain in a briefing from the section chief or medical leader.

Operations Section

Operations Section Chief:

- Reports to the Incident Commander
- Establishes tactical objectives
- Assigns deputies, e.g., medical leader
- Manages all operational activities
- Defines branches, divisions, groups, and resources

"Field medical personnel will usually function under the Operations Section Chief."

Personal Preparation

- Equipment and clothing
- Technical training
- Know the team
- Medical kit – team and personal
- Understand your role and limitations
- What protocols are you working under?

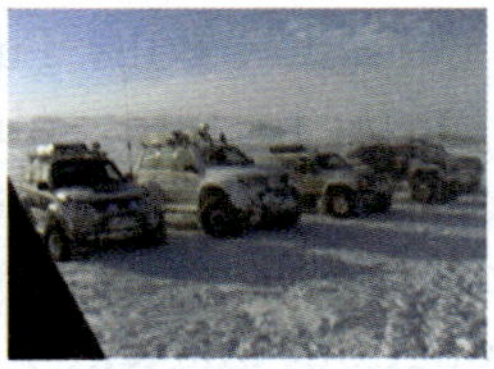

Risk Versus Benefit

Most emergency response to medical problems, from the street to the open ocean, generates risk well in excess of any benefit from speed. The reasons include the inability of people on the scene to distinguish serious from not serious, the reluctance of dispatchers and responders to trust people's judgment, and long-standing protocol that considers everything an emergency until proven otherwise. Most 911 calls result in an ambulance, often accompanied by a police cruiser and a fire department engine company, disturbing traffic and distracting drivers over miles of busy highway.

This emergent response strategy continues despite several good studies in urban areas that have demonstrated a substantial increase in risk with the routine use of lights and sirens on ambulances, but no overall improvement in medical outcome. Realistically, the default value should be *non-emergent until proven otherwise*. This simple baseline is far less likely to kill or injure somebody.

Type of Response

Known Location Known Medical	Known Location Unknown Medical
Known Medical Unknown Location	Unknown Location Unknown Medical

"Identifying the type of response can help you equip appropriately and set a reasonable level of urgency.

A SAR response, even an emergent one, is usually more careful, deliberate, and less exciting. Early involvement of the medical officer in mission planning can help determine the sense of urgency. Sometimes this must be based on scant information, but any communication directly between the medical officer and the scene or reporting party can be useful. A few direct questions, much like a scene survey and primary assessment, can give you a sense for serious or not serious: Is the scene safe for the next few hours? Is the patient awake and talking? Is the patient having any trouble breathing? Is the patient getting worse or getting better? It is much more likely for the responses to be reassuring than alarming. The mission profile can usually involve lower speed and less risk.

Although the data also suggest that aeromedical helicopters may not be worth the risk and expense in urban EMS, this is not the case in the backcountry. The benefit is seldom in speed of access, but more commonly in reducing risk to rescuers. A 20-minute flight with a crew of three may save 20 rescuers an overnight ground evacuation in avalanche terrain or a rescue vessel many hours underway in rough seas. This is a perfectly legitimate use of a helicopter, and if the medical officer can determine that the scene and patient are stable, the air crew can pick the best weather and time of day. This is an extremely valuable and appropriate application of critical thinking and risk management.

Chapter 34 Review:
The Medical Role in Search and Rescue

- It is often up to the medical officer to set the level of urgency and help develop a mission profile that keeps risk within the range of acceptable.
- Any communication directly between the medical officer and the scene or reporting party can be useful.
- Whatever the situation, and for any role to which you are assigned, you should know at a minimum who you are working for, who is working for you, what you are doing, and how long you are expected to do it.
- Supervision of field operations, where most medical personnel are deployed, is usually delegated to an operations section chief.
- If you are responding to an unfamiliar operation, look for the IC or the command post (CP). In the field, look for the operations section chief or medical leader.
- Your preparation and response will be determined by the type of incident that is involved.
- Most emergency response to medical problems, from the street to the open ocean, generates risk well in excess of any benefit from speed.
- The benefit of helicopter use is seldom in speed of access, but more commonly in reducing risk to rescuers.

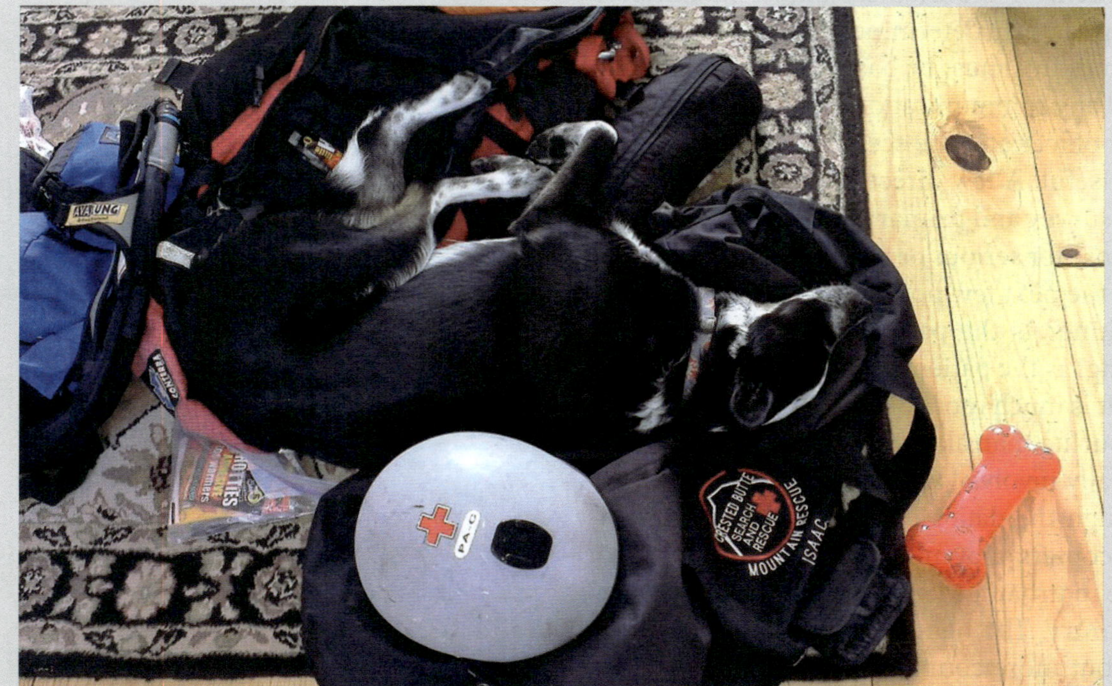

The Operations Section Chief.

Chapter 35: Appropriate Medical Technology

An emergency medical products website offers an unlimited opportunity to pack your bags with useless equipment. The cornucopia of gadgets, apps, and solutions looking for a problem can fill a truck, overload a med kit, and boggle the mind. Fortunately, the exercise of stuffing what you think you need into a pack and then carrying it for several miles uphill in a snowstorm can really help reset your priorities.

Some of the equipment and material used in the ambulance or emergency department will function well in the backcountry, but most will not. Appropriate medical technology for the offshore and wilderness environment is closer to that used by veterinarians and home health care nurses. You are looking for equipment that is simple and light with few moving parts. Bandages and dressings will need to survive harsh conditions but be simple to apply. Medications should not require close monitoring or prolonged administration, and they should not cause unacceptable side effects. Fortuitously, in all categories, the choices are limited.

Backcountry Medical Equipment

The size and weight of medical supplies and equipment carried will be determined by how you transport it, the role you fill, your level of training, and the number of people to be covered. There is no point in carrying anything that you don't know how to use, and no reason to carry anything that can be improvised from something else. Mariners and motorized rescuers can usually find space for dedicated splinting materials, irrigation solutions, and other bulky supplies. The practitioner who backpacks a medical kit will need to be much more discriminating.

A simple pocket mask connected to a helpful rescuer provides heated and humidified ventilations without the weight and complexity of an oxygen-powered system with an external heat source. Vet wrap, an elastic bandage originally designed for livestock, stands up to mud and rain much better than the white roller gauze found in the emergency department does. Pain medication that can be administered by mouth, transmucosal route, or intramuscular injection is easier to manage than anything that requires an intravenous (IV) line.

Carrying traction or long leg splints for the lower extremity is generally not necessary for a patient who is going to be carried anyway. A well-padded litter or vacuum mattress effectively splints everything from the neck through the tibia. Stabilization of ankle, wrist, hand, and forearm injuries can be accomplished with a simple malleable aluminum splint or any rigid object. Add a sling and you can include the elbow, upper arm, and clavicle.

Oxygen is administered for almost everything on the ambulance but in the wilderness setting you need a good reason to carry this relatively heavy and bulky equipment. You might choose to leave it behind when responding to an unknown problem at an unknown location. However, oxygen is certainly worth packing when responding to a known respiratory system problem at a known location.

The automated external defibrillator (AED) falls into the same category. You may choose to carry one when responding to a known cardiac problem. Otherwise, the likelihood of use does not justify its weight and bulk in your pack.

On most trips, it makes sense to arrange your kit in modules. Put the materials used for minor maintenance and repair like adhesive bandages and antibiotic ointment in a separate container. This module will have as much to do with preventing medical problems as treating them, and it should be easily accessible. It may work best for each member of the team to have their own. The more critical but less frequently used supplies can be kept elsewhere.

Medications

Medications should be repackaged to prevent damage from moisture and movement. A bottle of loose pills will turn into powder after a few hours on the trail or miles at sea. Pack the contents tight with cotton or gauze in a waterproof vial and add a few grains of dry rice to absorb any stray moisture. Any prescription medications should be accompanied by documentation from the prescribing practitioner, especially if you will be crossing international borders. Include written instructions for the use of the medication. For each medication, you should know the following:

Actions. A drug's action is how it works. Epinephrine, for example, constricts blood vessels and dilates bronchial tubes. Ibuprofen inhibits the chemical mediators of pain and inflammation.

Indications. The indication is what the drug is for. In the backcountry, epinephrine is used to treat asthma and anaphylaxis. Ibuprofen reduces pain, inflammation, and fever.

Contraindications. A contradiction indicates when a drug should not be used. Ibuprofen, for example, irritates the stomach and therefore should not be used when vomiting is an anticipated problem, or for anyone with a stomach problem.

Side effects. Side effects are the secondary effects of the drug that may or may not be desirable or acceptable. For example, drowsiness is a side effect of diphenhydramine/Benadryl. This may be useful or dangerous, depending on the situation. Allergies are an undesirable side effect that can occur with any medication.

Dosage and route. Dosage answers the question, how much is given, and how often? Medications can be administered by many routes, including by mouth, by injection, absorbed by the mucous membranes of the nose or mouth, absorbed through the skin, or given rectally.

You Should Know...

- Indications
- Contraindications
- Precautions
- Dosage
- Route
- Side Effects
- Interactions

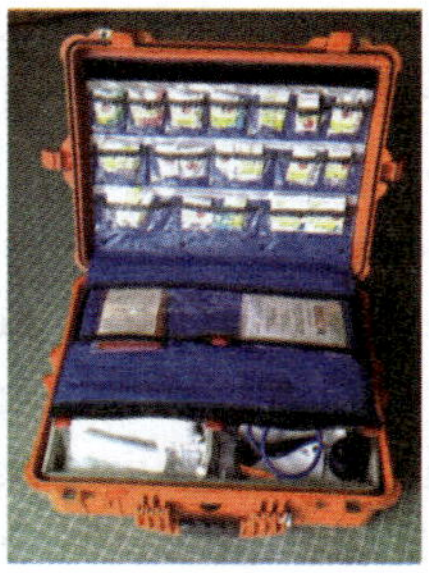

Fluid Replacement

In many cases where dehydration is the primary mechanism, rehydration in the field can make a carry-out evacuation unnecessary. IV fluid replacement is ideal, but not always practical. Oral fluid replacement with electrolyte solutions can be very effective if the patient can swallow safely and is not vomiting.

Subcutaneous fluid replacement (hypodermoclysis) is another option, but somewhat slower. This technique is very safe and low risk and can be easily accomplished with minimal training. It is a good option to consider aboard ship, for example, where carrying several liters of IV fluid is practical and the probability of dehydration from seasickness is high. Another example might be a vehicle supported bicycle or trekking trip.

If fluid replacement is required during evacuation a gravity-fed IV or subcutaneous drip will be difficult to maintain. There are various pressure and power infusers that can be packaged with the patient, eliminating the need to hang the fluid bag above the litter. A better option is to use periodic bolus infusions administered while the litter team is taking a rest. This can be accomplished through intermittent connection to an IV heparin lock or via an intact system with the IV line closed while the patient is being carried. Fluid bolus can also be given subcutaneously in the same way that veterinarians sometimes do for cats and dogs.

Aggressive fluid replacement for shock from uncontrolled bleeding can be dangerous when surgical care is not immediately available. The increase in blood pressure with volume expansion may dislodge clots causing bleeding to become worse. Additionally, too much fluid can dilute clotting factors. Current guidelines for hemorrhagic shock usually call for a limited bolus of up to 500 ml followed by a slow drip until hemostasis is confirmed. Considering its weight versus its potential for benefit, packing more than a liter of normal saline or lactated Ringer's into the backcountry is justified only when responding to a known medical problem where significant dehydration is likely to be on the problem list.

Risk Versus Benefit

The most basic risk in the use of any device is that it will take up space, weight, and money that could be better used for something more likely to reduce risk and improve outcome. The most obvious example is the EMS crew running into the backcountry loaded down with drugs, monitors, defibrillators, and jump kits but no head lamps, food, water, or rain gear. The corollary, of course, is the SAR crew arriving on scene fully prepared to weather the night, but without any way to treat the patient's open fracture and pain, or prevent a serious infection.

A more insidious form of risk is presented by technology in its tendency to distract you from good basic assessment and treatment. Your cardiac monitor may show normal sinus rhythm, but does it really change the field treatment of a 65-year-old man with substernal chest pain and sweating? Your pulse oximeter may read 75%, but does this really change your response to a patient with normal mental status, good skin color, and no apparent respiratory distress? In a field setting, diagnostic technology like this can confuse as often as confirm the pattern you've observed. A good question to ask when deploying diagnostic instrumentation is: *what am I going to do with the information it gives me, and what difference will it make in my treatment?* In the remote setting, the answer is often *not much*.

Chapter 35 Review: Appropriate Medical Technology

- You are looking for equipment that is simple and light with few moving parts.
- There is no point in carrying anything that you don't know how to use, and no reason to carry anything that can be improvised from something else.
- A simple pocket or intraoral mask connected to a helpful rescuer provides heated and humidified ventilations.
- Pain medication that can be administered by mouth, transmucosal route, or intramuscular injection is easier to manage than anything that requires an intravenous (IV) line.
- A well-padded litter or vacuum mattress effectively splints everything from the neck through the tibia.
- It may work best for each member of the team to have their own supply of frequently used items. The more critical but less frequently used supplies can be kept elsewhere.
- Any prescription medications should be accompanied by documentation from the prescribing practitioner, especially if you will be crossing international borders.
- For each medication, you should know the actions, indications, contraindications, side effects, dosage, and route.
- In many cases where dehydration is the primary mechanism, rehydration in the field can make a carry-out evacuation unnecessary. Oral fluid replacement can be very effective if the patient can swallow safely and is not vomiting.
- Aggressive fluid replacement for shock from uncontrolled bleeding can be dangerous when surgical care is not immediately available.
- The most basic risk in the use of any device is that it will take up space, weight, and money that could be better used for something more likely to reduce risk and improve outcome.
- A good question to ask when deploying diagnostic instrumentation is: what am I going to do with the information it gives me, and what difference will it make in my treatment?

Chapter 36: Training for Performance Under Stress

With thanks to author and instructor: Deb Ajango

The puzzle of who performs well under pressure, and why, has been studied extensively during the past two decades. The most recent findings, with the help of advances in neuroscience, could have a significant impact on the process of training for performance under pressure. Not only does this information offer a fascinating glimpse into the brain's automated systems for dealing with danger, but by applying the findings to the field of wilderness medicine, first responders and their trainers can better prepare for real-life crises.

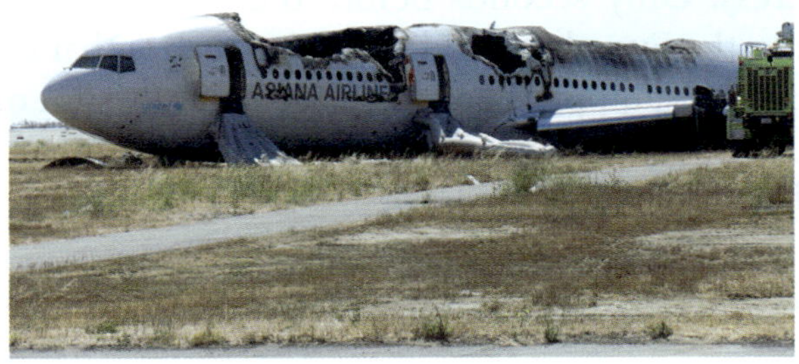

Asiana Flight 214

Stress and the Brain

On July 6, 2013, Asiana Flight 214 landed short of the runway in San Francisco, California. Within minutes, the Boeing 777 was engulfed in flames and destroyed, yet only two people died at the scene. Dramatic photos of the scorched fuselage left viewers dumbstruck as to how anyone could have survived.

How could more than 300 passengers and crew have exited the aircraft within 90 seconds of landing? And how is it that everyone could evacuate so quickly and efficiently under such duress?

After hearing news of the July 6 crash, many people undoubtedly wondered how they would have performed had they been on the flight that day. Although we often fantasize about what we would do or how we would act in an emergency, research shows that our imaginations rarely mirror reality. Many people wrongly assume, for instance, that the average person panics in a disaster. In fact, numbers show that only 10%–15% of people panic under pressure, while another 10%–15% will perform very effectively. The other 70%–80% of people, when confronted with a highly stressful and novel situation, will actually do very little to save themselves or others. This latter and larger group falls into what John Leach, author of Survival Psychology, calls a bewildered state. While this freeze response is not always dangerous it is certainly not ideal when a situation calls for immediate action.

As trained first responders know, the brain responds to any perceived threat by secreting chemicals that lead to an acute stress response. And although this response can be highly beneficial in certain emergencies, elevated levels of stress chemicals almost always negatively affect thought processes and performance. As stress levels rise, one's ability to recall information falls, decision-making becomes bogged down, and multi-tasking becomes almost impossible.

While untrained people are more likely to underperform in an emergency even experienced professionals can be affected. Consider the tragic case of Eastern Airlines Flight 401 where the flight crew became hyper-focused on a burned-out landing gear indication light. Their ability to take in environmental cues, sometimes referred to as situational awareness, naturally declined under stress. Only seconds before the plane crashed into the Everglades did the pilots realize that the aircraft's autopilot had been accidentally shut off and the plane had been in a long descent. More than 100 people died.

How We Respond

To some degree, how one performs in an emergency will be influenced by factors that cannot be modified through training. There is no doubt, for instance, that physiology and life experiences will affect how a person responds. Nonetheless, research consistently shows that by minimizing surprises and by modifying training techniques we can improve the chances that first responders will perform well when it counts.

To start, let us consider how the brain responds in a crisis. When the pre-frontal cortex (where decision-making and critical thinking take place) is presented with a sudden emergency that requires an immediate decision, it kicks into action by conducting a lightning fast "search" of sorts, scanning its databanks for prior knowledge that might be helpful. Relevant memories, impactful experiences, and applicable trainings pop up as search "hits," and each of these options are quickly assessed for their potential as viable options. If no "hit" is found, that is; if a person has no prior experiences or relevant training, then no alternatives pop up, and like the spinning computer icon, the person remains frozen (bewildered) as the brain considers what to do.

It is useful to know that bewildered people, although ineffective on their own, are often highly suggestible. When the crew of Asiana Flight 214 started giving instructions, people followed. Flight attendant Lee Yoon-Hye, downplayed the accolades and instead gave credit to her training. "I wasn't really thinking," she said, "but my body started carrying out the steps needed for an evacuation." In the year prior, she added, she and her colleagues had gone through timed trials set up by her employer. She had been required to shout over pandemonium and engine noise, she had confronted and given direction to actors frozen in fear, and she had repeatedly opened jammed doors and windows. For her and her colleagues the high-quality trainings and scenarios had created multiple "hits" providing the brain with a foundation for action.

Improving the Odds

For more than 50 years researchers have interviewed thousands of people who have faced extremely intense situations looking for trends or commonalities. In the 1940s, for instance, S.L.A. Marshall examined the behaviors of American soldiers who fought in WWII. Curious to know how the average man performed under the pressures of battle Marshall interviewed thousands of men. In his report, he suggests that 75 percent of frontline soldiers never fired their weapons. Instead, he said, those who were involved in intense gun battles often froze, hid, or ran.

Although the military leadership initially condemned Marshall's report and defended its training methods, the soldiers came to Marshall's defense. Many pointed to fact that they had been trained to shoot at stationary bull's-eye targets, not real people, as a problem. To highlight their points, many added "German soldiers look nothing like those targets."

Marshall theorized that the men's brains had been overwhelmed by extreme stress. Because real fighting was nothing like their training, and because shooting and killing people were unfamiliar tasks that only added to the pressure, Marshall pointed out that the amount of stress chemicals flowing through the soldiers must have been debilitating. As automated limbic responses usurped critical thinking, each man's instinct to survive took over.

Ultimately the U.S. military reevaluated its training methods and modified its techniques. Over time, drills became more realistic and more dangerous. Today highly realistic scenarios are routinely used to enhance performance.

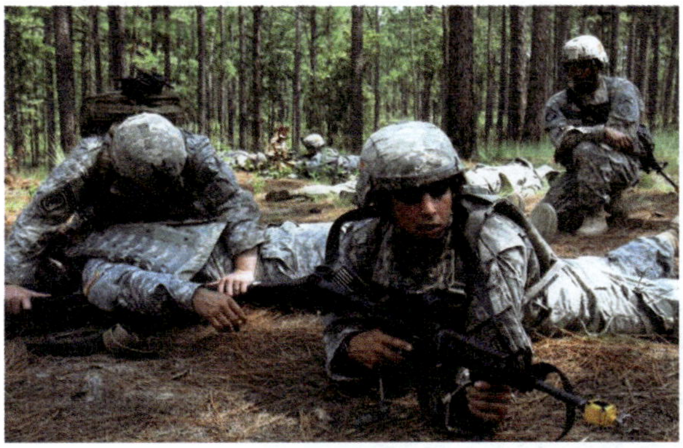

Stress Exposure Training, or SET, includes the use of scenarios that come as close as possible to what soldiers will actually see in wartime. Moulage, smoke, and pyrotechnics are used, and actors are brought in as role players. In some cases, actual fighting is allowed. To improve a soldier's progress, and as advised by experts who teach about "building expertise," trainers provide quality and timely feedback so that the soldier has the opportunity to modify decisions and change behaviors.

Marshall's work along with the work of his predecessors ultimately served as a catalyst for a myriad of other researchers who have focused on the concept of performing under pressure. Although the details of the various studies differ, nearly all the researchers reached similar conclusions that can be easily applied to first responders and their trainers:

People's abilities to think and reason deteriorate in highly stressful situations, and this reality should be expected and anticipated. First responders can use this information to plan ahead, to minimize surprises, and to anticipate the situational and behavioral challenges that they might face.

People perform as they practice, at best, and rarely does a person's proficiency improve when under pressure. Holding first responders to high-levels of performance during practice sessions is key, and the quality of practice matters. If possible, realistic scenarios and drills should be used to enhance habits and proficiency.

At Florida State's Human Performance Lab, Anders Ericsson—an expert in how to develop expertise—and his team of researchers work to create elaborate simulations to test police officers, medical professionals, firefighters, and other participants in taxing situations. Their findings offer convincing evidence of the efficacy of practicing while under realistic and stressful situations. Echoing this sentiment military training masters such as Alex Horton and Dave Grossman claim that the more you can approximate true-to-life circumstances the greater the carryover is likely to be. "From cops in mock shoot-outs to ordinary people stuck in fire drills," says Grossman, "in order for training to be effective, it must be as realistic as possible."

Risk Versus Benefit

Although realistic scenarios can be time consuming to create and implement, WMAI encourages first responders and their trainers to incorporate stress into their training regimens as much as possible, and rescue organizations should weigh the cost of time and labor against the verifiable benefits that can be achieved when drills and scenarios are realistic. Not only do high-stress drills help students learn to function under pressure, but they also provide the brain with relevant memories, or "search-engine hits," that can be used at a later date.

In addition, by teaching first responders about effective stress-control methods such as breathing techniques, self-talk, and imagery, medical trainers can help responders learn to better control their stress levels in emergencies. Not only might the techniques assist the medics, but the same techniques can be used to calm stressed-out bystanders and patients.

It is also useful for first responders and trainers to know that stress chemicals are released when someone is required to perform an unmastered skill in a crisis. In other words, novices in the use of satellite phones, beacons, or other rescue equipment commonly make mistakes in emergencies, unless very-user-friendly directions are included.

Once a crisis has passed it is common for people to want to congregate, to share stories, and to mill around. Many feel soothed by human touch—a warm embrace, a hand on a shoulder, or a light finger to one's forearm can reduce blood pressures and pulses almost immediately. First responders who are focusing their attentions on the injured are often unaware of the fear and anxiety they inadvertently add to scene when they ask loved ones and bystanders to stand back or step aside.

Recognizing these, and other behavioral characteristics, is as much a part of situational awareness as recognizing risks associated with stabilization, treatment and evacuation. Your own performance as a rescuer can be a hazard or a benefit depending on your response. By anticipating and training for the problems associated with high-intensity situations, you and your team can be better prepared for the realities associated with true crises.

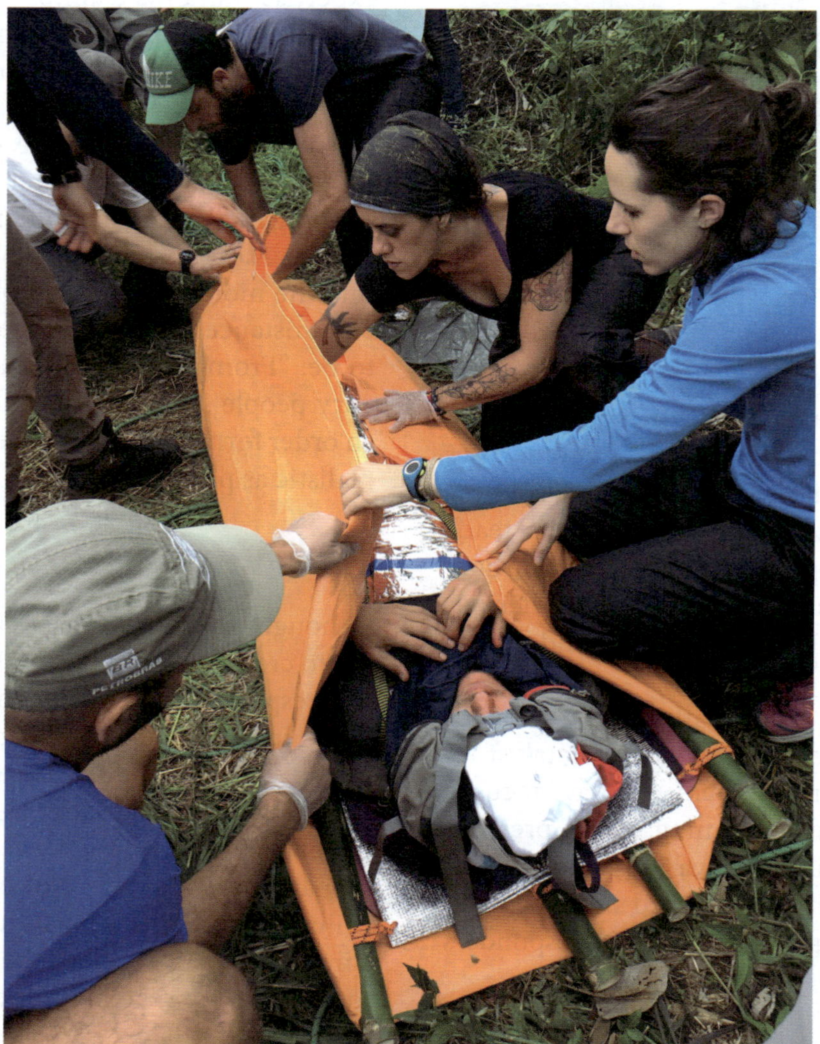

Chapter 36 Review:
Training for Performance

- Only 10%–15% of people panic under pressure, while another 10%–15% will perform very effectively. The other 70%–80% of people will actually do very little to save themselves or others.
- If a person has no prior experiences or relevant training the person remains frozen (bewildered) as the brain considers what to do.
- Research consistently shows that, by minimizing surprises and by modifying training techniques, we can improve the chances that first responders will perform well when it counts.
- People's abilities to think and reason deteriorate in highly stressful situations, and this reality should be expected and anticipated.
- People perform as they practice, at best, and rarely does a person's proficiency improve when under pressure.
- If possible, realistic scenarios and drills should be used to enhance habits and proficiency.
- First responders, who are focusing their attentions on the injured, are often unaware of the fear and anxiety they inadvertently add to scene when they ask loved ones and bystanders to stand back or step aside.
- Your own performance as a rescuer can be a hazard or a benefit depending on your response. By anticipating and training for the problems associated with high-intensity situations, you and your team can be better prepared for the realities associated with true crises.

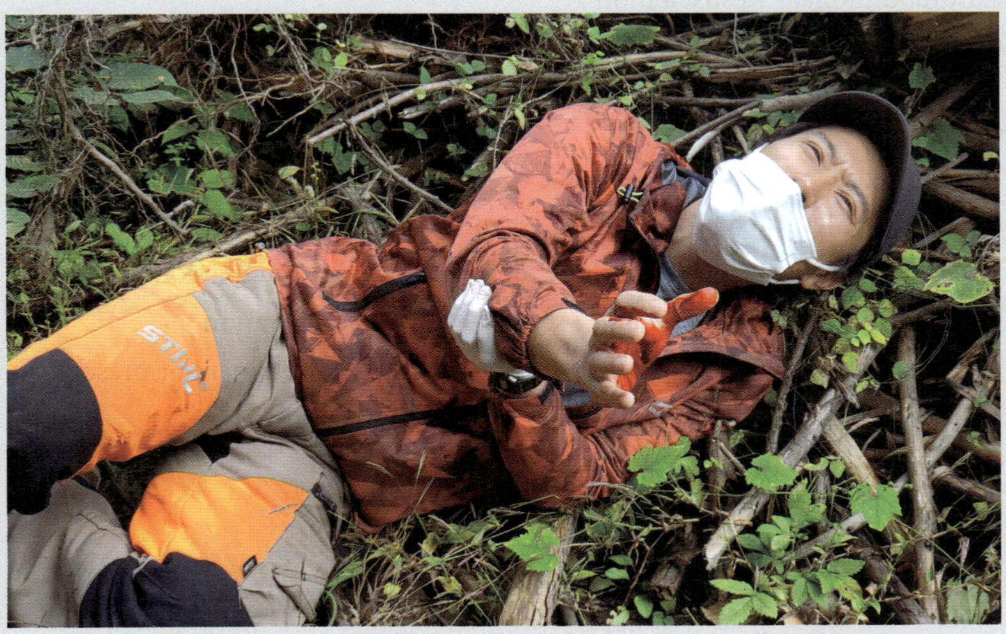

"...in order for training to be effective, it must be as realistic as possible."

Abbreviations, Acronyms, and Mnemonics

A	Problem List
A'	Anticipated Problem
A and O	Awake and oriented
APAP	Acetaminophen
AVPU	**A**wake **V**erbal stimulus response **P**ainful stimulus response **U**nresponsive
ALS	Advanced Life Support
ASA	Aspirin
BBP	Bloodborne Pathogen
BLS	Basic Life Support
BSA	Body Surface Area
c̄	With
CC	Chief Complaint
CHI	Close Head Injury
C/MS	Level of Consciousness and Mental Status
CNS	Central Nervous System
c/o	Complains of
CPR	Cardiopulmonary Resuscitation
CSM	Circulation, Sensation, and Movement
CVA	CerebroVascular Accident (stroke)
EMS	Emergency Medical Services
EMT	Emergency Medical Technician
HACE	High-Altitude Cerebral Edema
HAPE	High-Altitude Pulmonary Edema
Hx	History
ICP	Intracranial Pressure
IM	Intramuscular
IV	Intravenous
mcg	microgram; 1/1000 of a milligram
mg	milligram; 1/1000 of a gram
mmol/L	millimoles per liter
MI	Myocardial Infarction (heart attack)
MOI	Mechanism of Injury
MVA	Motor Vehicle Accident
NPO	Nothing by Mouth. From the latin *nil per os*.
NSAIDs	Non-Steroidal Anti-inflammatory Drugs
O	Objective
O_2	Oxygen
OM	*otitis media*; Ear Infection
P	Plan
PAS	Patient Assessment System
PCN	Penicillin
PEP	Post-Exposure Prophylaxis
PFA	Pain-Free Activity
po	*per os*; By Mouth
pr	Per rectum
prn	As needed
qd	Each day
q4h	Every 4 hours
RICE	**R**est **I**ce **C**ompression **E**levation
Rx	Treatment or prescription
S	Subjective

SAMPLE
- **S**ymptoms
- **A**llergies
- **M**edicines
- **P**ast history of medical problems
- **L**ast meal
- **E**vents leading up to injury

SAT Oxygen saturation

sc Subcutaneous; under the skin

sl Sublingual; under the tongue

SOB Shortness of Breath

SOAP
- **S**ubjective – Information gained by questioning
- **O**bjective – Information gathered during examination of the patient
- **A**ssessment – List of problems discovered
- **P**lan – What is to be done about each problem

STOPEATS
- **S**ugar
- **T**emperature
- **O**xygen
- **P**ressure
- **E**lectricity
- **A**ltitude
- **T**oxins
- **S**alts

sx Symptoms

s/sx Signs and symptoms

TBI Traumatic Brain Injury

TIP Traction into Position

TM Tympanic Membrane; Ear Drum

VS Vital Signs (with time recorded)
- **BP** – Blood Pressure
- **R** – Respiratory Rate
- **T** – Core Temperature
- **C** – Level of Consciousness (Mental Status if Awake)
- **S** – Skin
- **O** – Oxygen Saturation
- **P** – Pulse

WALS© Wilderness Advanced Life Support

WEMT Wilderness Emergency Medical Technician

WFR Wilderness First Responder

WOB Work of Breathing

Conversion Tables

Temperature: Fahrenheit to Celsius

°F	°C	°F	°C
107.6	42	82.4	28
105.8	41	68	20
104	40	59	15
102.2	39	50	10
100.4	38	41	5
98.6	37	32	0
95	35	23	-5
89.6	32	14	-10
87.8	31	5	-15
86	30	0	-18
84.2	29		

Kilograms to Pounds

Kilograms (kg)	Pounds (lbs)
1	2.204
20	44.092
40	88.184
60	132.277
80	176.369
100	220.462
120	264.554
140	308.647

Ounces to Milliliters

Ounces (oz)	Milliliters (mL)
1	29.57
8	236.58
33.81	1000

Glasgow Coma Scale

Eye Opening Response

- Spontaneous—open with blinking at baseline **4 points**
- To verbal stimuli, command, speech **3 points**
- To pain only (not applied to face) **2 points**
- No response **1 point**

Verbal Response

- Oriented **5 points**
- Confused conversation, but able to answer questions **4 points**
- Inappropriate words **3 points**
- Incomprehensible speech **2 points**
- No response **1 point**

Motor Response

- Obeys commands for movement **6 points**
- Purposeful movement to painful stimulus **5 points**
- Withdraws in response to pain **4 points**
- Flexion in response to pain (decorticate posturing) **3 points**
- Extension response in response to pain (decerebrate posturing) **2 points**
- No response **1 point**

Glossary

abrasion Superficial wound that damages only the outermost layers of skins or cornea.

abscess A localized infection isolated from the rest of the body by inflammation.

acute hypothermia Condition in which the patient has become hypothermic quickly, typically due to cold water immersion, resulting in less dehydration and less glycogen depletion.

acute stress reaction (ASR) Autonomic nervous system-controlled response to any stress, physical or emotional, that can cause severe but temporary and reversible changes in vital signs. ASR can mimic respiratory distress, shock, or brain failure.

advanced life support (ALS) The emergency treatment of major critical system problems using medications and advanced procedures.

afterdrop Condition in which the body core temperature continues to decrease even after rewarming has begun.

airway The passage for air exchange between the alveoli of the lungs and the outside. Most commonly refers to the upper airway, including the nose, mouth, and trachea.

alkalosis Abnormal drop in acidity of the blood. Can be caused by a decrease in carbon dioxide in the blood or by certain toxins.

allergy The body's exaggerated immune response to an internal or surface agent, causing the local or systemic release of the chemical histamine and other mediators producing local or systemic swelling, itching, and rash.

altitude illness The constellation of symptoms produced by altitude adjustment, high altitude cerebral edema, and high-altitude pulmonary edema. Can be mild, moderate, or severe.

alveoli Membranous air sacks in the lungs where gas is exchanged with the blood.

amnesia Loss of memory.

anaphylaxis Severe systemic allergic reaction capable of causing generalized edema, vascular and volume shock, and respiratory distress secondary to upper airway swelling and lower airway constriction.

angina The pain of myocardial ischemia. Also called *Angina pectoris.* May be stable or unstable.

antibiotic (ABX) A drug that selectively kills or interferes with the function or reproduction of bacteria.

Anticipated problems (A') Problems that may develop over time because of injury, illness, or the environment. Part of the SOAP note under Assessment (A).

antifungal A drug that selectively kills or interferes with the function or reproduction of pathogenic fungus.

antiviral A drug that selectively kills or interferes with the function or reproduction of viruses.

arrhythmia Abnormal heart rhythm. Also called a *dysrhythmia.*

artery Vessel carrying blood from the heart to the capillary beds in body tissues. Arteries have muscular walls, the constriction of which contribute to maintaining perfusion pressure. Carries blood under high pressure.

aspiration Inhaling foreign liquid or other material into the lungs.

Assessment (A) The part of the SOAP note giving a succinct list of medical, logistical, and environmental problems associated with an ill or injured patient. Also called problem list or diagnosis.

asthma A chronic inflammatory disease that can cause acute episodes of lower airway constriction and respiratory distress.

ataxia Uncoordinated voluntary movement.

automated external defibrillator (AED) A computerized device used by bystanders or medical personnel that can analyze heart rhythm and recommend and deliver an appropriate corrective electric shock.

AVPU A consciousness assessment tool that classifies patients as Awake, responsive to Verbal stimuli, responsive to Painful stimuli, or Unresponsive.

basic life support (BLS) The generic process of supporting the functions of the circulatory, respiratory, and nervous systems using CPR, bleeding control, and spine stabilization.

beta-agonist Drug that stimulates beta-adrenergic receptors in body cells. This is used primarily to relax the smooth muscle lining the bronchial tubes in the treatment of asthma and other causes of lower airway constriction. Examples include albuterol, salmeterol, and metaproterenol.

biphasic reaction Return of the symptoms of anaphylaxis after treatment caused by the continued presence of the antigen, and the metabolism and excretion of the emergency medications.

blood pressure cuff Also known as a sphygmomanometer. Used for measuring blood pressure.

brain failure Impaired brain function evidenced by altered mental status or reduced level of consciousness. May include inadequate nervous system control of other critical systems.

bronchospasm Contraction of the muscular walls of the bronchial tubes.

bronchi and bronchioles Tubes of the lower airway conducting air to the alveoli of the lungs.

capillaries The smallest blood vessels in body tissues where gases and nutrients are exchanged between tissue cells and the circulating blood.

cardiac arrest Loss of effective heart activity.

cardiogenic shock Shock due to inadequate pumping action of the heart.

cardiopulmonary resuscitation (CPR) A technique for artificially circulating oxygenated blood in the absence of effective heart activity. Includes positive pressure ventilation (PPV) and chest compressions.

carotid pulse The pulse felt on the side of the neck at the site of the carotid artery.

cartilage Connective tissue on the ends of bones at joints that provides a smooth gliding surface.

central nervous system (CNS) The brain and spinal cord.

cervical spine The section of the spine in the neck between the base of the skull and the top of the thorax.

chief complaint The problem or symptom that the patient is most concerned about.

clotting factors Chemicals in the blood contributing to the process of blood clotting.

cold challenge The combined cooling influence of wind, humidity, and ambient temperature.

cold diuresis The tendency of the body to produce more urine when shell/core compensation occurs.

cold response The normal body response to the cold challenge, including shell/core effect and shivering.

compartment syndrome Swelling within a confined body compartment, like the connective tissue compartments in the leg or inside the skull, that results in ischemia.

compensated volume shock (CVS) Condition in which the body is successfully maintaining pressure adequate to perfuse vital organs despite low blood volume. Evidenced by the volume shock pattern in an awake and responsive patient.

compensation Involuntary changes in body functions designed to maintain perfusion pressure and oxygenation of vital body tissues in the presence of injury or illness.

concussion Brain injury. May be mild or severe. Also called *closed head injury* or *traumatic brain injury*.

conjunctiva The membrane covering the white of the eye and the inner surfaces of the eye lids.

conjunctivitis Inflammation of the conjunctiva due to irritation, infection, or injury. Most often used in reference to infection (pink eye).

consciousness and mental status (C/MS) On of the six vital signs. C refers to level of consciousness while MS refers to mental status in an awake patient.

contusion Bruise or blunt injury to bone or soft tissue.

cornea The clear part of the eye over the iris and pupil.

cornice An overhanging drift of snow formed as wind blows over a ridge or mountaintop.

crepitus The feel or sound of bones or cartilage grating when moved. Typical at the site of an unstable fracture. Can also describe the feel or sound of subcutaneous air when palpated.

cyanosis The blue color seen in the lips and skin of a patient with poor tissue oxygenation. This is the color of de-oxygenated hemoglobin.

debridement Wound cleaning, including removal of foreign material and devitalized tissue.

decompensated shock Condition in which the body is unable to maintain adequate pressure to perfuse vital organs in the presence of low blood volume. Evidenced by the volume shock pattern in a patient with significantly altered mental status or reduced level of consciousness.

debris field The pile of snow and debris at the bottom of an avalanche where a buried victim is most likely to be found.

decompression sickness Hyperbaric injury caused by the accumulation of bubbles in the circulatory system as dissolved gasses are released from blood and body tissues; also called the bends.

definitive medical care Therapy that cures the disease or corrects the problem.

dental abscess Infection at the base of a tooth.

diagnosis (DX) The identification of a medical problem by name. May be generic or specific.

diaphragm Muscle at the lower end of the chest cavity, which contracts to create a vacuum that draws air into the lungs. The diaphragm works with muscles of the chest wall, shoulders, neck to perform ventilation.

diastolic blood pressure The standing pressure within the circulatory system remaining while the heart is between contractions. Documented as the second or lower number in blood pressure.

differential diagnosis (D/DX) The list of possible causes of a medical problem or symptom.

discharge Fluid escaping from the site of infection or inflammation. Also called exudate.

dislocation Disruption of normal joint anatomy.

distal An anatomical direction; away from the body center. The wrist is distal to the elbow.

dura Connective tissue and membrane lining of the cranium and brain.

dyspnea Also called shortness of breath, respiratory distress, or difficulty breathing.

dysrhythmia An abnormal heart rhythm. Also called arrhythmia.

edema Swelling due to leaking of serum from capillaries.

electrolyte Elements or molecules in the blood. Examples include sodium, potassium, chloride, and calcium.

embolus Object or substance traveling in the blood capable of lodging in the circulatory system and causing ischemia. Examples include bubbles of air, fat globules, and freely floating blood clots.

emphysema Chronic lower airway constriction leading to lung hyperinflation and the formation of cavities within lung tissue.

epinephrine The synthetic form of the hormone adrenalin. Used to constrict blood vessels and dilate airway tubes.

EpiPen Device that automatically injects 0.3 mg of epinephrine when armed and triggered. Epinephrine autoinjectors are also sold under a number of other brand or generic names.

etiology The cause of a disease or injury.

evacuation Transferring a patient from the scene of injury or illness to definitive medical care.

evisceration Injury that leaves abdominal or thoracic organs outside the body.

exercise-induced hyponatremia Condition of electrolyte dilution caused by over consumption of water in relation to electrolytes, and to a lesser extent, the loss of salt in sweat.

extension Movement at a joint that extends an extremity away from the center of the body. The opposite of flexion.

extracellular space Between and among the cells of body tissues.

extrication Removing or freeing a patient from entrapment or confinement.

exudate Discharge, usually from a wound or infection.

fascia A layer of tough connective tissue that lies below the fat and over the muscle, bone, organs, and joints.

femoral artery Large artery that travels along the femur in the thigh.

femur Long bone of the thigh.

flail chest The loss of rigidity of the chest wall due to multiple rib fractures.

flexion Bending of a joint. The opposite of extension.

fracture Broken bone, cartilage, or solid organ.

frostbite Frozen tissue. May be superficial or deep.

frostnip Loss of circulation due to the vasoconstriction of blood vessels in the skin during the early stages of tissue freezing.

glaucoma Disease or condition causing increased pressure within the globe of the eye.

Glasgow Coma Scale An assessment of level of consciousness and mental status resulting in a numeric score. See page 253.

glycogen Carbohydrate stored in the liver and muscles. Glycogen is converted into sugar for use as fuel during exercise.

guarding Protective tightening of the abdominal wall muscles in response to the pressure of abdominal palpation. Can be voluntary or involuntary.

closed head injury Injury to the brain. Also called concussion.

heart attack Heart muscle ischemia caused by a blood clot or spasm of the coronary arteries or by an arrhythmia, resulting in the necrosis (or infarction) of heart tissue.

heat challenge Combined effects of ambient temperature and metabolic activity that contribute to body heating.

heat exhaustion State of fatigue related to heat stress. May or may not include dehydration.

heat response The normal body response to the heat challenge, including sweating and vasodilation of the shell.

heat stroke Severe elevation of body temperature (over 105°F).

hemoglobin Molecule contained within red blood cells that binds to oxygen during its transport to body cells.

hemothorax Blood in the chest cavity as a result of injury, usually collecting between the chest wall and lung tissue.

hemotoxin Toxins that destroy body cells, causing inflammation, pain, and swelling. Also called tissue toxins.

high-altitude cerebral edema (HACE) The accumulation of fluid in brain tissue due to hypoxia at altitude, capable of producing elevated intracranial pressure.

histamine Hormone released by various processes causing, among other effects, vasodilation and bronchoconstriction.

hollow organs The stomach, intestines, bladder, and other organs enclosing space occupied by fluid and/or gas.

hormones Chemical compounds released by glands to have specific effects of specific body tissues.

hyperextension To extend a joint beyond its normal range of motion.

hyperventilation syndrome Respiratory alkalosis. The nervous system symptoms of numbness, visual field contraction, and light-headedness caused by reduced carbon dioxide in the blood due to excessive ventilation, usually associated with acute stress reaction.

hypodermoclysis Injecting IV fluid, usually normal saline, into the subcutaneous space where it can be absorbed by the circulatory system.

hypoglycemia A condition characterized by a low blood glucose level, capable of causing brain failure.

hyponatremia A condition in which the body has insufficient sodium and other salts, usually because of excess water intake.

hypothermia Low body core temperature.

hypoxia Lack of oxygen.

infarction Tissue death; also called necrosis.

infection Pathologic colonization of body tissues by bacteria, virus, fungus, or other microorganisms.

inflammation A generic body response to illness or injury resulting in redness, swelling, warmth, and tenderness.

intoxication Altered level of consciousness or mental status due to the influence of chemicals such as drugs, alcohol, and inhaled gasses.

intracellular space Inside the cells of body tissues.

intracranial Inside the skull (cranium).

intravenous fluids (IV) Fluids infused directly into the circulatory system through a hypodermic needle inserted into a vein, usually used to temporarily increase the volume of circulating blood or restore fluid lost to sweating or diarrhea.

intubation Placing an endotracheal tube into the trachea.

involuntary guarding Refers to abdominal muscle spasm to protect the abdomen from painful movement. Considered a sign of peritoneal irritation.

ischemia Local loss of perfusion due to swelling, deformity, or obstruction; can result in infarction.

level of consciousness (LOC) Describes the level of brain function in terms of responsiveness to specific stimuli: (The AVPU Scale) **A** = Awake, **V** = responds to Verbal stimuli, **P** = responds to Painful stimuli, **U** = Unresponsive to any stimuli.

ligaments Tough connective tissue joining bone to bone across joints.

local effects Effects that are restricted to the immediate area of injury or infection (versus systemic effects).

local toxins Toxins that affect only the immediate area of contact.

long bones Bones that have a long structural axis such as leg and arm bones as opposed to flat bones such as ribs and shoulder blades.

lower airway trachea, bronchi, and alveoli.

lumbar spine The lower section of the spine between the thorax and the pelvis.

lymphangitis Spread of a local infection into the lymph system. The early stage of a systemic infection. Symptoms include red streaks running centrally from the site of a local infection.

mechanism of injury (MOI) What caused the problem. The MOI can be non-specific, such as "fall from a cliff," or very specific, such as "compensated volume shock due to vomiting and dehydration."

mental status Describes the level of brain function in an awake patient (A on AVPU) in terms of memory, orientation, level of anxiety, and behavior.

middle ear barotrauma Condition in which the air pressure in the middle ear does not match the air pressure outside the middle ear, injuring the ear drum.

mid-range position Position in a joint's range of motion between full extension and full flexion. Also called neutral position.

myocardial ischemia Loss of perfusion to heart muscle, usually due to a clot or plaque in a coronary artery.

myocardial infarction (MI) Loss of perfusion to heart muscle resulting in death of muscle tissue.

neurotoxins Toxins that interfere with the function of the nervous system, capable of causing muscle spasm, paralysis, altered sensation, and respiratory distress.

neurovascular bundle An artery, vein, and nerve combination routed though the body together.

neutral position The position approximately half way between flexion and extension. Also called the mid-range position.

normal saline (NS) A fluid used for volume replacement or wound irrigation having the same percentage of salt as the blood and body tissues.

Objective (O) The part of the SOAP note describing physical exam findings, including Vital Signs.

open fracture Fracture with an associated break in the skin. Also called a compound fracture.

oxygenation To saturate blood with oxygen in the lungs. Also describes the transfer of oxygen from the blood to body cells (cellular oxygenation).

pain out of proportion Pain that is significantly greater than would be expected from a particular injury or illness. Sometimes a sign of an undetected serious problem such as compartment syndrome.

paresthesia Neurological deficit usually described as numbness and tingling.

patella An isolated bone imbedded as a fulcrum in the quadriceps tendon.

pathologic Harmful to the body. Usually used to describe bacteria, fungus, or virus.

patient assessment system A system of surveys including scene size-up, primary assessment, and secondary assessment designed to gather information about an injured or ill patient and the environment in which the patient is found.

percussion Examination technique using tapping to elicit tenderness or sounds. For example, tapping teeth gently with a stick to elicit tenderness or percussing the abdomen to evaluate distention.

perfusion The passage of blood through capillary beds in body tissues.

peripheral nerves The nerves running between body tissues and the spinal cord.

peristalsis The wave of muscular contraction in the stomach and intestine used to move food and fluid.

peritoneal signs Signs and symptoms associated with irritation of the peritoneal lining of the abdomen.

photophobia Eye pain or headache caused by bright lights.

Plan (P) A succinct list of actions to be taken to treat problems and prevent anticipated problems. Can include protection and evacuation.

plasma The liquid portion of the blood consisting of water, proteins, and other compounds.

pneumonia Infection of lung tissue resulting in the accumulation of fluid in the alveoli.

pneumothorax Free air in the chest cavity, usually from a punctured lung or chest wall.

poison Toxins that are encountered by surface contact, inhalation, or ingestion. There is no delivery mechanism.

polypro Slang for polypropylene clothing.

positive mechanism of injury Any event that could cause injury or illness.

post-concussive syndrome Signs and symptoms associated with traumatic brain injury, including headache, photophobia, nausea, sleep disturbance, and dizziness.

posturing Global extensor or flexor muscle contraction resulting from severe brain injury. An indication of severe increased intracranial pressure.

problem list (A) A succinct list of medical, logistical, and environmental problems associated with an ill or injured patient. Includes anticipated problems that may develop as a result of existing problems. Also called the assessment or diagnosis.

prognosis The expected course or outcome of a medical problem.

prophylaxis Treatment initiated to prevent a problem from developing. For example, prophylactic antibiotics to prevent infection in high-risk wounds.

pulmonary edema Swelling of lung tissue resulting in the collection of fluid in the alveoli.

pulse oximeter Device that measures the percentage of the hemoglobin in the blood that is saturated with oxygen.

rales Fine crackles. The noise produced by pulmonary edema. Sounds like crinkling cellophane or air being sucked through a wet sponge.

red blood cells (RBC) Cells floating in the blood that contain hemoglobin. Primarily responsible for carrying oxygen.

reduction The process of restoring a dislocated joint or deformed fracture to its normal anatomical position.

respiratory arrest Absence of effective respiration.

respiratory distress Difficulty breathing, but the respiratory system is still able to adequately oxygenate the blood to maintain brain function. The patient remains awake and responsive. Any mental status changes are mild or primarily due to ASR.

respiratory failure Difficulty breathing where the respiratory system is not able to adequately oxygenate the blood to maintain brain function. The patient will have altered mental status or reduced level of consciousness.

rhabdomyolysis A condition in which the breakdown of damaged and ischemic muscle cells release myoglobin, enzymes, and electrolytes that can cause kidney failure.

rhonchi Coarse crackles. The sound produced by mucous or fluid in the lower airways.

rule out (r/o) Used as a verb for the act of determining that a condition or problem does not exist.

seizure Uncoordinated electrical activity in the brain.

sepsis Systemic infection.

serum The liquid portion of the blood, as distinguished from blood cells and platelets.

sexually transmitted infection (STI) Infection transmitted from person to person by sexual activity.

shell/core compensation Vasoconstriction in the skin and gut to shunt blood to vital body organs. Occurs as compensation for volume shock and cold response.

shell/core effect A compensation mechanism seen in shock and cold response that reduces blood flow to the body shell to preserve perfusion and warmth in the vital organs of the core. Can also be reversed in core/shell effect.

shock Inadequate perfusion pressure in the circulatory system, resulting in inadequate tissue oxygenation.

signs Response elicited by examination, e.g., pain when the examiner touches an injured area (tenderness).

sinus Hollow spaces in the bones of the skull.

sinusitis Inflammation of the membranous lining of the sinuses due to infection, allergy, or toxic exposure. Usually used in reference to infection.

solid organs Liver, spleen, pancreas, kidneys and other organs without significant hollow space.

spasm Involuntary contraction of muscle.

spinal cord The cord-like extension of the central nervous system encased within the bones of the spinal column, running from the base of the brain to the mid-lumbar spine.

spine The column of bony vertebrae extending from the base of the skull to the pelvis. Includes the bones, ligaments, cartilage, and spinal cord.

spine assessment A systematic examination of the spinal column and spinal cord function looking for evidence of injury. Also called Focused Spine Assessment.

static rope A rope with very limited stretch. Often used in rescue work. In contrast to a dynamic rope that can stretch and absorb shock-loading.

stethoscope An instrument used to transmit body sounds directly to the ears of the examiner via rubber tubes.

STOPEATS A mnemonic used to summarize the various factors that can affect brain function: Sugar, Temperature, Oxygen, Pressure, Electricity, Altitude, Toxins, Salts.

stridor Stuttering, raspy, or coarse wheezing sound heard on inspiration. Caused by partial obstruction of the upper airway.

stroke Localized brain ischemia, typically caused by a clot or bleed, that results in partial loss of brain function. Capable of causing elevated intracranial pressure.

subacute hypothermia A slow-onset hypothermia in which glycogen stores and blood glucose are depleted and the patient becomes dehydrated.

Subjective (S) The part of the SOAP note describing what was learned from the scene, bystanders, and the patient history.

sublingual Under the tongue. Usually refers to a route of medication administration such as a sublingual tablet of nitroglycerine or morphine.

submersion Occurs when somebody goes under water.

survey A systematic examination of the scene or patient.

swelling Abnormal fluid accumulation in body tissues due to bleeding or edema.

symptomatic treatment Therapy that relieves symptoms but does not necessarily treat the cause.

Symptoms (Sx) Conditions described by the patient, e.g., pain on swallowing.

synovial fluid Joint fluid, lubrication inside a joint.

systemic Involving the entire body such as a systemic infection or systemic allergy.

systemic toxins Toxins that affect the body as a whole.

systolic blood pressure The pressure within the circulatory system generated by contraction of the heart.

tamponade Bleeding within a confined space such that blood loss stops when the space if full.

tendon Fibrous tissue connecting muscle to bone.

tetanus Nervous system spasm and paralysis cause by the toxin released by Clostridium tetani bacteria. Also called lock jaw.

thorax The chest or chest cavity.

tissue toxins Toxins that destroy body cells, causing inflammation, pain, and swelling. Also called hemotoxins.

tourniquet A constricting band used to prevent or restrict the flow of blood to an extremity.

toxins Chemicals that have a damaging effect on body tissues or the function of the nervous system.

toxin load The combined systemic effect of numerous small toxic exposures such as a large number of insect bites or man-of-war stings.

traction Tension applied along the long axis of an extremity.

traction splint A splinting device designed to maintain traction on an extremity, primarily used for femur fractures in the field setting.

trauma Injury.

traumatic brain injury (TBI) Injury to brain tissue caused by trauma. Also called closed head injury (CHI), or concussion.

treatment (Tx) Can be used interchangeably with Plan (P), however more commonly refers specifically to medical interventions.

trench foot Inflammation due to ischemia and necrosis caused by cold-induced vasoconstriction during prolonged exposure to cold and wet conditions.

umbilicus Navel, belly button.

upper airway Mouth, nose, throat (larynx).

vacuum mattress A patient stabilization device consisting of a vinyl bag filled with plastic beads that coalesce to form a rigid package when the air is evacuated from the device.

vapor barrier A vapor-proof wrap or covering that prevents evaporative cooling.

vascular bundle A grouped nerve, artery, and vein following the same pathway.

vascular shock Shock due to dilation of blood vessels.

vascular space Inside the blood vessels.

vasodilation Dilation of blood vessels.

vasodilator A drug that stimulates blood vessel dilation.

vein Vessel returning blood from body tissues to the heart. Equipped with one-way valves to enhance flow. Carries blood under low pressure.

ventilation The movement of air in and out of the lungs.

ventricular fibrillation Uncoordinated contraction of heart muscle. An example of a dysrhythmia.

vertebrae The bones of the spine.

vital signs (VS) Measurements of body function including blood pressure, pulse, respiration, level of consciousness, skin color, and body core temperature.

volume shock Inadequate blood volume resulting in inadequate perfusion pressure in the circulatory system leading to inadequate cellular oxygenation.

voluntary guarding Voluntary contraction of abdominal muscle as the patient protects themself from the pain caused by palpation.

wilderness context A situation where access to definitive medical care is delayed by distance, logistics, or danger.

Index

F

G

H

I

J

K

L

M

N

O

P

R

S

T

U

V

W

Photo and Image Credits

Section 1
Chapter 3
pg 20: Jeff Isaac, PA-C

Section 2
Chapter 6
pg 46: Amol Kulkarni
pg 47: Jeffrey Isaac, PA-C

Case Study 3
pg 51: Jeffrey Isaac, PA-C

Section 3
Chapter 7
pg 61: Jeffrey Isaac, PA-C
pg 61: United States Coast Guard

Chapter 8
pg 64: Atlas Dermatologico
pg 64: Jeffrey Isaac, PA-C
pg 65: Jeffrey Isaac, PA-C
pg 66: Jeffrey Isaac, PA-C

Section 4
Chapter 11
pg 79: Tom Clausing
pg 81: United States Army

Chapter 12
pg 87: Jobi Hansen

Chapter 13
pg 90: Amol Kulkarni
pg 91: Jeffrey Isaac, PA-C
pg 91: Jeffrey Isaac, PA-C
pg 93: Jeffrey Isaac, PA-C
pg 93: United States Army
pg 93: Jeffrey Isaac, PA-C
pg 94: Jeffrey Isaac, PA-C
pg 94: David Johnson, MD
pg 95: Jeffrey Isaac, PA-C
pg 95: Paul Roche, MD
pg 96: Jeffrey Isaac, PA-C
pg 98: Tom Clausing
pg 100: Jeffrey Isaac, PA-C
pg 100: Jeffrey Isaac, PA-C

Chapter 14
pg 102: Jeffrey Isaac, PA-C
pg 103: Jeffrey Isaac, PA-C
pg 104: WMAI
pg 107: Jeffrey Isaac, PA-C
pg 109: Jeffrey Isaac, PA-C
pg 109: Jeffrey Isaac, PA-C

Chapter 16
pg 120: Jeffrey Isaac, PA-C
pg 122: Jeffrey Isaac, PA-C
pg 122: Jeffrey Isaac, PA-C
pg 131: Jeffrey Isaac, PA-C
pg 131: Jeffrey Isaac, PA-C

Case Study 9
pg 134: Jeffrey Isaac, PA-C

Section 5
Chapter 17
pg 139: Ben Greene
pg 140: WMA Japan

Chapter 18
pg 147: Jeffrey Isaac, PA-C
pg 148: Rob Weisbaum
pg 148: Peter Goth, MD
pg 148: Wilderness Medical Society
pg 152: Jeffrey Isaac, PA-C

Chapter 19
pg 156: Jeffrey Isaac, PA-C

Chapter 20
pg 163: Jeffrey Isaac, PA-C

Chapter 21
pg 165: Jobi Hansen
pg 165: WMA Japan
pg 168: WMA Brazil

Chapter 22
pg 171: Ross Orton

Chapter 23
pg 184: Luke O'Neill
pg 188: Jeffrey Isaac, PA-C

Case Study 11:
pg 192: Sea Education Association

Section 6
Chapter 24
pg 196: Jeffrey Isaac, PA-C

Chapter 25
pg 198: Jeffrey Isaac, PA-C
pg 205: Jeffrey Isaac, PA-C

Chapter 26
pg 208: Jeffrey Isaac, PA-C

Chapter 31
pg 229: Jeffrey Isaac, PA-C
pg 229: Atlas Dermatologico
pg 230: Jeffrey Isaac, PA-C
pg 231: Jeffrey Isaac, PA-C
pg 232: Jeffrey Isaac, PA-C

Section 7
Chapter 33
pg 243: Jeffrey Isaac, PA-C
pg 244: WMA Japan

Chapter 34
pg 248: Jeffrey Isaac, PA-C

Chapter 36
pg 255: United States Army
pg 256: WMA Brazil
pg 257: WMA Japan